Sociology as applied to medicine

Commissioning Editor: Michael Parkinson
Project Development Manager: Hannah Kenner
Project Manager: Nancy Arnott
Designer: Erik Bigland, Keith Kail
Illustrator: MTG

Sociology as applied to medicine

Edited by

Graham Scambler BSc PhD

Professor of Medical Sociology,
Centre for Behavioural Sciences and Social Sciences in Medicine,
University College London,
London, UK

FIFTH EDITION

SAUNDERS

EDINBURGH   LONDON   NEW YORK   PHILADELPHIA   ST LOUIS   SYDNEY   TORONTO   2003

SAUNDERS

An imprint of Elsevier Science Limited

© W. B. Saunders Company Limited 1997
© Harcourt Publishers Limited 2000
© 2003, Elsevier Science Limited. All rights reserved.

First edition 1982
Second edition 1986
Third edition 1991
Fourth edition 1997
Fifth edition 2003

ISBN 0 702 02665 4

British Library Cataloguing in Publication Data
A catalogue record for this book is available from the British Library

Library of Congress Cataloging in Publication Data
A catalog record for this book is available from the Library of Congress

The
publisher's
policy is to use
**paper manufactured
from sustainable forests**

Printed in China

Foreword to the first edition

Students of medicine and of other related disciplines may be forgiven for feeling that their schools and colleges insist that they learn more and more about an increasing number of aspects of the human condition in health and illness. There was a halcyon time, not so long ago, when the pre-clinical curriculum consisted of one course in human anatomy and another in physiology; the clinical phase involved merely learning the skills needed to recognize the signs and symptoms of a wide but ultimately limited range of diseases. Moreover, there was little institutional pressure on students to study since they were free to repeat examinations until they passed them.

The picture is very different today. Knowledge of the molecular structure of living beings and the factors which determine natural and pathological growth and decay has expanded exponentially in the last fifty years and continues to do so. Students are expected to know a good deal about the theories and research methods of the scientific disciplines, the 'ologies', which have led to this increased knowledge, as well as about the implications of their findings for medical practice. More and more disciplines claiming relevance to medical knowledge and practice jostle each other for a place in the pre-clinical curriculum; new clinical specialities want medical students to be exposed at some time during their clinical studies to what they have to offer. All make claims to the indispensable nature of their own contribution to the curriculum. Meanwhile, medical students are no longer free to work at their own pace. Examinations weed out those who cannot satisfy their teachers after a maximum of two failures. The pressures are those of the institution. Students of other health professions, such as nursing, dentistry, pharmacy and optometry, are exposed to broadly comparable pressures in the process of qualifying as practitioners.

Sociology is one of the disciplines which has recently claimed the attention of the medical and other related health professions and their students. Its formal introduction into the curriculum as a basic medical science, which by the 1980s had taken place in most of the medical schools of the United Kingdom, was a radical innovation. Compared with most of the other new subjects it involves a break away from the traditional preparation for medicine based exclusively on the detailed study of parts of the biological organism which we call the human body. Its focus is not on the human individual *per se:* it is on the two-way relationships between the individual and society. Sociology as applied to medicine is concerned specifically with those aspects of the relationship which influence the experiences of health and illness in individuals and the response to them of others – relatives, doctors, nurses, administrators and governments.

Not surprisingly, not all those already involved in medical education welcomed the advent of sociological teaching. Some of the staff involved in teaching the traditional laboratory based or clinical subjects saw in it an intrusion of a largely unknown and untested quantity competing for the students' limited span of attention time. They were unfamiliar with its methods or potential and sceptical about its contribution to the making of a good practitioner. Some students, expecting the medical curriculum to resemble in essence the pre-medical natural science courses they had taken prior to entry, also needed to be persuaded that sociology was relevant to their preparation as future doctors, especially when they felt themselves to be under pressure to absorb all that the teachers of subjects which were more thoroughly examined put before them.

Such early doubts have not entirely disappeared, but they have substantially diminished. Indeed, the General Medical Council's recommendations for medical education in the 1980s are even more insistent than earlier recommendations on the necessity for broadening the students' basic understanding of the social context of health and illness and of social determinants of medical practice and health service provision. This then is the major task and challenge for those responsible for the teaching of sociology as applied to medicine, and the contributors to this book are to be congratulated for providing a concise introduction to the subject.

In this book, which will form an admirable basic text upon which teachers and students can build, the contributors have shown how some of the theories, concepts and methods developed by sociologists can illuminate aspects of human experience in health and illness. They look at how such socially determined factors as marital status, social class and family composition influence the pattern of morbidity and mortality. They show that medical perceptions of what constitutes mental or physical illness are not necessarily shared by the populations served and that the absence of shared perceptions may frustrate much medical effort. They look at the variety of ways in which old age, death and ethnicity are regarded and treated and the dilemmas which such variety can pose for practitioners. They explore the social origins of contemporary systems of health care in order to obtain greater understanding of their present problems. They examine too the various interpretations which can be placed upon the collective and individual behaviour of members of the medical profession, and on the expansion of medical concern and metaphors into many aspects of social life. This list does not exhaust their concerns and there are many other developments in the sociology of health and illness which cannot be covered in a volume of this size.

It seems to me impossible to argue that acquaintance with such findings and with the methods and conceptual frames of the discipline on which they are based is not an essential ingredient in the preparation of the doctor for medical practice whether it be in general practice, an age-band or body-system speciality, or community medicine. He or she needs it at the very least for protection against the very real hazard of frustration and unhappiness when it proves difficult to implement medical measures; but above all it is needed if the medical and other health-related professions are to make their greatest potential contribution to the welfare of the populations they are privileged to serve.

Margot Jefferys
August 1981

Preface

The first edition of 'Sociology as Applied to Medicine' was published two decades ago in 1982, since when there have been innumerable changes not only to the contents of health, professional and social science courses, but also to the health professions, the healthcare system and society itself. We have tried to keep abreast of these changes, many of which are represented and commented on in this fifth edition of a textbook that has survived longer and fared better than we dared anticipate when we first met, as teachers based in London medical schools, in recognition of a dire student need for guidance in what was then a new discipline informing the education of health professionals.

Each edition of 'Sociology as Applied to Medicine' has occasioned a rethink, to take account not only of ongoing change but also of feedback from colleagues and, more importantly, students. We are grateful to all those who have taken the trouble to engage with us in this way. Once again, there are new faces among the contributors. This always invigorates and gives new slants to areas and topics, and for the fifth edition the new blood has not displaced the old, because all the contributors to the fourth edition remain. Annette Scambler has joined the team to contribute a chapter on gender and health; Ian Rees Jones has taken over responsibility for the chapters on the health professions and health promotion; and Fiona Stevenson has brought a new perspective to the chapter dealing with issues of community care.

It is appropriate, finally, to recall once more the roles of Donald Patrick, co-editor of the first two editions, and of Margot Jefferys, whose support was so vital to the project from its conception. Sadly, Margot passed away in early 1999. She was instrumental in many ways in establishing the sociology of health and illness in the recognized curricula of medical schools. She was also a wise and shrewd teacher and counsellor to generations of medical sociologists. Her Foreword to the first edition of 'Sociology as Applied to Medicine' is included here. Our project bears modest testimony to her influence, warmth and generosity.

Graham Scambler 2003

Contributors

David Blane, Department of Social Science and Medicine, ICSTM Charing Cross, St Dunstan's Road, London W6 8RP

Ray Fitzpatrick, Department of Public Health, Institute of Health Sciences, University of Oxford, Old Road, Headington, Oxford OX3 7LF

Paul Higgs, Centre for Behavioural and Social Sciences in Medicine, University College London, Wolfson Building, 48 Riding House Street, London W1N 8AA

Sheila Hillier, Institute of Community Health Sciences, Barts and the London School of Medicine and Dentistry, Turner Street, London E1 2AD

David Locker, Faculty of Dentistry, University of Toronto, 124 Edward Street, Toronto, Ontario M56 1G6, Canada

Nicholas Mays, Department of Public Health and Policy, London School of Hygiene and Tropical Medicine, Keppel Street, London WC1E 7HT

Myfanwy Morgan, Department of Public Health Sciences, King's College London (Guy's Campus), Capital House, Weston Street, London SE1 3QD

Ian Rees Jones, Faculty of Health and Social Care Sciences, St George's Hospital Medical School, Cranmer Terrace, London SW17 0RE

Annette Scambler, 58 South Street, Epsom, Surrey DT18 7PQ

Graham Scambler, Centre for Behavioural and Social Sciences in Medicine, University College London, Wolfson Building, 48 Riding House Street, London W1N 8AA

Fiona Stevenson, Department of Primary Care and Population Sciences, Royal Free and University College Medical School, Rowland Hill Street, London NW3 2PF

Contents

CONTENTS

Social Aspects of Disease

1

Society and Changing Patterns of Disease

Ray Fitzpatrick

One of the most important recent developments in ideas about health care and illness has been the widespread recognition that social and economic conditions have a major effect on patterns of disease and death rates. A wide range of sources – historical, medical and sociological – have provided the evidence for such influences. This chapter considers how lines of influence from society and the economy can be traced to patterns of disease.

The starting-point of this analysis is the dramatic variation to be found in death rates both in the past and at present. For example, the death rate per annum has virtually halved in England and Wales over the past 150 years: in 1851 it was 22.7 per 1000 population and by 1999 it had fallen to 10.6. Another way to express the difference over this period is in terms of the average number of years an individual could expect to live at birth, i.e. life expectancy. A man or woman born in 1840 could, on average, expect to live to 40 and 43 years, respectively, whereas by 1999 life expectancy had risen to 75 and 80 years, respectively. However, such differences in overall mortality rates disguise a more complex picture if we look at particular age groups. The higher death rates of the mid-nineteenth century were much more severe in particular age groups, especially in infancy and childhood. Thus, future life expectancy for those who have reached the age of 45 years has improved only slightly over the last 100 years, and not nearly as dramatically as has the life expectancy of a child at birth.

The higher death rates and lower life expectancies are not of course simply an historical phenomenon. At present, many under-developed countries have much lower life expectancies than England; for example, in 1999, life expectancies for men and women in Ethiopia were 41 and 43 years, and for Sierra Leone 33 and 35 years, respectively. Under-developed countries with higher death rates resemble nineteenth-century England and Wales in that infant and child mortality are one of the main reasons for lower life expectancy.

VARIATION IN DISEASE PATTERNS IN HUMAN SOCIETY

The diseases encountered by humans have not remained the same over time. The history of humans might be viewed as a progressive victory over disease, but this is an over-simplification. Although some diseases are less important than in the past, others have become more important. Complex social and biological processes have altered the balance between humans and disease. A number of authorities (McKeown 1979, Powles 1973) now agree on three characteristic disease patterns in historical sequence.

Preagricultural disease patterns

Before about 10 000 BC, indeed for most of the evolution of humans as a distinct species, humans lived as hunter–gatherers, that is, without any form of settled agriculture for subsistence. Although conclusions based on such early evidence are somewhat speculative, anthropologists and epidemiologists have argued that the infectious diseases that were later to become major causes of illness and death were relatively uncommon at this stage of social evolution. Furthermore, diseases that are sometimes described as diseases of civilization, such as heart disease and cancer, were less common than at the present time (Powles 1973). It is likely that mortality in adults arose from environmental and safety hazards, for example hunting accidents and exposure.

Diseases in agricultural society

Knowledge of the diseases that plagued agricultural societies is more certain. These were predominantly the infectious diseases, which for purposes of discussion can be divided into the following:

1. air-borne diseases, such as tuberculosis
2. water-borne diseases, such as cholera
3. food-borne diseases, such as dysentery
4. vector-borne (i.e. carried by rats or mosquitoes) diseases, such as plague and malaria.

In England and Wales, and in Europe generally, the plague was a particularly important cause of death and at its most virulent, in the Black Death of 1348, it killed one-quarter of the English population. It last occurred on any large scale in England and Wales in 1665, and disappeared from Europe shortly after. The plague was spread by the fleas carried by black rats. Its disappearance was due to the replacement of the black rat by the brown rat, which was much less prone to infest human habitations.

Malaria was never as great a health problem in England and Wales as it has been in the tropics, where conditions are ideal for the natural life cycle of both vector and parasite. By the mid-nineteenth century, when reliable vital statistics were available in England and Wales and the country's economy was changing from agricultural to industrial, the major causes of death were tuberculosis, bronchitis, pneumonia, influenza and cholera.

The modern industrial era of disease

By the mid-twentieth century, infectious diseases had become relatively unimportant causes of death in England and Wales and in the western world in general, although some infectious diseases, such as influenza, remained common causes of death, particularly in the elderly. The infectious diseases have been replaced as major causes of death by the so-called degenerative diseases, cancer and cardiovascular disease.

Because of these changes in patterns of death, the major medical problems of today are chronic illnesses such as atherosclerosis, diabetes and osteoarthritis. These are all problems involving multiple risk factors, rather than a single cause. Their onset is quite early in life; they tend to be progressive; and they appear in all modern societies. Fries (1983) argues that there appear to be quite definite limits to the extension of the human lifespan, so that life expectancy at age 100 years has barely changed in the past 80 years. However, if one looks at such indices as age at first heart attack or age-specific lung cancer rates in the USA, there have been quite definite improvements in recent years. Fries concludes that health policy should make the compression of morbidity a major objective. Combining medical and social approaches to reducing the risk factors for chronic illnesses such as atherosclerosis would result in a life in which serious illness and decline in functioning were increasingly confined to later ages and the years of vigorous life extended.

This dramatic increase in importance of the chronic degenerative diseases is characteristic of almost all countries that have undergone industrialization, although the exceptions and the variations in rates from one country to another provide important and intriguing problems for the medical and social scientist. Japan, for example, has a much lower incidence of heart disease than comparable industrialized societies. On the other hand, the level of stomach cancer is considerably higher in Japan than, for example, the USA.

Explaining changes in disease prevalence

It would be all too easy to regard changes in disease patterns as the inevitable consequences of medical and technical progress without further explanation. Close examination of the major influences on disease patterns, however, uncovers a complex picture that is increasingly recognized as important for the understanding of disease in the contemporary world. The study of how disease patterns have changed indicates the pervasive influence of social and economic factors on disease prevalence.

Three main factors seem important in the changes in disease patterns that followed the transition from nomadic hunting and gathering to agricultural life. First, the development of cereals such as wheat allowed agricultural societies to feed more mouths and hence support higher population densities. Evidence from epidemiological studies, however, shows that many infectious organisms thrive when human populations grow above certain densities. Second, agricultural work necessitated permanent settlement, whereas hunter–gatherers moved settlement periodically in search of fresh food sources. However, in the absence of sanitation and awareness of its importance, permanent settlement often led to the contamination of water supplies by waste products, which increased the risks of infection from a number of organisms. Third, the development of cereals as the major source of food, although supporting greater numbers of people, paradoxically narrowed the range and quality of diet, a factor that crucially reduced resistance to infection.

More careful examination is needed to explain the remarkable changes in death rates and the decline in significance of mortality from infectious disease that occurred with the transition from agricultural to industrial economies. The victory over death and diseases in the nineteenth and twentieth centuries still represents the most dramatic improvement in health in the history of human kind. Death rates for the various infectious diseases did not decline simultaneously. Tuberculosis, the most common cause of death in the nineteenth century, began to decline in the first half of that century, as indicated in Fig. 1.1.

There are a limited number of possible explanations for such a marked decline in mortality from an infectious organism. Box 1.1 shows the competing explanations that have been offered, not only for the decline of tuberculosis but for the wide range of infectious diseases for which mortality rates declined dramatically in the course of the nineteenth century in Britain and other parts of western Europe. It is possible that a change occurred in the virulence of the organism itself or that the genetic immunity of the

6

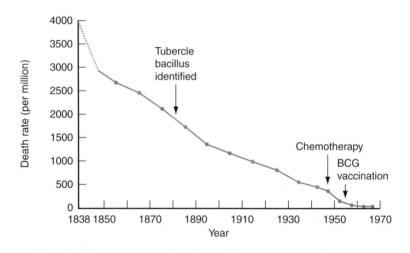

Fig. 1.1 Pulmonary tuberculosis: annual death rates for England and Wales, 1838–1970. (*Reproduced with permission from Mckeown 1979*).

BOX 1.1	Possible Explanations for the Decline of Mortality from Infectious Disease in Britain in the Nineteenth Century

- Decline in virulence of organisms: organisms responsible for diseases, for example tuberculosis and bronchitis, became less lethal as a result of changes in their biological properties
- Reduction in exposure of humans to infectious organisms: for example, through changes in domestic housing and urban planning or through reduced contamination of food and water supplies
- Genetically induced increase in resistance of humans to infection: human genes associated with resistance to infection might be favoured by Darwinian selection processes and thus individual and population resistance increased over time
- Acquired resistance of humans to infection: general fitness brought about by improved nutrition resulted in greater resistance in terms of probability of: (1) being infected; and/or (2) recovering from infection
- Specific medical interventions: rates of recovery from infectious diseases were improved by developments in medical treatment and therefore mortality rates were reduced

population improved. Both these possibilities are generally discounted. There is no theoretical reason why the organisms responsible for tuberculosis and a number of other infectious diseases should fortuitously change in their virulence at approximately the same period. It is very unlikely that genetic immunity could improve in such a short time as the selection processes implied would require dramatic increases in mortality rates across a range of diseases. For these reasons, the first and third explanations in Box 1.1 are normally rejected as unlikely. The most convincing explanation for the decline in mortality from tuberculosis and, later in the century, from air-borne diseases such as pneumonia, is that of greater acquired resistance. An increased resistance to infection resulted from improvement in nutritional intake as agricultural techniques improved and transportation of produce became faster and more efficient. Much of the nineteenth century also saw unprecedented increases in real wages and the standard of living in Britain. It is also possible to argue for the significance of nutrition with contemporary evidence. In many third world countries today, diseases such as measles or tuberculosis have a much higher fatality, especially among the very young in populations whose resistance is reduced by malnutrition. McKeown cites the conclusion of the World Health Organization report that one-half to three-quarters of all statistically recorded deaths of infants and young children are attributed to a combination of malnutrition and infection (McKeown 1979). However, the role of the second possible explanation in Box 1.1 – reduced exposure to infectious organisms – is also of importance. The incidence of illness and mortality from water-borne diseases such as cholera declined somewhat later in the nineteenth century, largely as the result of concerted efforts by the public health movement to prevent the contamination of drinking water supplies by sewage; gastroenteric infectious diseases came under control by the beginning of the twentieth century, resulting in a dramatic impact on infant mortality. The sterilization and more hygienic transportation of milk in particular, and improved food hygiene in general, constitute another form of environmental change that produced the decline in infectious disease mortality.

Thus, most of the decline in death rates achieved in Britain and in the western world generally by the Second World War can be attributed to environmental factors such as improvements in food and hygiene, which were the products of economic development. Other social changes, such as the decline in the birth rate, reduced the demand for food and housing resources. Improved housing and better personal hygiene also played their role in reducing mortality rates.

Historians still dispute the precise nature of the changes that brought about the decline in mortality rates just described. The nature of that debate can, with some simplification, be termed one between the 'public health' form of explanation and the 'invisible hand' version of events (Box 1.2). The debate is of more than purely historical interest because it mirrors and has implications for current debates. Even now, some would argue that improvements in the economy and wealth are the most effective ways of producing improvements in the health of modern populations ('the invisible hand' (Guha, 1994)). Others would argue that more direct and political intervention is required by a modern public health movement to address the ills described later in this chapter (Szreter, 1988). Box 1.2 shows how difficult it is to disentangle claims, even with historical hindsight!

The global burden of disease

There is a danger of focusing excessively on changing patterns of disease in developed countries. A ranking of the top ten causes of death and disability combined for the world as a whole in 1999 shows that five of the top ten causes primarily affect younger children: lower respiratory tract infections, conditions arising during the perinatal period, diarrhoeal diseases, childhood vaccine-preventable diseases and nutritional deficiencies (Michaud et al 2001). Two further causes are infectious diseases largely associated with poverty in developing countries: malaria and HIV. There is an unfinished agenda of childhood and infectious diseases responsible for the majority of ill-health in the modern world.

THE HISTORICAL ROLE OF MEDICINE

To this point nothing has been said about the role that medical intervention (the last possible explanation listed in Box 1.1) has played in the relationship between man and disease. At first glance, this might seem an important omission, given that medical knowledge was accumulating throughout the period and that hospitals had grown in number since the latter part of the eighteenth century. The evidence that McKeown and others have gathered, however, suggests that very little of the decline in mortality rates can be attributed to improvements in medical care. They list a range of evidence against the role of specific medical interventions having a substantial effect on mortality:

● Hospitals and surgical procedures were actually harmful. When Florence Nightingale began to reform the hygienic conditions in hospitals, it was widely thought that hospitals constituted a risk to health; in other words, one stood a high risk of cross-infection – contracting a disease from other patients – because wards were unsegregated as well as unhygienic. Similarly, despite the advances in surgery made possible by the development of anaesthetics, there is little evidence that surgical procedures made any impact on life expectancy in the nineteenth century (McKeown & Brown 1969).

● Drugs were largely ineffective. Before the twentieth century a large armoury of medicines appears to have been available to the Victorian doctor. However, only a few, such as digitalis, mercury and cinchona, used in the treatment of heart disease, syphilis and malaria, respectively, would be recognized by modern standards as having specific efficacy and, in any case, dosages were unlikely to have been appropriate.

The first drugs that can be shown to have influenced mortality rates did not appear until the end of the 1930s. Antibiotics, which are used in the treatment of a wide range of bacterial infections, were developed in the 1930s and 1940s. Prophylactic immunization against

BOX 1.2 The Debate Between 'Public Health' and 'The Invisible Hand' to Explain Improved Life Expectancy in Nineteenth Century Britain

The 'public health' explanation emphasizes deliberate government interventions:
● The public health movement improved water supplies, housing standards, regulation of food sold to public
● Increased income of working classes sometimes coincided with deteriorating death rates because of migration into more unhygienic industrial towns

The 'invisible hand' explanation emphasizes benefits of rising incomes:
● Some areas of London enjoyed improved death rates in the nineteenth century before reforms to water supplies
● Studies of claims to insurance societies show that while working class sickness rates due to infectious disease were stable, deaths from the same causes declined
● In some nineteenth century towns, such as Mansfield, deaths from infectious disease remained high despite excellent water supplies
● The greatest benefit of improved diet is upon the capacity of infants and children to survive infectious disease

such diseases as whooping cough and polio date from the 1950s. In the case of these medical breakthroughs, however, it is easy to overstate the contribution that they made to mortality rates. The decline in mortality for most infectious diseases took place before the introduction of antibiotics. The period of decline for tuberculosis can be seen in Fig. 1.1, and the mortality rates for bronchitis, pneumonia and influenza are shown in Fig. 1.2. Moreover, it is difficult to distinguish between the improvements in disease mortality that can be attributed to the introduction of treatment or immunization and those due to the continuing influence of improving social and economic conditions. The immunization programmes for diphtheria and polio probably brought about the greatest improvements that can be attributed to specific medical intervention.

DISEASE RATES AND SOCIAL FACTORS IN MODERN SOCIETY

The association between diseases and social and economic circumstances is not a purely historical phenomenon. In many parts of the third world life expectancy at birth is much lower than in Europe or North America. Many aspects of the environment in the third world provide much more favourable conditions for the spread of infectious diseases than those that prevailed in historical Europe. For example, tropical ecology is particularly favourable for the vectors of diseases such as malaria (the mosquito) and sleeping sickness (tsetse fly). Nevertheless, it is the extremely low standard of living above all else that produces high mortality rates in countries such as Bangladesh and Ethiopia.

In countries like Britain, the social and environmental factors that are responsible for many kinds of commonly occurring disease are somewhat different and will require different explanation. The association between standard of living and the risk of disease, however, is still apparent in the social-class differences in illness and mortality rates discussed in Chapter 8. It is evident that environmental factors, whether in the home or at work, continue to play an important role in influencing the risks of illness and mortality.

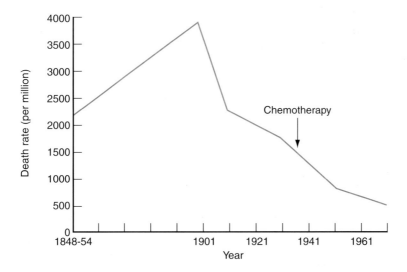

Fig. 1.2 Bronchitis, pneumonia and influenza: death rates for England and Wales, 1848–1971. (Reproduced with permission from Mckeown 1979).

The report of the Research Working Group on Inequalities in Health (DHSS 1981) makes clear in many of its recommendations which aspects of the social and economic environment it considers responsible for inequalities in health in Britain. Its proposed strategy largely targets poverty and low income:

● Benefits such as the maternity grant and child benefits need to be increased to reduce child poverty.

● Major programmes are needed in housing improvement, the prevention of accidents to children and the provision of school meals.

● More action is needed to prevent accidents in the work place, largely in manual occupations.

These recommendations are a clear reminder that, for large sections of society, health is harmed by material deprivation in terms of income, diet and housing, rather than because of the 'diseases of affluence'.

Although environmental conditions associated with poverty increase the risk of disease, many kinds of disease are now associated with behaviour that might have little or nothing to do with poverty. Increasingly, the mass media focuses attention on the role that over-eating or inappropriate diet, smoking and excessive alcohol consumption have in a wide variety of disorders such as heart disease, diabetes, lung cancer and cirrhosis of the liver.

The association between smoking and lung cancer has been established beyond all reasonable doubt. It is important to recognize, however, that contemporary health risks associated with behaviour are just as certainly a function of current social conditions as were the infectious health risks associated with the social conditions of the nineteenth century. This is an essential point to grasp, because it is all too easy to view behaviour such as smoking as simply reflecting an individual's decisions and preferences. To focus on an individual smoker would not only lead to erroneous and oversimplified explanations of the causes of his or her behaviour but, more importantly, it might lead to misguided or naive attempts to change that behaviour (Box 1.3).

| **BOX 1.3** | Smoking: A Product of the Economy as Much as of Individual Behaviour? |

Who smokes is socially patterned:
● 13% of men and 14% of women in social class 1 are smokers (see Chapter 8 for the definition of the five social classes)
● 44% of men and 33% of women in social class V are smokers
● Attitudes and behaviour are influenced by:
  – advertising and marketing strategies
  – governmental health warnings
  – taxation
● Effective health policies require evidence of social factors; there is no point in increasing spending on health education to alter the behaviour of groups who do not respond to such influences.

Economic significance of cigarettes:
● An analysis of smoking should include political, economic and health issues
● An increase in taxation would make cigarettes cost-prohibitive to some, but this would result in a decline in revenue
● A reduction in smoking would lead to a decrease in National Health Service costs but an increase in pensions, as greater numbers would live to old age
● A reduction in the tobacco industry would reduce the amount of sickness absence but lead to unemployment in areas dependent on the industry

The example of smoking illustrates that disease is as much a reflection of the economy today as it has been in the past. Diet is another example. It has been estimated (Lock & Smith 1976) that 56% of women and 52% of men in Britain over the age of 40 years are at least 15% overweight. The mortality risks of men who are 10% overweight are one-fifth higher than average, especially in mortality associated with diabetes and vascular disease. Clearly, over-eating is a major health risk. Burkitt (1973) and others have argued that inappropriate diet is also a problem. He argues that diverticular disease, cancer of the bowel, diabetes and indeed various venous diseases such as varicose veins and deep vein thrombosis, can all be linked to lack of fibre. Populations that have diets with a high fibre content seem relatively free of many such diseases. In Britain, the daily fibre intake from bread has been reduced to about one-tenth of its level in 1850, and the consumption of sugar and other refined carbohydrates has almost doubled. Again, the statistics of change do not reveal the causal links. Changes in diet have reflected changes in the food-producing industries, which are now concentrated in a small number of multinational companies whose main concern is to produce standardized, well-accepted and easily transported commodities: nutritional values have taken second place to the expansion of profits.

Another essentially modern form of health hazard can be identified in the 6000 deaths and 80 000 serious injuries that occur annually as a result of road traffic accidents. Doll (1983) makes the point that the rate per million of deaths on the roads is actually lower now than it was in the 1930s and is in this sense a testament to the beneficial effects of legislation with regard to prevention. Nevertheless, some 2000 hospital beds are occupied every day by the victims of road traffic accidents (Butler & Vaile 1984), which places a considerable demand on healthcare resources. The risk of having an accident as a motorcyclist is 18 times higher than the risk to car drivers, and much more still could be achieved to prevent accidents to this group by, for example, legislation on training and testing riding ability.

It might seem that an analysis of the relationship of social and economic factors to health is unhelpful because it points to features of our economic system that are central, firmly established and difficult to change. If this is the case, then another parallel is suggested with the nineteenth-century problems of environmental disease. The changes in sanitation, urban planning and building that were required to transform the pattern of infectious diseases in Victorian times were similarly regarded as unrealistic and resisted for long periods by politicians and business interests; but the reforms were adopted slowly and growing awareness of the relationship between commercially promoted behaviours such as smoking and unhealthy eating in our own time should help to speed the process of securing reforms.

A multidisciplinary committee has produced a major report to assess the effectiveness of existing public health policies and to stimulate new national strategies (Smith & Jacobson 1988). Six areas of current lifestyles that influence health were identified, for which research evidence of harmful effects is strong and support for the feasibility of action is clear cut:

1. tobacco
2. diet
3. physical activity
4. alcohol
5. sexuality
6. road safety.

Similarly, five areas of preventive services were identified where evidence is very strong that public health interventions could now produce dramatic improvements:

1. maternity services

2. dental health

3. immunization

4. early cancer detection (breast and cervix)

5. detection of high blood pressure.

The approach in each of these 11 priority areas is to identify precise quantitative targets and make specific recommendations to public bodies and institutions. Thus, one of a number of specific nutritional targets is to increase the total dietary fibre intake from 20 g per person per day to 30 g. The list of agencies to which nutritional targets and specific actions are recommended includes the food industry, local authorities, health authorities and government. The committee's view is that agencies need specific targets to stimulate action and to provide a ready means of monitoring results.

THE ECONOMY AND HEALTH POLICY IN MODERN SOCIETY

Some of the most recent research on the relationship between the economy and health suggests that, even in modern societies, economic factors play the predominant role in determining patterns of illness, and that the role of health services is negligible by comparison. Four different views of how the economy generally, and patterns of employment and income in particular, can affect health are evaluated here (Box 1.4).

Unemployment and health

Brenner (1977) has argued that most of the variation in annual overall mortality rates for the USA can be explained statistically in terms of changes in the annual level of employment, provided that a time lag of 5 years is allowed for unemployment to have its effect on health. This impact is produced in two ways: first, unemployment reduces family income and, therefore, the material standard of living; second, the individual loses a sense of meaning and purpose found at work and experiences increased fears about the future and tension at home. This results in greater vulnerability to ill health. From USA data, Brenner concluded that a 1% increase in unemployment, if sustained for 5 years, was statistically responsible for nearly 37 000 extra deaths. Similar results have been found from analyses of data collected in England and Wales and in Sweden (Brenner 1979).

Rapid economic growth and health

This work has been challenged by Eyer (1977), who argues that the influence on health of experience such as unemployment generally occurs within a much shorter time than the 5-year lag that Brenner allows. If this is the case, the association between unemployment and mortality is considerably reduced. Instead, Eyer argues that death rates increase at the time of business booms, when employment rates are high. He explains the association between employment and mortality in terms of four connected social factors that attend business cycles.

1. Economic booms increase workers' migration, which weakens the social networks that normally protect individuals against disease.

2. 'Stress' through overwork in times of business peaks increases ill health.

BOX 1.4   Alternative Models of the Economy and Health

- Unemployment is major cause of ill health
- Rapid economic growth is a major cause of ill health
- Particular forms of employment are causes of ill health:
  - 'job-strain' model
  - 'effort–reward imbalance' model
- Income distribution is a major cause of ill health

---

3. The unhealthy consumption of alcohol and tobacco increases.

4. Conversely, during low periods of the economy, social networks are strong and act to protect individuals.

Similar deleterious effects upon health of rapid economic growth have been detected in history. To return to the evidence of nineteenth century Britain, it can be argued that it was the disruption caused by rapid economic growth that resulted in little or no overall increase in life expectancy in the middle of that century. Mortality rates were particularly poor in the rapidly growing industrial cities such as Manchester, Glasgow and Liverpool. Rapid economic growth was associated with large-scale immigration of the rural poor into cities, growing social divisions between rich and poor within cities and a decline in willingness of those in power to fund environmental and public health protection (Szreter 1999). Szreter argues that the 'invisible hand' of rapid economic growth alone proved harmful to health and that only a deliberate public health movement in the second half of the nineteenth century restored the improving trends in life expectancy associated with economic growth.

Forms of employment and health

It is increasingly argued that the nature of work processes need to be examined for possible health effects. One very influential theory is associated with the work of Karasek & Theorell (1990). According to the 'job–strain' model, individuals who have very demanding jobs but who see themselves as having very little control over their work, experience not only higher levels of stress than others but also elevated cardiovascular disease. A number of studies have been carried out in Sweden and the USA to support this approach. A related model – the effort–reward imbalance model – argues rather similarly that those whose work is demanding and stressful, but who perceive themselves as insufficiently rewarded for their efforts, are also more prone to distress as well as to cardiovascular disease (Siegrist et al 1990). Rewards are not primarily monetary but prospects of status enhancement or promotion. Both models, when tested on work forces, have been found to demonstrate the highest levels of risk in semi- and unskilled manual workers.

Income distribution and health

One final model of the effects of the economy on health argues that it is the relative degree of inequality in incomes within a country that influences health (Wilkinson 1994). The evidence to support this model comes from international comparisons of countries where it is claimed that countries with the smallest spread and least inequality of incomes from top to bottom (e.g. Japan and Sweden) have higher life expectancies than those with large income differentials (such as the USA and the UK). The emphasis of the model is, therefore, not on how absolute income influences health but how people attach meaning to disadvantage in ways that actually harm them.

Of the four models outlined, only the role of unemployment has been researched to any great extent. The other three need further investigation. Bunn (1979) examined national statistics for the incidence of ischaemic heart disease in Australia. He found that economic recessions and their associated problems of high unemployment were associated not only with subsequently higher levels of heart disease mortality, but also with increased rates of drug prescribing. The latter he interpreted as a potential indicator of the stress of the recession, which resulted in increased general practitioner (GP) prescribing. One of the most convincing pieces of statistical evidence to support this research is the Office of Population Censuses and Surveys (OPCS) Longitudinal Study (OPCS 1984). This found that men who were unemployed in 1971, and their wives, experienced a 20% higher mortality rate than those men employed in the following 10 years (Moser et al 1987).

Other studies, instead of looking at correlations in national statistics, have examined at close hand the experiences of unemployed families. Fagin (1981) examined in detail a small sample of families in which the male breadwinner had been without work for at least 16 weeks. In many families the breadwinners developed clinical depression, loss of self-esteem, insomnia and suicidal thoughts, much of which necessitated psychotropic drug treatment by their GP. Physical symptoms included asthmatic attacks, backache and skin lesions. The health of younger children in some families also seemed to be affected.

MODERN MEDICINE AND HEALTH

The issues raised by these contrasting approaches are far from being resolved. All four models at least agree in placing the main responsibility for health and illness on economic policy rather than on the health services. This controversial position is partly shared by more radical writers who are more concerned with analysing directly the contribution of modern medicine to health. Perhaps the best known is Illich (1977), who argues that medicine has played a very small role in improving health and that its contribution has actually been negative, insofar as it has:

● raised public expectations of 'wonder cures', which in reality are ineffective

● extended too far the kinds of problem that are thought to be medical

● been responsible for large amounts of iatrogenic (medically induced) illness

● decreased the ability of individuals to cope with their own illness by fostering a debilitating dependency on the expert (see Chapter 12).

Illich's own solution is first to break down the monopoly of medicine in health care, so that there is a 'free market' in which anyone can practise healing, and second to reverse the social trend towards dependency by restoring the value of personal responsibility.

This approach, which is attractive to many advocates of 'alternative medicine' and self-help groups, is rejected as mistaken and utopian by writers such as Navarro (1975) because it wrongly blames the medical profession and a 'gullible' public for aspects of ill health that are best understood as products of a capitalist economy. It is this that directly creates much illness, maintains an unequal distribution of illness and encourages a very inappropriate healthcare system for treating illness once it has occurred. Hence, Navarro advocates radical political changes in society as the only solution to the kinds of problems that have been identified in this chapter.

Other writers, such as McKeown and Powles, place more emphasis on the need to reform health care rather than concerning themselves with wider issues of social change. First, they argue that, because much disease is caused environmentally, preventive medicine in teaching, research and practice should concentrate on the prevention of disease rather than treatment after it has occurred. Not only has prevention had a significant impact in the past, it appears to be a simple, more humane and sound means of reducing disease for the present.

Second, these analysts also maintain that healthcare resources and energy have become too concentrated on high technology and hospital-based acute medicine at the expense of preventive and community resources. In the light of the evidence reviewed above, it seems that there is an unwarranted faith in technological medicine. With the possible exception of antibiotics and immunization, few improvements in health can be attributed to breakthroughs in laboratory medicine. Cochrane (1972) argues that all too few medical procedures have been submitted to rigorous evaluation of their effectiveness (see Chapter 18).

Third, it is argued that another shift in the emphasis of medicine is needed, that from cure to care. Because medicine can claim few cures to be effective, it must confront the task of caring for the sick with greater zeal and effectiveness. Caring necessitates concern with the quality of life of the ill and reduction in any handicap or disadvantage consequent to disease. However, financial and other resources, reflecting medical values, are at present spent more in efforts in acute medicine than in the psychiatric or geriatric units. Medical education perpetuates such values because it is conducted predominantly in acute hospitals where consultants maintain traditional values in their teaching.

Clearly, these arguments are controversial and have not gone unchallenged. Lever (1977) has argued that inferences about current health planning based on historical patterns are hazardous. To prove that environmental factors were the most important determinants of mortality in the past does not necessarily prove that environmental measures will produce such beneficial effects in the present. Given limited funds for health services, a major shift towards environmental and preventive health care would be a major gamble. Whatever the merits of such points, it has to be acknowledged that at present insufficient resources have been committed to such preventive services as health education and occupational medicine, compared with expenditure on hospital technology, to allow any serious examination of their potential role.

It might also be argued that analysts like McKeown are too pessimistic in their interpretation of the impact of medical treatments, which have been shown to have led to markedly improved survival rates for many forms of childhood cancers and Hodgkin's disease and cancer of the testis amongst adult cancers (Doll 1990). Moreover, the debate has tended to focus on death rates, thereby ignoring substantial benefits that could have been derived from medical treatments in improving individuals' quality of life, for example by mitigating symptoms of pain, discomfort or disability (see Chapter 18). There is now very firm evidence that rates of physical disability among the elderly are declining in the USA (Cutler 2001). This is very striking evidence of movement towards the 'compression of morbidity' discussed earlier in this chapter, given the popular assumption (supported by some evidence) that longer life expectancy will be associated with increased levels of disability. The 25% reduction in disability in the elderly observed since 1982 cannot easily be explained but is almost certainly due to a combination of:

- improved medical treatments such as drugs and joint replacement surgery for arthritis and cataract surgery for visual impairment
- behavioural changes such as reduced smoking and improved diet that, as well as improving mortality, also reduce disability from respiratory disease, stroke and heart disease

- greater availability of adaptive devices such as devices to aid walking and walk-in showers that reduce the disabling consequences of chronic disease.

Such analyses challenge the excessively negative critiques of modern medicine. However, they do so by showing the limitations of opposing medical with social interventions (both are involved) and by demonstrating the need to move beyond mortality as the sole outcome of interest.

At present, much work remains to be done regarding the influence that social and economic factors exert on health. At the same time, controversial debates continue unresolved about the priorities in efforts and expenditure that are most appropriate to modern patterns of illness.

References

Brenner M 1977 Health costs and benefits of economic policy. International Journal Health Services 7:581–623

Brenner M 1979 Mortality and the national economy. Lancet ii:568–573

Bunn A 1979 Ischaemic heart disease mortality and the business cycle in Australia. American Journal of Public Health 69:772–781

Burkitt D 1973 Some diseases characteristic of modern Western civilization. British Medical Journal 1:274–278

Butler J, Vaile M 1984 Health and health services. Routledge & Kegan Paul, London

Cochrane A 1972 Effectiveness and efficiency: random reflections on the health service. Nuffield Provincial Hospitals Trust, London

Cutler D 2001 The reduction in disability among the elderly. Proceedings of the National Academy of Sciences USA 98:6546-6547

Department of Health and Social Security (DHSS) 1981 Inequalities in health. HMSO, London

Doll R 1983 Prospects for prevention. British Medical Journal 286:81–88

Doll R 1990 Are we winning the fight against cancer? An epidemiological assessment. European Journal of Cancer 26:500–508

Eyer J 1977 Does unemployment cause the death rate peak in each business cycle? International Journal of Health Services 7:625–662

Fagin L 1981 Unemployment and health in families. Department of Health and Social Security (DHSS), London

Fries J 1983 The compression of morbidity. Milbank Memorial Fund Quarterly 61:397–419

Guha S 1994 The importance of social intervention in England's mortality decline: the evidence reviewed. Social History of Medicine 7:89–114

Illich I 1977 Limits to medicine. Medical nemesis: the expropriation of health. Penguin, Harmondsworth

Karasek R, Theorell T 1990 Healthy work. Basic Books, New York

Lever A 1977 Medicine under challenge. Lancet i:353–355

Lock S, Smith T 1976 The medical risks of life. Penguin, Harmondsworth

McKeown T 1979 The role of medicine: dream, mirage or nemesis, 2nd edn. Blackwell Scientific, Oxford

McKeown T, Brown R 1969 Medical evidence related to English population changes in the eighteenth century. In: Drake M (ed) Population in industrialisation. Methuen, London

Michaud CM, Murray CJ, Bloom BR 2001 Burden of disease – implications for future research. Journal of the American Medical Association 285:535–539

Moser K et al 1987 Unemployment and mortality: comparison of the 1971 and 1981 longitudinal study census samples. British Medical Journal 294:86–90

Navarro V 1975 The industrialization of fetishism or the fetishism of industrialization: a critique of Ivan Illich. International Journal of Health Services 5:351–371

Office of Population Censuses and Surveys (OPCS) 1984 Mortality statistics. HMSO, London

Powles J 1973 On the limitations of modern medicine. Science, Medicine and Man 1:1–30

16

Siegrist J et al 1990 Low status control, high effort at work and ischaemic heart disease: prospective evidence from blue-collar men. Social Science and Medicine 31:1127–1139

Smith A, Jacobson B (eds) 1988 The nation's health: A strategy for the 1990s. Kings Fund, London

Szreter S 1988 The importance of social intervention in Britain's mortality decline c. 1850–1914: a reinterpretation of the role of public health. Social History of Medicine 1:1–38

Szreter S 1999 Rapid economic growth and 'the four Ds' of disruption, deprivation, disease and death: public health lessons from nineteenth-century Britain for twenty-first century China. Tropical Medicine and International Health 4:146–152

Wilkinson R 1994 The epidemiological transition: from material scarcity to social disadvantage? Daedalus 123:61–78

2

Social Determinants of Health and Disease

David Locker

Chapter 1 presented evidence to indicate that the improvements in health observed during the eighteenth and nineteenth centuries were the product of rising standards of living and sanitary reform. This illustrates the general principle that the health of a population is closely tied to the physical, social and economic environment. This chapter expands on this point of view by examining some of the social factors that have been linked to health and disease. Research in this field has grown significantly over the past 40 years, with relatively new disciplines such as social epidemiology and psychophysiology devoted to the investigation of the links between the social environment, psychological and emotional states, physiological change and disease. The broad implication of this work, and the view of health it embodies, is that health and illness are social, as well as medical, issues.

THEORIES OF HEALTH AND DISEASE

Before the rise of modern medicine, disease was attributed to a variety of spiritual or mechanical forces. It was interpreted as a punishment by God for sinful behaviour or the result of an imbalance in body elements or 'humours'. Many infectious diseases were ascribed to a life of vice or to a weak moral character, or believed to be due to 'miasma', that is, bad air arising out of dirt and decaying organic matter. The ancient Greeks rejected the notion that disease was a punishment for sin or the consequence of witchcraft and saw it as being related to the natural environment or the way in which human populations lived and worked. However, they failed to recognize that many diseases were contagious. The idea that disease could be passed from person to person arose in the Middle Ages and coexisted with the belief that disease was linked to evil behaviour. For example, by the mid-nineteenth century there was good evidence that cholera could be transmitted by close personal contact with a cholera victim. The observation that outbreaks occurred at great distances from exiting cases lead to the idea that the disease could also be transmitted in the water supply. John Snow, a physician who investigated the London cholera epidemics of 1848–9 and 1853–4, provided convincing evidence that the disease was spread by water contaminated by the excretions of cholera victims. Although this provided a means to control epidemics of the disease, it was not for another 40 years that the organism causing cholera was identified. However, Snow's work did illustrate the important principle that epidemics of disease could be controlled without knowing the biological mechanisms involved.

The ideas about disease that emerged during the late nineteenth century were influenced by two developments that provided a philosophical and empirical basis for the biomechanical approach characteristic of modern medical practice. These developments were the 'Cartesian revolution', which gave rise to the idea that the mind and body were independent, and the doctrine of specific aetiology, which flowed from the discovery of the microbiological origins of infectious disease. These effectively denied the influence of social and psychological factors in disease onset. Rather, the body was viewed as a machine, to be corrected when things went wrong by procedures designed to neutralize specific agents or modify the physical processes causing disease. These ideas have been progressively challenged as the monocausal view of disease has been modified by multicausal models of disease onset. The key features of these theories of health and disease are summarized in Box 2.1.

The germ theory of disease

During the second half of the nineteenth century, the work of Ehrlich, Koch and Pasteur revealed that the prevailing health problems of the time were the product of living organisms that entered the body via food, water, air or the bites of insects or animals. In 1882, Koch identified and isolated the bacillus causing tuberculosis and, between 1897 and 1900, the organisms responsible for 22 infectious diseases were identified. This work gave rise to the idea that each disease had a single and specific cause. This was embodied in Koch's postulates, a set of rules for establishing causal relationships between a microorganism and a disease. These state that, to be ascribed a causal role, the agent must always be found with the disease in question and not with any other disease. This doctrine and its monocausal approach came to dominate medical research and practice. As a result, research effort moved from the community to the laboratory and concentrated on the identification of the noxious agents responsible for a given disease, whereas medical practice became devoted to the destruction or eradication of that agent from individuals already affected (Najman 1980).

Multicausal models of disease

Although the infectious organism theory of disease made a significant contribution to explaining and solving the major health problems of its time, it has serious limitations in terms of our understanding of disease processes. The most important of these is that not all those exposed to pathogens become ill: an organism or other noxious agent is a necessary,

19

BOX 2.1   Theories of Disease Causation: Key Ideas

Germ theory:
- Disease is caused by transmissible agents
- A specific agent is responsible for one disease only
- Medical practice consists of identifying and neutralizing these agents

Epidemiological triangle:
- Exposure to an agent does not necessarily lead to disease
- Disease is the result of an interaction between agent, host and environment
- Disease can be prevented by modifying factors that influence exposure and susceptibility

Web of causation:
- Disease results from the complex interaction of many risk factors
- Any risk factor can be implicated in more than one disease
- Disease can be prevented by modifying these risk factors

General susceptibility:
- Some social groups have higher mortality and morbidity rates from all causes. This reflects an imperfectly understood general susceptibility to health problems. This probably results from the complex interaction of the environment, behaviours and life-styles

Socioenvironmental approach:
- Health is powerfully influenced by the social and physical environments in which we live
- Risk conditions integral to those environments damage health directly and through the physiological, behavioural and psychosocial risk factors they engender
- Improving health requires political action to modify these environments

---

but not a sufficient, cause of disease. The epidemiological triangle approach sees disease as the product of an interaction between an agent, a host and the environment. Agents are biological, chemical or physical factors whose presence are necessary for a disease to occur. Host factors include personal characteristics and behaviours, genetic endowment and predisposition, immunological status and other factors that influence susceptibility, whereas environmental factors are external conditions, other than the agent, that influence the onset of disease. These can be physical, biological or social in nature. For example, the extent of HIV transmission in a population is the result of multiple agent, host and environmental factors (Box 2.2). In this respect, all diseases, including infections, are multifactorial and have multiple causes. One of the benefits of this broader view is that the health of a population can be promoted by procedures that modify susceptibility and exposure, as well as by procedures that attack the agent involved in the disease. That is, disease can be prevented as well as cured.

The epidemiological triangle is useful in understanding infectious disorders, but is less useful with respect to chronic, degenerative disorders such as heart disease, stroke and arthritis, for here no specific agent can be identified against which individuals and populations can be protected. Many contemporary medical problems are better understood in terms of a web of causation. According to this concept, disorders such as heart disease develop through complex interactions of many factors, which form a hierarchical causal web of events. These factors can be biophysical, social or psychological and can promote or inhibit the disease at more than one point in the causal process. Ultimately, they determine the level of disease in a community. This is illustrated with respect to heart disease in Fig. 2.1. As many of these factors can be modified, prevention offers better prospects for health than

---

BOX 2.2   Agent, Host and Environmental Factors in HIV transmission

Agent:
- HIV subtype (A, B, C, D, E)
- Phenotypic differences
- Genotypic differences
- Antiretroviral drug resistance

Host:
- Host genetics
- Stage of infection
- Antiretroviral therapy
- Reproductive tract infections
- Cervical ectopy
- Male circumcisions
- Contraception
- Menstruation and pregnancy

Environment:
- Social norms
- Average rate of sex partner change
- Local prevalence/probability of exposure
- Social and economic determinants of risk behaviours such as unsafe sex

Source: Royce et al (1997).

21

cure. It is also important to note that many of the factors implicated in heart disease have been identified as increasing the risk of other disorders, such as stroke and cancer.

The theory of general susceptibility

The theory of general susceptibility has emerged over the past 20 years and departs in important ways from monocausal and multicausal models of disease. It is not concerned with identifying single or multiple risk factors associated with specific disorders, but seeks to understand why some social groups seem to be more susceptible to disease and death in general. For example, numerous studies have shown that social class, measured by occupation, education, income or area of residence, is closely related to health, even in countries with nationalized and egalitarian healthcare systems such as the National Health Service (NHS) in the UK (see Chapter 8).

The socioenvironmental approach

During the late 1980s, the theory of general susceptibility became more explicitly formulated as the socioenvironmental approach. This approach is not so much concerned with the causes of disease, but rather seeks to identify the broad factors that make and keep people healthy. In its concern with populations rather than individuals, it forms the basis for the health promotion strategies described in Chapter 17. One framework concerning the determinants of health identifies five broad factors that can be targeted in order to improve population health: (1) the social and economic environment; (2) the physical environment; (3) personal health practices; (4) individual capacity and coping skills; and (5) health services. An expanded list, along with a rationale for each broad factor is presented in Box 2.3. Other

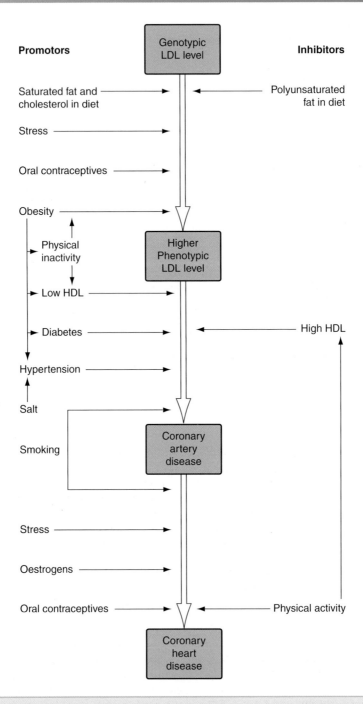

Fig. 2.1 The web of causation: risk factors for heart disease. HDL, high density lipoproteins; LDL, low density lipoproteins.
(*Reproduced with permission from Mausner & Kramer 1985*).

BOX 2.3   Social and Environmental Determinants of Health

- **Income and social status**: there is a close association between income and health so that health improves at each step up the income and social hierarchy. In addition, societies with a high standard of living in which wealth is more equally distributed are healthier, irrespective of the amount spent on health services.
- **Social support networks**: support from family, friends and social organizations is associated with better health. Moreover, people living in communities with higher levels of social cohesion tend to be healthier.
- **Education**: higher levels of education are associated with better health. Education increases opportunities for income and job security and equips people with the means to exert control over their life circumstances.
- **Employment and working conditions**: hazardous physical working environments and the injuries they induce are important causes of health problems. Moreover, those with more control over their work, and who have jobs that involve fewer stress-inducing demands, are healthier. However, unemployment, particularly if long term, is associated with poorer health.
- **Physical environments**: the quality of air and water influence the health of populations. So do features of the constructed physical environment, such as housing, roads and community design.
- **Personal health practices and coping skills**: social environments that encourage healthy choices and healthy lifestyles are key influences on health, as are the knowledge, behaviours and skills that influence how people cope with challenging life issues and circumstances.
- **Healthy child development**: prenatal and early childhood experiences can have a powerful effect on development and health throughout the life span.
- **Health services**: although not a major determinant of population health, health services can, if organized and delivered appropriately, prevent disease and help promote and maintain health.

Source: Federal, Provincial and Territorial Advisory Committee on Population Health (1994).

---

factors that have been cited as determinants of health include social exclusion in the form of racism and discrimination, food and transportation (Wilkinson & Marmot 1998).

According to Labonte (1993), social and environmental factors constitute risk conditions that have a direct effect on health and well-being and also affect health through the numerous psychosocial, behavioural and physiological risk factors that they engender (Fig. 2.2). One implication of the model presented in Fig. 2.2 is that material deprivation and a lack of control over important dimensions of one's life are the main issues that need to be addressed in promoting the health of the population. It is no accident that those countries where the income gap between the rich and the poor is narrowest have the lowest overall mortality rates. As a consequence, social and political change, including income redistribution, might be necessary to modify the health experience of lower socioeconomic groups.

These theories of the causes of disease have been presented in a more or less historical sequence. From the brief descriptions offered it is clear that the role ascribed to the physical, social and psychological environment increases as we progress from the germ theory of disease to socioenvironmental models of health. The latter completely overturns the doctrine of specific aetiology central to the former, for broad non-specific social and psychological factors are seen to be associated with a variety of disease outcomes, and ultimately the health and well-being of the population.

It would, however, be a mistake to assume that the role of social and psychological factors as causes of disease has been realized only in modern times. Many of the so-called 'prescientific' explanations of disease gave recognition to the part played by such factors. In many

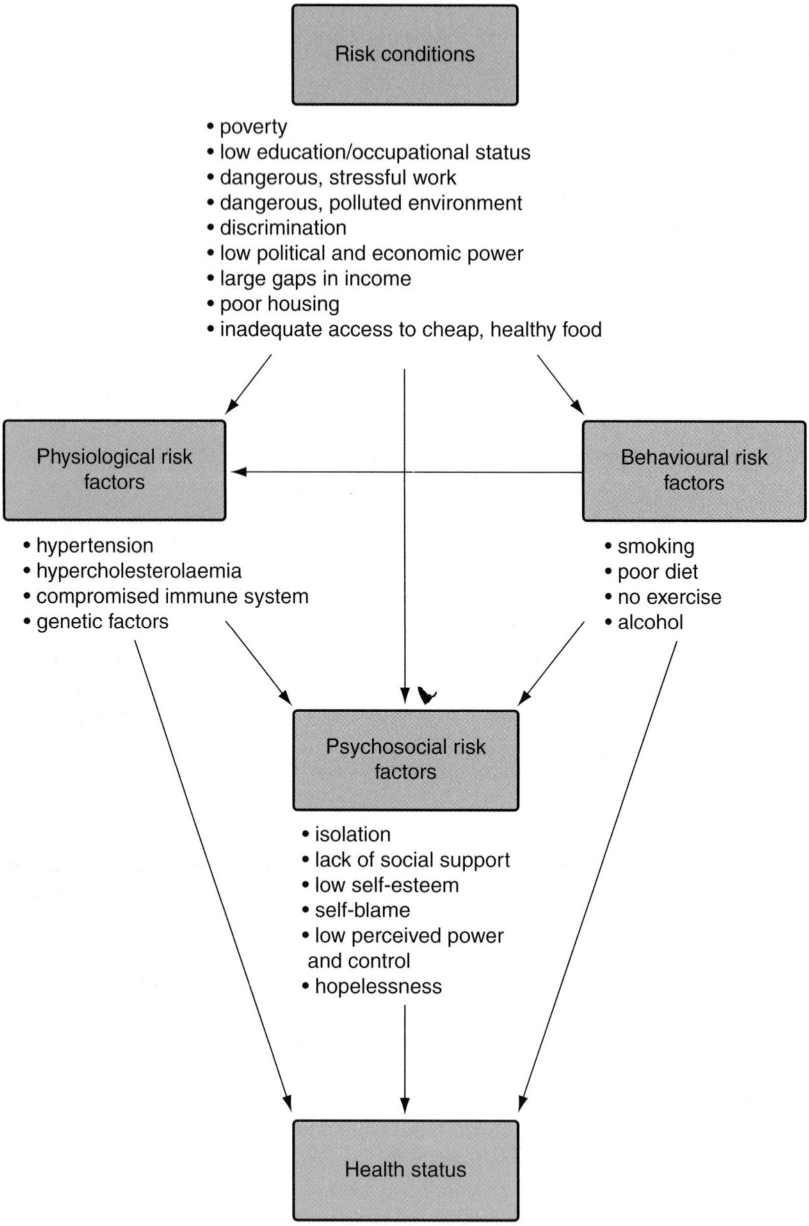

24

Fig. 2.2 The socioenvironmental approach.
(*Reproduced with permission from The University of Toronto from Labonte 1993*).

cultures, disease is still seen in social terms, as the outcome of a lack of harmony in social relationships. In the context of modern medical history, the idea that disease can be brought about by psychological influences was integral to the work of Freud, who explained disorders such as asthma and gastric ulcers as the product of unresolved psychological conflict. Freud's work gave rise to the notion that some diseases were 'psychosomatic' whereas others were not. The contemporary view is that social and psychological factors are implicated in all diseases, although the mechanisms by which they influence health are complex and variable.

SOCIAL AND PSYCHOLOGICAL FACTORS AND HEALTH

The research effort invested in studies of social and psychological factors and health is substantial and the body of work that has been produced is difficult to summarize. One reason for this is that a wide variety of factors with a potential influence on health and disease have been studied. As the discussion of theories of disease indicated, these factors fall into three broad types: socioenvironmental, behavioural and psychological.

25

Clearly, there are close links between many of these factors, and contemporary models of illness attempt to specify how and when they are involved in the mechanisms leading to disease. Even though behaviours such as smoking are individual acts, a number of social and cultural factors influence whether someone will become a smoker and continue to smoke. These factors include 'cultural themes associated with smoking such as relaxation, adulthood, sexual attractiveness and emancipation; the socioeconomic structure of tobacco production, processing, distribution and legislation; explicit and continual advertising by the tobacco companies and the influence of peers, siblings and significant others' (Syme 1986).

Some of the social and psychological factors having an influence on health and explanations of their role as causes of disease are reviewed below.

Social and cultural change

Most of the early studies of social factors and disease onset were concerned with the effects of social and cultural change. They included studies of industrialization and urbanization, migration and social, occupational and geographical mobility. The major disease outcome studied was coronary heart disease, because this is predominantly a disease of industrialized, urbanized nations. Some populations isolated from western culture have low blood pressure that does not rise with age. However, blood-pressure levels and coronary heart disease rates increase when these populations move to urban settings.

A number of studies conducted during the 1960s and early 1970s found higher rates of disease among people who changed jobs, place of residence or life circumstances. For example, one study found that men reared on farms who moved to urban centres to take middle-class jobs had higher rates of coronary heart disease than men who continued to work on the farm or who took up labouring jobs in cities (Syme et al 1964). Similar observations have been made with respect to cancer.

A number of mechanisms might be responsible for the negative effects of social and cultural change on health. The adverse effects might be the direct result of change itself, a product of the circumstances to which individuals move or the product of personal characteristics that predispose individuals to both mobility and poor health. One study that attempted to evaluate these explanations compared rates of heart disease among Japanese immigrants to California and Hawaii with those of Japanese men still living in Japan (Marmot et al 1975). Coronary heart disease and mortality rates were highest among those living in California and lowest in Japan. Among those living in California, some had become 'acculturated' and had adopted western lifestyles, whereas others retained traditional Japanese ways. The former had disease rates up to five times as high as the latter. This suggests that being mobile is not, in itself, the important factor, rather it is the change in the environment in which these people lived that explained the increase in disease risk.

Social support

One of the earliest studies of the relationship between social environment and health was undertaken by the French sociologist Emile Durkheim and published in 1897. In this work Durkheim pioneered the use of statistical methods for exploring and explaining differences in suicide rates across different social groups. Although suicide is an individual act, these differences in rates have persisted over time and across cultures. Durkheim explained suicide in terms of the social organization of these groups, particularly the extent to which individuals were integrated into the group, and the way in which this encouraged or deterred individuals from suicide. High rates of suicide were associated with groups that had very high and very low levels of integration.

More recent studies of social ties and health have focused on the relationship between social support and well-being. Some of this early work looked at differences in health according to marital status. The single, widowed and divorced have higher mortality rates than the married, the differences being much larger for men than for women (Table 2.1). These differences, which were first observed and reported in the mid-nineteenth century, have been remarkably consistent over time, and are consistent across cultures and health-care systems. Only a small part of the differences in mortality rates can be explained by the selective effects of marriage (Morgan 1980).

One possible explanation of these differences is that marital status has an influence on psychological states and lifestyles (Gove 1979). Studies have shown that people who are married tend to be happier and more satisfied with life than unmarried people, they are less likely to be socially isolated and have more social ties. In a society in which marriage and family life are a central value, being married gives meaning and significance to daily life, promotes a sense of well-being and is a source of social and emotional support. This explanation tends to be supported by data on marital status and specific causes of death. Variations in mortality rates are large where psychological states or aspects of lifestyle play a direct role in death, as in suicide or death from accidents, or are associated with acts such as smoking or alcohol consumption. Large differences are also observed with respect to

TABLE 2.1	Mortality, all causes: ratio of mortality rate of the unmarried to the mortality rate of the married; whites aged 25–64 years, USA 1960		
Maritial status	**Sex**	**Ratio**	
Single	Male	1.96	
	Female	1.68	
Widowed	Male	2.64	
	Female	1.77	
Divorced	Male	3.39	
	Female	1.95	

Reproduced with permission from the University of Chicago Press from Gove (1979).

diseases such as tuberculosis, where family factors can influence entry into medical care, willingness to undergo treatment or the availability of help and support.

An influential study, which clearly demonstrated that integration into the community has a direct effect on health, was undertaken by Berkman & Syme (1979). They followed a random sample of adults over a 9-year period. At the start of the study a social network score was calculated for each subject based on marital status, contacts with friends and relatives and membership of religious and other social groups. Over the 9-year period of the study those with low network scores were more likely to die than those with high network scores. After controlling for other factors such as weight, cigarette smoking, alcohol consumption, physical activity, health practices and health status at baseline, mortality rates for the socially isolated were two to three times higher than those with extensive social networks. These early findings have been confirmed in a number of other longitudinal studies. For example, a 6-year study of men in Finland found that risk of death was highest among those who reported having few persons to whom they gave or from whom they received support. Lack of participation in social organizations, having few friends and not being married were associated with mortality after taking into account baseline health and other risk factors including income (Kaplan et al 1994).

Other evidence suggests that social integration and social support have a broad influence on health. Early studies found that they were linked to heart disease, complications of pregnancy and emotional illness. More recent studies have found that social integration exerts a protective effect on the incidence of non-fatal myocardial infarction in men aged 50 and over (Vogt et al 1992) whereas social isolation increased the risk of stroke in a study of male health professionals in the US (Kawachi et al 1996). There is also strong and consistent evidence to show that lack of social support, social isolation and not being married have an influence on long-term survival among men following an initial myocardial infarction (Williams et al 1992). Other studies have found that social support was related to levels of residual disability following a stroke and to the onset of depression and degree of disability among rheumatoid arthritis patients (Fitzpatrick et al 1991). A 2-year follow-up study of people with disabilities found that people with few social contacts were more likely to deteriorate in physical and psychosocial functioning than people with high levels of contact with others (Patrick et al 1986). However, the greatest and most significant difference between those with and without social support occurred among those reporting an adverse life event during the period of the study.

Social support refers to a fairly broad category of events and includes practical assistance, financial help, the provision of information and advice and psychological support. The mechanisms by which it enhances or protects health are not known. One hypothesis concerning this mechanism has emerged in the context of studies of the negative health impact of stressful life circumstances. This research suggests that social support acts as a buffer against adverse events that would otherwise have health-damaging effects. In their research on the social origins of depression, Brown & Harris (1978) found that social support was protective only in the context of a severe life event. Although this and other studies strongly suggest that social support enhances coping and the ability to tolerate stressful life circumstances, it is also possible that it exerts an influence via psychological, hormonal and neurophysiological pathways.

Life events

A more comprehensive attempt to assess the influence of life experiences such as bereavement and unemployment is to be found in studies of life events and health. This approach emerged at the end of the 1960s with the development of instruments such as the Social

Readjustment Rating Scale (SRRS). This scale consists of a list of 42 events, each of which involves personal loss or some degree of change in roles or personal relationships. Each event is given a score depending on how much life change it involves. Scores for an individual are totalled to give a numerical estimate of the amount of life change experienced in a defined period, usually the past year. A number of studies have shown that there is some relationship between scores on this scale and future changes in health.

There have been a number of criticisms of this method of measuring the frequency and severity of life events. Perhaps the most important is that scales such as the SRRS fail to take account of variations in the meaning and significance of life events. The birth of a child, for example, will be a positive event for some women but a negative event for others, depending on the social context in which it occurs. More sophisticated measures of life events have been developed to take account of variations in the meaning of life events based on contextual factors (Brown & Harris 1978).

A second criticism of the SRRS is that it focuses on major life events and ignores less severe but more common life difficulties. A measure that attempts to assess such difficulties is the Hassles Scale (Kanner et al 1981). Its proponents claim that measures of life stress based on daily 'hassles' are better predictors of changes in physical and psychological health than measures based on major life events.

Clearly, the measurement of life stress is a complex issue and establishing a relationship between such stress and negative health outcomes is challenging. Many studies showing such a relationship have design weaknesses making interpretation of their results difficult.

One particularly noteworthy study is that conducted by Brown & Harris (1978), which was mentioned above in connection with social support. This was an investigation of the social and economic circumstances causally implicated in the onset of depression in women. Using measures that were context sensitive, Brown & Harris were able to show a clear relationship between life events with long-term threatening implications and the onset of depression in women. Events with short-term implications, no matter how stressful, were not associated with depression. However, whether or not a woman became depressed after an event involving long-term threat depended on the presence of four 'vulnerability factors'. These were: (1) the absence of a close, confiding relationship with a spouse or other person; (2) loss of mother before age 11 years; (3) lack of employment outside the home; and (4) having three or more children under the age of 15 living at home. The greater the number of these factors present, the greater was the likelihood of depression following an event with long-term threatening implications. Brown & Harris (1978) believe that these vulnerability factors produce ongoing low self-esteem and an inability to cope with the world. These interact with life events to produce generalized feelings of hopelessness and, subsequently, depression.

Life events have also been implicated in the mechanisms leading to physical disorders. They have been linked to disturbances in the control of diabetes, to diseases such as duodenal ulcer, and to abdominal pain leading to appendectomy (Creed 1981).

Occupational hierarchies and the organization of work

The physical environments in which people work are often hazardous and damaging to health. Air pollution at work, exposure to carcinogens, working with machinery and industrial accidents take a large toll on the health of manual workers. However, the psychosocial environments in which we work can also have a negative impact on health. Two models that identify important aspects of the psychosocial work environment are the demand–control model and the effort–reward imbalance model (Marmot et al 1999). The former suggests that jobs that combine a high level of psychological demands with low levels of control and skill utilization lead to stress and increase the risk of illness such as coronary heart disease. The latter suggests that jobs that combine a high degree of effort but low levels of gain in the form of financial or emotional rewards, employment security or career advancement also lead to emotional distress, job strain and illness.

Evidence in support of the demand–control model comes from a study of British civil servants, which explored the links between the organization of their work and health outcomes (Marmot & Theorell 1988). None of the subjects in the British study were living in poverty; nevertheless, there were differences in health status according to occupational grade. Those in the lowest grade had a mortality rate three times that of those in the highest grade, higher rates of onset of heart disease and higher rates of sickness absence. These differences were directly related to the degree of control in the workplace. Another noteworthy finding was that although blood pressure levels were similar for low- and high-grade civil servants when at work, they declined much more for the latter than the former when they were at home. This study concluded that a lack of freedom to make decisions at work, particularly when jobs are stressful or psychologically demanding, is linked to at-risk behaviours such as smoking, physiological risk factors such as high blood pressure and health outcomes such as heart disease.

Recent studies from Sweden have also found a higher risk of myocardial infarction among men in high demand/low control jobs, with this association being particular evident among manual workers (Hallqvist et al 1998).

To date, few studies have explored the effort–reward imbalance model. However, those available indicate that chronic stress associated with an effort–reward imbalance results in a two- to six-fold increase in the risk of onset of heart disease (Bosma et al 1998, Siegrist et al 1990). This increased risk could not be explained by other biomedical or behavioural risk factors. Other studies have documented adverse effects on mental health, musculoskeletal and gastrointestinal disorders, sleep disturbance and sickness absence.

Unemployment

Although the physical and social environments in which we work can have a negative effect on health, so can unemployment. There are two main reasons why unemployment could conceivably affect health (Marmot & Madge 1987). First, it is related to standards of living and the material conditions of life, and second it is a stressful event that can become chronic and deprive an individual of a social role, meaningful daily existence and contact with others.

Two approaches are evident in studies of unemployment and health and both are subject to problems in interpretation, largely because it is difficult to separate the effects of unemployment from the effects of other social and economic conditions (Marmot & Madge 1987). The first of these approaches attempts to demonstrate an association between unemployment rates and mortality rates and the way these co-vary with the ups and downs of the economic cycle. The most recent of this work was conducted by Brenner (1979) and is reviewed in Chapter 1. The second approach attempts to assess the health of people who are, or have recently become, unemployed. Because ill health can lead to unemployment, as well as vice versa, such studies need to be conducted carefully before it can be concluded that unemployment is a cause of poor health. Nevertheless, evidence from well-designed research does suggest that the unemployed experience more illness, have higher blood pressure, poorer psychological health and increased mortality (Jin et al 1996, Montgomery et al 1999, Turner 1995). Poverty, stress and insecurity, particularly housing insecurity, have all been implicated in the onset of the health problems following unemployment (Nettleton & Burrows 1998).

Health behaviours

Many behaviours can have a positive or negative impact on health. Diet, exercise, drinking, smoking and the use of illegal drugs are examples that have been the subject of numerous investigations. Although these behaviours are often characterized as being the result of individual choice and personal responsibility, it is more useful to see them as the product of social circumstances (Jarvis & Wardle 1999). Evidence that they are linked to social contexts is to be found in data showing that behaviours likely to promote health are less common in groups subject to poverty and social deprivation, whereas behaviours likely to damage health are more common. For example, smoking among both men and women is inversely related to occupational class and education. However, many circumstances are related to smoking (Jarvis & Wardle 1999). Rates are higher among the unemployed, those living in rented accommodation, those without access to a car and those who are divorced, separated or single parents. Clearly, material deprivation and factors that indicate stressful social and personal circumstances all predict whether an individual will smoke. The highest rates of all are found among groups characterized by combinations of these factors. There is also evidence to suggest that rates of smoking cessation are substantially lower in deprived than in non-deprived groups, even though there appears to be little difference between these groups in terms of wanting to quit smoking. One reason for this might be that nicotine dependence is strongly related to deprivation. Another reason is that the social environments in which deprived groups live and work are less conducive to quitting. One implication of this research is that smoking rates among the deprived are unlikely to decline unless the social circumstances that foster smoking and nicotine dependence are addressed.

PEOPLE, PLACES AND HEALTH

Although a great deal has been made of the links between social and physical environments and health, it is rare for these environments themselves to be the focus of research. The overwhelming tendency has been to look at the characteristics of individuals rather than the characteristics of the places in which they live. However, as evidence begins to accumulate, it is clear that the immediate neighbourhood in which one lives can have an impact on health. Simply put, poor people living in wealthier neighbourhoods have better health than similarly poor people living in poor neighbourhoods (Blaxter 1990). MacIntyre et al (1993) have argued that findings such as these indicate a need for research to discover precisely which features of local areas either damage or promote health. Although there has been some research trying to link aspects of the physical environment, such as air pollution or water hardness, to diseases such as bronchitis and cancer, very little work has tried to identify the social, cultural or economic characteristics of areas that affect health. The importance of such work is clear; we might be able to improve health by changing places rather than people.

As an example of this kind of research, MacIntyre et al (1993) compared two areas of Glasgow to identify differences in the living environments they provided. One was in the north-west of the city and had relatively low mortality rates; the other was in the south-west of the city and had high mortality rates. They found differences between the areas, such that living in the north-west would be more conducive to good health than living in the south-west. Healthy foodstuffs were more available and cheaper in the north-west, there were more sporting and recreational facilities, better transport services, better health services, less crime and a less hostile environment. Even though two people might have the same personal characteristics (the same income, family size and composition, and housing tenure, for example) the one living in the north west would be advantaged compared with the one in the south-west in ways likely to be related to physical and mental health.

Social cohesion

One community-level factor that does appear to be related to health is that of social cohesion. This is a difficult idea to grasp but essentially refers to the existence of mutual trust and respect between different sections of a community. Cohesive communities are ones in which there is a high level of participation in communal activities and high levels of membership of community groups (Stansfield 1999). Important components of social cohesion seem to be the friendliness and support of neighbours, opportunities for interaction with other members of the community and the fear of violence and crime. Emerging evidence suggests that these characteristics are linked to health and mortality (Wilkinson 1996). Certainly, interventions that improve the physical characteristics of a community so that they promote feelings of safety and perceptions of the friendliness of an area have resulted in improvements in the mental health and self-esteem of residents (Halpern 1995).

The main conclusion to be drawn from this and the other research summarized above is that patterns of health and disease are largely the product of social and environmental influences. Although health and illness involve biological agents and processes, they are inseparable from the social settings in which people live. Ultimately, it is these that influence the challenges people encounter in daily life and their capacity to manage them. Changing these environments is one way in which the health of a community can be improved.

THE SOCIAL CAUSES OF DISEASE: BIOLOGICAL PATHWAYS

Although the evidence linking socioenvironmental factors and health is compelling, the question remains as to how social factors operate to influence health and disease. Psychoneuroimmunology, an emerging and sometimes controversial field of knowledge, is beginning to provide evidence of the biological pathways linking social factors and disease and filling in the gaps in the social-stress–illness model. Although there are a number of formulations of this model, most assume that stressors (threatening environmental circumstances) give rise to strains (psychological and physiological changes) that increase an individual's susceptibility to disease. There is evidence to suggest that stress, or its outcome in the form of depression, leads to a number of changes in the human body. It interferes with the normal functioning of neuroendocrine, autonomic metabolic and immune systems, leads to increased heart rate and respiration, dilatation of blood vessels to the muscles and alterations in gastrointestinal function. These changes are believed to cause disease directly or render an individual more prone to disease (Brunner & Marmot 1999).

As some of the research reviewed above suggests, this essentially simple model is more complex than it seems. Clearly, the link between stressors and illness is mediated by a number of factors that can increase or decrease an individual's vulnerability when faced with a stressor. Social factors (such as social support) and psychological variables (such as personality characteristics, perceptual processes and coping styles) interact in complex ways to affect health outcomes. Moreover, as the socioenvironmental approach suggests, behavioural responses to environmental stressors in the form of health-damaging activities such as smoking also play an important role (Najman 1980). However, whereas the specification of these biological and behavioural pathways strengthens the credibility of the research evidence, the implications of that evidence are clear. Changing the social circumstances of deprived groups is necessary to improve population health.

References

Berkman L, Syme S 1979 Social networks, host resistance and mortality: a nine-year follow-up of Alameda County residents. American Journal of Epidemiology 109:186–204

Blaxter M 1990 Health and lifestyles. Tavistock-Routledge, London

Bosma H, Peter R, Siegrist J, Marmot M 1998 Alternative job stress models and the risk of heart disease. American Journal of Public Health 88:68–74

Brenner M 1979 Mortality and the national economy. Lancet ii:568–573

Brown G, Harris T 1978 The social origins of depression. Tavistock, London

Brunner E, Marmot M 1999 Social organization, stress and health. In: Marmot M, Wilkinson R (eds) Social determinants of health. Oxford University Press, Oxford

Creed F 1981 Life events and appendicitis. Lancet i:1381–1385

Federal, Provincial and Territorial Advisory Committee on Population Health 1994 Strategies for population health: investing in the health of Canadians. Minister of Supply and Services Canada, Ottawa

Fitzpatrick R, Newman S, Archer R, Shipley M 1991 Social support, disability and depression: a longitudinal study of arthritis and depression. Social Science and Medicine 33:605–611

Gove W 1979 Sex, marital status and mortality. American Journal of Sociology 79:45–67

Hallqvist J et al 1998 Is the effect of job strain on myocardial infarction due to interaction between high psychological demands and low decision latitude. Results from the Sweden Heart Epidemiology Program. Social Science and Medicine 46:1405–1415

Halpern D 1995 Mental health and the built environment. More than bricks and mortar? Taylor and Francis, London

Jarvis M, Wardle J 1999 Social patterning of health behaviours: the case of cigarette smoking. In: Marmot M, Wilkinson R (eds) Social determinants of health. Oxford University Press, Oxford

Jin RL, Shah CP, Sroboda TJ 1996 The impact of unemployment on health: a review of the evidence. Canadian Medical Association Journal 153:529–540

Kanner A, Coyne J, Schaefer C, Lazarus R 1981 Comparison of two modes of stress measurement: daily hassles and uplifts versus major life events. Journal of Behavioural Medicine 4:1–39

Kaplan G et al 1994 Social functioning and overall mortality: prospective evidence from the Kuopio ischemic heart disease risk factor study. Epidemiology 5:495–500

Kawachi I, Colditz G, Ascherio A 1996 A prospective study of social networks in relation to total mortality and cardiovascular disease in men in the USA. Journal of Epidemiology and Community Health 50:245–251

Labonte R 1993 Health promotion and empowerment: practice frameworks. Issues in Health Promotion no 3. Centre for Health Promotion, University of Toronto

MacIntyre S, MacIver S, Soomans A 1993 Area, class and health: should we be focusing on places or people? Journal of Social Policy 22:213–234

Marmot M, Madge N 1987 An epidemiological perspective on stress and health. In: Kasl S, Cooper C (eds) Stress and health: issues in research methodology. Wiley, Winchester

Marmot M, Theorell T 1988 Social class and cardiovascular disease: the contribution of work. International Journal of Health Services 18:37–45

Marmot M, Syme L, Kagan A 1975 Epidemiological studies of heart disease and stroke in Japanese men living in Japan, Hawaii and California. Prevalence of coronary and hypertensive disease and associated risk factors. American Journal of Epidemiology 102:514–525

Marmot M, Siegrist J, Theorell T, Feeny A 1999 Health and the psychosocial environment at work. In: Marmot M, Wilkinson R (eds) Social determinants of health. Oxford University Press, Oxford

Mausner J, Kramer S 1985 Epidemiology: an introductory text. WB Saunders, Philadelphia

Montgomery S, Cook D, Bartley M, Wadsworth M 1999 Unemployment in young men predates symptoms of depression and anxiety resulting in medical consultation. International Journal of Epidemiology 28:95–100

Morgan M 1980 Marital status, health, illness and service use. Social Science and Medicine 14A:633–643

Najman J 1980 Theories of disease causation and the concept of general susceptibility: a review. Social Science and Medicine 14A:231–237

Nettleton S, Burrows B 1998 Mortgage debt, insecure home ownership and health: an exploratory analysis. Society, Health & Illness 20:731–753

Patrick D, Morgan M, Charlton J 1986 Psychosocial support and change in the health status of physically disabled people. Social Science and Medicine 22:1347–1354

Royce R et al 1997 Sexual transmission of HIV. New England Journal of Medicine 336:1072–1078

Siegrist J et al 1990 Low status control, high effort at work and ischemic heart disease: prospective evidence from blue collar men. Social Science and Medicine 31:1127–1134

Stansfield S 1999 Social support and social cohesion. In: Marmot M, Wilkinson R (eds) Social determinants of health. Oxford University Press, Oxford

Syme S 1986 Social determinants of health and disease. In: Last J (ed) Public health and preventative medicine. Appleton-Century-Crofts, Norwalk, CT

Syme S, Hyman M, Enterline P 1964 Some social and cultural factors associated with the occurrence of coronary heart disease. Journal of Chronic Diseases 17:277–289

Turner JB 1995 Economic context and the impact of unemployment. Journal of Health and Social Behaviour 35:213–219

Vogt T et al 1992 Social networks as predictors of ischemic heart disease, cancer, stroke and hypertension: incidence, survival and mortality. Journal of Clinical Epidemiology 45:659–666

Wilkinson R 1996 Unhealthy societies: from inequality to well-being. Routledge, London

Wilkinson R, Marmot M (eds) 1998 Social determinants of health: the solid facts. WHO Regional Office for Europe, Copenhagen

Williams R, Barefoot J, Califf R 1992 Prognostic importance of social and economic resources among medically treated patients with angiographically documented coronary heart disease. Journal of the American Medical Association 267:520–524

Social Factors in Medical Practice

3

Health and Illness Behaviour

Graham Scambler

Definitions of 'health' and 'illness' vary within cultures, subcultures and communities, and even within households – between generations for example. There can also be gaps between lay and medical concepts. The primary focus of this chapter is on lay beliefs about, and attitudes towards, health and illness, and on the various ways in which these, together with a host of other social factors, can influence people's behaviour when faced with what they perceive to be threats to their well-being.

Consideration is given first to differences in people's perspectives on health and illness. A brief review is then given of studies of the prevalence of illness and disease in the community. Special attention is paid to those factors known to influence help-seeking behaviour, and especially to those known to affect whether or not people who define themselves as ill consult a physician, usually a general practitioner. Finally, self-help and sources of help other than allopathic medicine are considered, ranging from informal lay networks to alternative therapies.

PERCEPTIONS OF HEALTH AND ILLNESS

The modern study of how lay people define health and illness was pioneered by Herzlich (1973) with her research with 80, largely middle-class, adults in France. Analysing their accounts of health and illness, she found that illness was generally perceived as external and as a product of a way of life, notably urban life. This covered not merely pathological agents such as germs, but also accidents and diseases like cancer and various mental disorders. Health, on the other hand, was perceived as internal to the individual, with three different and discernible dimensions: (1) an absence of illness ('health in a vacuum'); (2) a 'reserve of health', determined by constitution and temperament; and (3) a positive state of well-being or 'equilibrium'.

Several studies in Britain have since led to similar distinctions. Pill & Scott (1982) interviewed mothers from working-class backgrounds with young children. They encountered definitions of health in terms of the absence of illness. A functional definition of health was also common, that is, in terms of the capacity to perform or cope with normal roles. As in Herzlich's study, a positive definition of health was apparent as well, although among Pill & Scott's sample it was associated with being cheerful and enthusiastic rather than with a state of equilibrium.

Such a positive dimension was missing, however, from the accounts of mothers and daughters in socially disadvantaged families questioned by Blaxter & Paterson (1982). References were made to health as the absence of illness, but the majority seemed to have a functional definition of health. They also had a functional definition of illness, many of them distinguishing between normal illness, which they accommodated, and serious illness, like cancer, heart disease and tuberculosis, which called for radical adjustment and change. These conceptions of health and illness, especially the lack of a positive definition of health, clearly reflected the high prevalence of health problems among the sample.

Reviewing these and other studies, Blaxter (1990) writes: 'Health can be defined negatively as the absence of illness, functionally, as the ability to cope with everyday activities, or positively, as fitness and well-being'. She adds that health also has moral connotations, which are as salient in modern urban communities as they are among pre-modern or primitive societies. There is a sense in which people feel a duty to be healthy and experience illness as failure. Health can be seen in terms of will-power, self-discipline and self-control.

Increasingly relevant too, it might be added, is an emphasis on what has been called 'body maintenance'. This is linked to innovative forms of entrepreneurial activity and to 'consumerism'. The body becomes a site of pleasure and a representation of happiness and success. As Nettleton (1995) puts it, 'to look good is to *feel* good'. Health education echoes the commercialization of body maintenance. Thus, Featherstone (1991) argues that common to the media treatment of body maintenance and to health education is the 'encouragement of self-surveillance of bodily health and appearance as well as the incentive of lifestyle benefits'. He goes on to refer to the 'transvaluation' of activities like jogging and slimming, which have been re-evaluated in light of their putative health benefits. The most conspicuous example of the commercialization of healthy life-styles is probably the 'fitness industry', its products ranging from exercise machines and videos to special stylish clothing.

Monaghan (2001) takes this line further to consider what he calls the 'vibrant pleasures'. He too argues that only recently has the body been linked to health as opposed to illness. In his ethnographic study of bodybuilding, he emphasizes the importance to participants of 'looking good' and 'feeling good'. As one interviewee put it: 'It's all to do with looks, and I would rather look good on the outside. That's what bodybuilding is. It's not for fitness reasons, it's all visual'. Monaghan maintains that 'a crucial point of overlap between "risk-inducing" bodybuilders and "health conscious" fitness enthusiasts more generally (e.g. weight-trainers, joggers, participants in step aerobics) is a shared attempt to *embody* and *display* a sense of empowerment and self-mastery'. It is simplistic to stereotype bodybuilding as injurious to health and as intimately associated with drug use. Rather, 'embodied pleasures', epitomized in the gym by 'the rush', and the perceived psychosocial benefits of anaerobic exercise, together with the imagery of muscle, are more directly relevant in sustaining people's consumption of (risky) bodybuilding technologies.

ILLNESS AND DISEASE IN THE COMMUNITY

The national 'Health and lifestyles' survey (Blaxter 1990) found that 71% of participants defined their health as at least 'good'. This did not mean that none of these people had symptoms of illness or, indeed, medically defined disease. For example, many disabled and/or elderly people defined their health as 'excellent', clearly meaning 'my health is excellent despite my disability/considering my advanced years'. Comparisons were made between participants' own assessments of their health and a series of objective measures. Although there was a general correspondence between the two, most obviously at the extremes, 10% of men and 7% of women in the top category of health, objectively measured, described their health as only 'fair' or 'poor'; and as many as 40% of those with undoubted health problems, objectively measured, described their health as 'good' or 'excellent'.

In a more recent survey of adults aged 16 or more in England in 1998, 22% of the men and 26% of the women reported 'less than good' general health, and 20% of men and 24% of women reported having a limiting longstanding illness (ONS 2000). Predictably, these self-reports were positively associated with age. Only in the youngest age group were women significantly more likely than men to report 'less than good' general health, and only in the oldest age-group were they significantly more likely than men to report a limiting longstanding illness.

Interestingly, the findings of a recent Swedish study of self-rated health suggested a strong relation between poor self-rated health and mortality in all the subgroups investigated, greater at younger ages, and similar among men and women and among people with and without chronic illness. The authors put forward the idea that self-rated health might be a useful outcome measure (Burstrom & Fredlund 2001).

The rate of reporting of individual symptoms of illness is high. The findings by Wadsworth et al (1971) remain typical of retrospective studies in this area. Of their sample of 1000 adults, 95% had experienced symptoms in the 14 days prior to interview and only one in five had consulted a doctor. In a prospective study (Scambler et al 1981) a sample of women aged 16–44 years kept 6-week health diaries in which they recorded any disturbances in their health. Symptoms were recorded on an average of one day in three. Table 3.1 shows the 10 most frequently recorded symptoms and also how often these precipitated medical consultations and the ratio of medical consultations to symptom episodes. Overall, there was one medical consultation for every 18 symptom episodes.

It might be thought that most symptoms not precipitating consultations are mild and not indicative of disease requiring medical intervention. Ingham & Miller (1979) found that symptom severity for seven selected symptoms was indeed greater in consulters than in non-consulters. There is convincing evidence, however, that general practitioners are often not consulted for disease that would undoubtedly respond to treatment. Epsom (1978) carried out a seminal investigation of the health status of a sample of adults using a mobile health clinic. Of the 3160 people investigated, 57% were referred to their general practitioners for further tests and possible treatment. Major diseases detected included seven instances of preinvasive cervical cancer, one confirmed case of carcinoma of the breast and one active case of pulmonary tuberculosis. A follow-up study of those referred to their general practitioners indicated that 38% of the findings had not previously been known to the general practitioners and that 22% of the findings made known to the general practitioners for the first time were judged serious enough to warrant hospital referrals. Thus a significant clinical iceberg exists: the professional health services treat only the tip of the sum total of ill health.

The existence of a clinical iceberg has important implications. Most obviously there is the problem of unmet need: many people of all ages are enduring avoidable pain, discomfort

TABLE 3.1	Symptom episodes and medical consultations recorded in health diaries				
Main types of symptom recorded	No. of symptom episodes	Percentage of total number of symptom episodes	Mean length of symptom episodes (days)	No. of occasions on which symptom episode precipitated medical consultation	Ratio of consultations to symptom episodes
Headache	180	20.9	1.3	3	1:60
Changes in energy, tiredness	109	12.6	1.4	0	–
Nerves, depression or irritability	74	8.6	1.7	1	1:74
Aches or pains in joints, muscles, legs or arms	71	8.2	1.6	4	1:18
Women's complaints like period pain[a]	69	8.0	1.7	7	1:10
Stomach aches or pains	45	5.2	1.5	4	1:11
Backache	38	4.4	1.6	1	1:38
Cold, flu, or running nose	37	4.3	4.1	3	1:12
Sore throat	36	4.2	2.4	4	1:9
Sleeplessness	31	3.6	1.5	1	1:31
Others	173	20.0	1.9	21	1:8
Total	863	100.0	1.7	49	1:18

Reproduced with permission from Scambler et al (1981).
[a] Stomach aches and pains and backache were classified as period pains if so defined by the women themselves.

and handicap. There is a gap in other words between the need for and the demand for health care. It must be remembered, however, that any substantial increase in the existing level of demand would swamp the primary care services. Many general practitioners also argue that there is currently a widespread tendency for people to consult for trivial, unnecessary or inappropriate reasons: in one national study, one-quarter of the general practitioners questioned felt that half or more of their surgery consultations fell into this category (Cartwright & Anderson 1981). Basic to these issues, of course, is the question of how to define 'need'.

UNDERSTANDING ILLNESS BEHAVIOUR

A number of studies have documented the sociodemographic characteristics of users and non-users of medical services. It is known, for example, that women consult more than men, children and the elderly more than young adults and the middle-aged. Social class, ethnic origin, marital status and family size are other factors that have been shown to be related to utilization. These studies tell us who does and does not make use of the services, rather than why. To begin to answer the more complex question of why people seek or decline to seek professional help is to begin to theorize about illness behaviour.

It is crucial to recognize that whether or not people consult their doctors does not depend only on the presence of disease, but also on how they, or others, respond to its symptoms. Mechanic (1978) has listed 10 variables known to influence consulting behaviour (Box 3.1). Mechanic acknowledges that this list is far from exhaustive and that, in reality, different variables tend to interact together. He also introduces a basic underlying distinction between 'self-defined' and 'other-defined' illness: the major difference is that, in the latter, individuals tend to resist the definitions that others attempt to impose upon them, and it might be necessary to bring them into treatment under great pressure, even involuntarily. As it is not possible to explore all the multifarious and interrelated influences on illness and consulting behaviour here, six broad categories have been selected for emphasis.

Cultural variation

The significance of cultural factors in determining how symptoms are interpreted has been well documented, perhaps most convincingly in studies of ethnicity and the experience and reporting of pain. In a pioneering study conducted in New York, Zborowski (1952) found that patients of Old-American or Irish origin displayed a stoical, matter-of-fact attitude towards pain and, if it was intense, a tendency to withdraw from the company of others. In contrast, patients of Italian or Jewish background were more demanding and dependent and tended to seek, rather than shun, public sympathy. Subsequent research has both corroborated Zborowski's findings and afforded support for the more general view that there is a marked cultural difference in the interpretation of and response to symptoms between so-called Anglo-Saxon and Mediterranean groups. It is tempting to assume that such cultural variation is explicable in terms of socialization alone, namely that differences

---

BOX 3.1   Mechanic's Variables Known to Influence Illness Behaviour

1. Visibility, recognizability or perceptual salience of signs and symptoms
2. The extent to which the symptoms are perceived as serious (that is, the person's estimate of the present and future probabilities of danger)
3. The extent to which symptoms disrupt family, work and other social activities
4. The frequency of the appearance of the signs or symptoms, their persistence, or their frequency or recurrence
5. The tolerance threshold of those who are exposed to and evaluate the signs and symptoms
6. Available information, knowledge and cultural assumptions and understandings of the evaluator
7. Basic needs that lead to denial
8. Needs competing with illness responses
9. Competing possible interpretations that can be assigned to the symptoms once they are recognized
10. Availability of treatment resources, physical proximity, and psychological and monetary costs of taking action (not only physical distance and costs of time, money and effort, but also such costs as stigma, social distance and feelings of humiliation)

Reproduced with permission of The Free Press from Mechanic (1978).

in illness behaviour merely reflect different culturally learned styles of coping with the world at large. The authors of a study of Anglo-Saxon, Anglo-Greek and Greek groups in Australia, however, have suggested that other factors might also be important. They found, for example, that immigrant status and, relatedly, the stress of adapting to a majority culture, played a significant part in accounting for the different patterns of illness behaviour among the Anglo-Saxon and Mediterranean groups (Pilowski & Spence 1977). In short, cultural patterns might vary, depending on the social context.

Symptoms and knowledge of disease

Studies have indicated that symptoms that present in a 'striking' way, for example, a sharp abdominal pain or a high fever, are more likely to be interpreted as illness and to receive prompt medical attention than those that present less dramatically. Consultation in such

circumstances might simply be a function of the pain or discomfort; alternatively, it might be a function of the degree of incapacitation or disruption engendered by the pain or discomfort (see 'Triggers' below). Many distressing symptoms are not indicative of serious disease; but, equally, some serious diseases, for example, some cancers, rarely appear in a striking fashion: their onset can be slow and insidious. The actions of potential patients are thus also dependent on their knowledge of disease and on their capacity to differentiate between diseases that are threatening/non-threatening and that can/cannot be effectively treated.

Triggers

Although many of the symptoms people experience are recognized as indicating disease processes, it is not necessarily the case that treatment is sought. What, when and if action to resolve any problems is undertaken often depends on a number of other factors. Zola (1973) has looked at the timing of decisions to seek medical care. He found that most people tolerated their symptoms for quite a time before they went to a doctor, and that the symptoms themselves were often not sufficient to precipitate a consultation: something else had to happen to bring this about. He identified five types of trigger:

1. the occurrence of an interpersonal crisis (e.g. a death in the family)
2. perceived interference with social or personal relations
3. 'sanctioning' (pressure from others to consult)
4. perceived interference with vocational or physical activity
5. a kind of 'temporalizing of symptomatology' (the setting of a deadline, e.g. 'If I feel the same way on Monday...', or 'If I have another turn...').

The decision to seek professional help is, then, very much bound up with an individual's personal and social circumstances. Zola also found that, when doctors paid insufficient attention to the specific trigger that prompted an individual or that an individual used as an excuse to seek help, there was a greater chance that the patient would eventually break off treatment.

Perceptions of costs and benefits

Doctors and other healthcare personnel tend to assume that a rational individual will report any symptoms that are causing him or her distress or anxiety; in other words, they take it for granted that the restoration of 'good health' is a natural first priority. Good health, however, is one goal among others; it is not always supreme. At any given time a person might deem obtaining treatment, which might involve hospitalization, to be less important or urgent than, for example, looking after young children or a dependent mother at home, preparing for an examination, being at work or going on holiday. Thus the value an individual attaches to good health varies in accordance with his or her perception of the benefits versus the costs of its accomplishment. The 'health belief model' represents one sustained attempt to bring together all those factors – from the demographic to the psychological – that influence an individual's assessment of the costs and benefits involved in seeking help.

Lay referral and intervention

It is comparatively rare for someone to decide in favour of a visit to the surgery without first discussing his or her symptoms with others. Scambler et al (1981) found that three-quarters of those participating in their study discussed their symptoms with some other person, usually a relative, before seeking professional help. Freidson (1970) has claimed that, just as doctors have a professional referral system, so potential patients have lay referral systems: 'the whole process of seeking help involves a network of potential consultants from the intimate confines of the nuclear family through successively more select, distant and authoritative laymen until the "professional" is reached'. Freidson has himself produced a model in terms of: (1) the degree of congruence between the subculture of the potential patient and that of doctors; and (2) the relative number of lay consultants interposed between the initial perception of symptoms and the decision whether or not to go to the doctor. Thus, for example, a situation in which the potential patient participates in a subculture that differs from that of doctors and in which there is an extended lay referral system would lead to the 'lowest' rate of utilization of medical services. In line with this example, one Scottish study reported that a high degree of interaction with interlocking kinship and friendship networks might well have 'inhibited' women in social class V from using antenatal care services (McKinlay 1973).

Occasionally, lay persons might take it upon themselves to intervene and to initiate medical consultations (see Mechanic's other-defined illness, above). This is most common when symptoms are perceived to be serious or life-threatening or when the sufferer is temporarily incapable of self-help: parents might take action on behalf of a child, a wife on behalf of a husband who is psychotic or who has experienced a tonic–clonic seizure. Scambler (1989) found that four out of five first consultations for epilepsy were other-initiated, many of them involving the calling of an ambulance. It has been suggested, however, that lay persons who are not members of the sufferer's family might be less likely than those who are to tolerate delays in help-seeking resulting from the normalization or denial of symptoms. Finlayson & McEwen (1977), for example, have described how the wives of some men tried in vain to persuade their husbands to see a doctor in the hour preceding myocardial infarction.

Access to healthcare facilities

Ease of access to healthcare facilities has obvious implications for usage. Tudor-Hart (1971) has argued that what he terms an 'inverse care law' applies in Britain; that is, the provision of health care is inversely related to the need for it (i.e. poor facilities in depressed areas characterized by high morbidity and good, or better, facilities in affluent areas characterized by low morbidity). He relates this to the market economy: the more prosperous areas attract the most resources, including skilled health workers, in both primary and secondary care.

The degree of equity of access to healthcare services is in fact not easy to determine (Goddard & Smith, 2001). In one recent study of the coverage of minor surgery, child health surveillance and chronic disease management for asthma and diabetes in relation to both population need and to key organizational features of general practice in the 481 primary care groups (PCGs) in England, the authors found little evidence of poorer service availability for PCGs with higher population need; but they did find evidence that the inverse care law might be geographically specific, and particularly pronounced for London PCGs (Baker & Hann 2001). It has often been shown that, as the distance between home and general practice increases, the likelihood of consultation diminishes; this is particularly true for elderly or disabled people, who are relatively immobile (Whitehead 1992).

SELF-CARE, SELF-HELP AND ALTERNATIVE THERAPY

The fact that only a small minority of all symptoms are presented to a doctor suggests that self-care, and especially self-medication, could be of considerable importance. Wadsworth et al (1971) found that self-treatment with non-prescribed medicines and home remedies is indeed extremely common. Dunnell & Cartwright (1972) found lower consultation rates among people who reported self-medication. They also found that in a 2-week period the ratio of non-prescribed to prescribed medicines taken by adults was approximately two to one; 67% of their sample had taken one or more non-prescribed medicines during this period. Moreover, only one in 10 of the non-prescribed medicines consumed had been first suggested by a doctor; most were recommended by members of lay referral systems. The data suggested that adults tended to use self-medication as an alternative to medical consultation. Anderson et al (1977) provide support for this interpretation, but add that whereas self-medication seems to be more popular among non-users than among users of the primary-care services, non-users are also less inclined than users to obtain medical help for potentially serious symptoms. Dunnell & Cartwright (1972) found that, for children, self- or parent-medication seemed to be used more as a supplement to medical consultation.

Of particular interest too is the rapid growth of self-help groups. Some, like Alcoholics Anonymous, have been established for a long time and are well known, but there are many newer and less well-known groups – for people with schizophrenia, skin diseases, depression, hypertension, cancer, the parents of handicapped children, victims of disasters, and so on. Some of these were the brainchildren of health workers who are still active within them, but many operate quite independently of the formal health services; in fact, the impetus for the formation of a number of groups has been the lack of adequate understanding, care, treatment or support from the various health professions. Some commentators regard self-help groups as a poor substitute for people who are starved of 'real' services. Others, like Robinson (1980), argue that 'it is the professional health services which should be seen as specific technical, organizational or expert assistance'; they contend that self-help should be regarded as one of the basic components of primary health care.

Kelleher (1994) notes that although many of the activities of self-help groups can be seen as complementary to the work of health professionals, some also reflect 'a subversive readiness to question the knowledge of doctors and to assert that experiential knowledge has value'. Developing this theme, he suggests that self-help groups might constitute a new social movement. His argument is that modern medicine, like other 'expert systems', has become increasingly limited in its capacity to comprehend human suffering and to engage with patients; it pays far too little attention, for example, to how people with chronic illnesses define their own situations experientially and 'cope' on an everyday basis. Self-help groups, whether or not they comprise a social movement, allow people to diverge from the medical perspective and, if necessary, to challenge and interrogate it. Kelleher (2001) has also argued that some self-help groups at least afford participants a genuine opportunity to construct their own personal and/or joint narratives, thereby 're-socializing people to see themselves as normal people with diabetes/epilepsy/schizophrenia'.

Apart from simply ignoring symptoms, another alternative to consulting a doctor or pursuing some form of self-care or self-help is to rely on alternative, complementary or non-orthodox therapies. Thomas et al (1991) estimated that in 1987 there were 1909 registered, non-medical practitioners of non-orthodox health care, that is, of acupuncture, chiropractic, homoeopathy, medical herbalism, naturopathy and osteopathy, working in Britain (Table 3.2). The same authors report that of the 70 600 patients seen by this group of practitioners in an average week, 78% were attending for musculoskeletal problems. About 36% of the patients had not received previous medical care for their main problem; 18% were receiving concurrent non-orthodox and medical care.

Alternative, complementary or non-orthodox medicine is growing much more rapidly than orthodox allopathic medicine. If non-registered practitioners offering therapies beyond those considered by Thomas and his colleagues are included, then it has been estimated that there are approximately 50 000 practitioners at work in the UK (that is, 60% more than the number of GPs) (Fulder 1996). A series of *Which?* surveys in Britain found that one in seven of the magazine's readers had used some form of alternative or complementary practice in 1986, one in four in 1992, and one in three in 1995; findings supported by regional studies funded by health authorities (Emslie et al 1996). Studies in other European countries and the USA reveal these British figures as fairly typical. Users are, it seems, more likely to be women, middle-aged, middle class and conscious of their health and of healthy living (Cant & Sharma 1999).

The increasing popularity of non-orthodox therapy might in part be a function of people's disillusionment with biomedicine. Practitioners themselves stress their longer consultations and a holistic orientation that concerns itself 'with complete wellness, not just symptomatology' (Bakx 1991). However, Saks (1994) cautions that although alternative therapists, like self-help groups, are now offering a real challenge to the mode of

TABLE 3.2	Main treatments and multiple treatments offered by registered non-orthodox practitioners (estimated numbers (%))			
Main treatment	**Registered practitioners (%)**		**Practitioners in each group offering multiple treatments and having membership of only one association**	
Acupuncture	507	27	100	20
Chiropractic	290	15	6	2
Homoeopathy	93	5	12	13
Medical herbalism	115	6	45	39
Naturopathy with osteopathy	128	7	41	32[a]
Osteopathy	680	36	34	5
Member of more than one association	96	5	–	
Total	1909	100	238	12

Reproduced with permission from Thomas et al (1991).
[a] Practitioners offering at least one treatment in addition to naturopathy and osteopathy.

practice of orthodox medicine, there is little evidence as yet that the legitimacy of medical authority is being seriously undermined.

To summarize, it has been shown that very often the decision whether to consult a doctor is not simply a function of the degree of pain or disability associated with symptoms, or of their perceived seriousness. What Hannay (1980) has termed 'incongruous referral behaviour' is commonplace. The heterogeneous assembly of factors that are known to influence decisions about medical consultation has been indicated. It has been stressed too, however, that the study of illness behaviour is not concerned exclusively with whether or not people visit doctors. On the basis of anthropological work, Kleinman (1985) suggested that there are typically three major arenas of care in what he calls 'local health care systems': popular, folk and professional (Fig. 3.1).

Most health care takes place in the popular sector, which embraces self-care, including self-medication, and those self-help groups that function independently of professional health workers. The folk sector comprises non-professional 'specialists' who offer some form of alternative or non-orthodox therapy. Professionalization, Kleinman contends, has a tendency to distance practitioners from patients and to lead to a focus on (medically defined) disease as opposed to (patient defined) illness. Of the professional sector in western societies he writes: 'Western-oriented biomedicine seems to be the more extreme example of this trend, perhaps because biomedical ideology and norms are more remote from (one almost wants to say estranged from) the life world of most patients' (Kleinman 1985).

Scambler (2002) associates Kleinman's popular, folk and professional sectors of local healthcare systems with different and distinctive 'relations of healing' (Table 3.3).

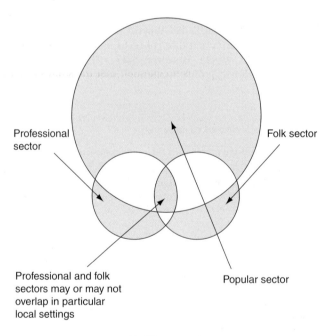

Fig. 3.1 Local healthcare systems.
(Reproduced with permission from Tavistock Publications from Kleinman 1985).

TABLE 3.3	Sectors of local healthcare systems and their relations of healing (adapted from Scambler 2002)
Sector	**Relations of healing**
Popular	Caring
Folk	Restoring
Professional	Fixing

The popular sector, he suggests, is characterized by relations of caring. He makes the point that it remains largely women who assume day-to-day responsibility for looking after those who are ill in this sector, not only those who are chronically or permanently ill but also children and partners who have mundane illnesses like flu. Arguably, the 'unpaid health work' done here underwrites the more specialist 'paid health work' on offer in the other sectors (see Chapters 9 and 16). The folk sector is characterized by relations of restoring, reflecting the holist philosophies that often underpin the endeavours of alternative or complementary practitioners. Finally, the professional sector gives rise to relations of fixing. The emphasis here is on the onus placed on doctors to treat disease within the confines of the 'sick role' (Chapter 4) so that people can resume their normal responsibilities as expeditiously as possible. Needless to say, this differentiation of relations of healing does not imply, for example, that doctors cannot or do not either care or restore, merely that Kleinman's sectors of local healthcare systems are distinguished in part by their own specific paradigms, modes or relations of healing.

Kleinman (1985) considers that the major challenge is to 're-work medicine's paradigm of clinical practice to make it more responsive to indigenous patient values, beliefs and expectations'. Agree or disagree, there is no question that the study of illness behaviour must address itself to the popular and folk as well as to the professional sectors of local healthcare systems.

References

Anderson J, Buck C, Danaher K, Fry J 1977 Users and non-users of doctors – implications for care. Journal of the Royal College of General Practitioners 27:155–159

Baker D, Hann M 2001 General practitioner services in primary care groups in England: is there equity between service availability and population need? Health and Place 7:67–74

Bakx K 1991 The 'eclipse' of folk medicine in Western society. Sociology, Health and Illness 13:20–57

Blaxter M 1990 Health and lifestyles. Tavistock/Routledge, London

Blaxter M, Paterson E 1982 Mothers and daughters. Heinemann Educational, London

Burstrom B, Fredland P 2001 Self rated health: is it as good a predictor of subsequent mortality among adults in lower as well as higher social classes? Journal of Epidemiology and Community Health 55:836–840

Cant S, Sharma U 1999 A new medical pluralism? Alternative medicine, doctors, patients and the state. UCL Press, London

Cartwright A, Anderson R 1981 General practice revisited: a second study of patients and their doctors. Tavistock, London

Dunnell K, Cartwright A 1972 Medicine-takers. Prescribers and hoarders. Routledge & Kegan Paul, London

Emslie M, Campbell M, Walker K 1996 Complementary therapies in a local health care setting. Part 1: is there a public demand? Complementary Therapies in Medicine 4:39–42

Epsom J 1978 The mobile health clinic: a report on the first year's work. In: Tuckett D, Kauffert J (eds) Basic readings in medical sociology. Tavistock, London

Featherstone M 1991 The body in consumer culture. In: Featherstone M, Hepworth M. Turner B (eds) The body: social processes and cultural theory. Sage, London

Finlayson A, McEwen J 1977 Coronary heart disease and patterns of living. Croom Helm, London

Freidson E, 1970 Profession of medicine. Dodds Mead, New York

Fulder S 1996 The handbook of alternative and complementary medicine, 3rd edn. Oxford University Press, Oxford

Goddard M, Smith P 2001 Equity of access to health care services: theory and evidence from the UK. Social Science and Medicine 53:1149–1162

Hannay D 1980 The iceberg of illness and trivial consultations. Journal of the Royal College of General Practitioners 30:551–554

Herzlich C 1973 Health and illness. Academic Press, London

Ingham J, Miller P 1979 Symptom prevalence and severity in a general practice. Epidemiology and Community Health 33:191–198

Kelleher D 1994 Self-help groups and their relationship to medicine. In: Gabe J, Kelleher D, Williams G (eds) Challenging medicine. Routledge, London

Kelleher D 2001 New social movements in the health domain. In Scambler G (ed) Habermas, critical theory and health. Routledge, London

Kleinman A 1985 Indigenous systems of healing: questions for professional, popular and folk care. In: Salmon J (ed) Alternative medicines: popular and policy perspectives. Tavistock, London

McKinlay J 1973 Social networks, lay consultation and help-seeking behaviour. Social Forces 53:255–292

Mechanic D 1978 Medical sociology, 2nd edn. Free Press. New York

Monaghan L 2001 Looking good, feeling good: the embodied pleasures of vibrant physicality. Sociology of Health and Illness 23:330–356

Nettleton S 1995 The sociology of health and illness. Polity Press, Cambridge

Office for National Statistics (ONS) 2000 Social trends 30. HMSO, London

Pill R, Scott N 1982 Concepts of illness causation and responsibility: some preliminary data from a sample of working-class mothers. Social Science and Medicine 16:43–52

Pilowsky I, Spence N 1977 Ethnicity and illness behaviour. Psychological Medicine 7:447–452

Robinson D 1980 The self-help component of primary care. Social Science and Medicine 14A:415–421

Saks M 1994 The alternatives to medicine. In: Gabe J, Kelleher D, Williams G (eds) Challenging medicine. Routledge, London

Scambler G 1989 Epilepsy. Routledge, London

Scambler G 2002 Health and social change: a critical theory. Open University Press, Buckingham

Scambler A, Scambler G, Craig D 1981 Kinship and friendship networks and women's demand for primary care. Journal of the Royal College of General Practitioners 26:746–750

Thomas K, Carr J, Westlake L, Williams B 1991 Use of non-orthodox and conventional health care in Great Britain. British Medical Journal 302:207–210

Tudor-Hart J 1971 The inverse care law. Lancet i:405–412

Wadsworth M, Butterfield W, Blaney R 1971 Health and sickness: the choice of treatment. Tavistock, London

Whitehead M 1992 The health divide, 2nd edn. Penguin, London

Zborowski M 1952 Cultural components in response to pain. Journal of Social Issues 8:16–30

Zola I 1973 Pathways to the doctor: from person to patient. Social Science and Medicine 7:677–889

CHAPTER

4

The Doctor–Patient Relationship

Myfanwy Morgan

The essential unit of medical practice is the occasion when, in the intimacy of the consulting room, or sick room, a person who is ill, or believes him- or herself to be ill, seeks the advice of a doctor whom he or she trusts. Such meetings are a frequent and regular occurrence, with over half a million consultations occurring between general practitioners and their patients in the UK every working day and a large number also taking place at a hospital level. Their success or otherwise depends not only on the doctors' clinical knowledge and technical skills, but also on the nature of the social relationship that exists between doctor and patient.

This chapter first examines the general societal expectations that influence the behaviours of doctors and patients in the medical consultation. It then describes some of the conflicts that can be experienced by doctors and different forms and determinants of the relationship between doctors and patients. Finally, the chapter examines the new partnerships that are developing involving shared treatment decision-making between doctor and patient and considers technical aspects of communication including new sources of information and decision aids.

SOCIAL ROLES OF DOCTORS AND PATIENTS

Parsons (1951) was one of the earliest sociologists to examine the relationship between doctors and patients. His interest arose from a broader theoretical concern with how society is able to function smoothly and respond to problems of deviance. Parsons regarded social functioning as partly achieved through the existence of institutionalized roles with socially prescribed patterns of behaviour. We are, therefore, all aware how people are likely to behave when they occupy the role of father, teacher, shop assistant, and so on, and of their expectations of us when we occupy the complementary role of child, pupil or customer. Parsons regarded illness as a form of social deviance because it impairs normal role performance and, if it occurs on a large enough scale, the smooth functioning of society (e.g. families caring for children, educational system, transport system, etc.) will be put at risk. Parsons believed that the amount of illness is controlled through the socially prescribed roles for doctors and patients, which facilitate interaction, and ensure both parties work together to return people to a state of health and normal role performance as quickly as possible.

◼ Parsons' model of the sick role and doctor's role

Parsons' description of the roles of doctor and patient is presented as an 'ideal type' model. This abstracts and presents what are regarded as the fundamental features of a particular social organization or social role and is an important method of analysing and describing very complex social phenomena. Parsons depicted the role of sick people as involving four general expectations. First, sick people are allowed, and might even be required, to give up some of their normal activities and responsibilities, such as going to work or playing football. Second, they are regarded as being in need of care. These two expectations and privileges are, however, contingent on the sick person fulfilling the third obligation of wanting to get well as quickly as possible, and the fourth of seeking professional medical advice and, most importantly for the doctor–patient relationship, cooperating with the doctor (Table 4.1).

Parsons points out that the specific expectations of the sick person, such as the number and type of activities the person is expected to give up, will be influenced by the nature and severity of the condition. It is also recognized that not all illness requires people to relinquish their normal social roles and occupy the status 'sick'. For example, much minor illness is coped with without recourse to the doctor and does not require any changes to a person's everyday life (see Chapter 3). Similarly, people with a chronic illness might need to consult the doctor regularly, but rather than occupying a permanent sick role they are generally expected to try to achieve their maximum level of functioning and to occupy the status 'sick' only if they experience a change in their usual health. Parsons thus viewed the sick role as a temporary social role that has been instituted by society with the aim of returning sick people to a state of health and restoring them to fully functioning members of society as quickly as possible. The sick role is also regarded as a universal role, in that its obligations and expectations apply to all sick people, whatever their age, gender, ethnicity, occupation or status in other spheres.

Parsons viewed the role of the doctor as complementary to the role of patient. Just as the patient is expected to cooperate fully with the doctor, doctors are expected to apply their specialist knowledge and skills for the benefit of the patient, and to act for the welfare of the patient and community rather than in their own self-interest. Doctors are also expected to be objective and emotionally detached, and to be guided by the rules of professional practice. Conformity with these general expectations is an essential requirement for carrying out the tasks of diagnosis and treatment, especially when this involves the need to know

TABLE 4.1	Parsons' analysis of the roles of patients and doctors
Patient: sick role	**Doctor: professional role**
Obligations and privileges:	**Expected to:**
1. Must want to get well as quickly as possible	1. Apply a high degree of skill and knowledge to the problems of illness
2. Should seek professional medical advice and co-operate with the doctor	2. Act for welfare of patient and community rather than for own self-interest, desire for money, advancement, etc
3. Allowed (and may be expected) to shed some normal activities and responsibilities (e.g. employment and household tasks)	3. Be objective and emotionally detached (i.e. should not judge patients' behaviour in terms of personal value system or become emotionally involved with them)
4. Regarded as being in need of care and unable to get better by his or her own decisions and will	4. Be guided by rules of professional practice
	Rights:
	1 Granted right to examine patients physically and to enquire into intimate areas of physical and personal life
	2. Granted considerable autonomy in professional practice
	3. Occupies position of authority in relation to the patient

Reprinted with permission from The Free Press from Parsons (1951).

intimate details about the patient that are not usually shared between strangers or the conduct of an intimate physical examination. Parsons also viewed doctors as enjoying considerable autonomy in executing their professional skills and occupying a position of authority in relation to the patient.

Parsons' analysis identifies the general expectations that guide the behaviour of doctors and patients, and shows how these roles facilitate interaction in the consultation, as both parties are aware how each other is expected to behave. The institutionalized roles of sick person and doctor also function to reduce the potentially disruptive effects of illness in society. This is partly achieved through the role of the doctor in officially legitimating illness and acting as a gatekeeper to the sick role, thus preventing inappropriate occupancy and enjoyment of the privileges of the sick role, such as time off work or financial benefits, when this is not justified by the patient's medical condition. In addition, the expectations placed on both doctors and patients ensure that people who are officially sanctioned as sick are returned to a state of health and normal role performance as quickly as possible (see Chapter 13).

Conflicts in the doctor's role

Although Parsons' analysis emphasizes the consensual nature of the roles and relation-ships between doctors and patients, in reality, tensions and strains often exist. One set of tensions arises from conflicts between doctors' own values and those of some of their patients. This is particularly likely to occur in relation to abortion, homosexuality, AIDS and other conditions or behaviours invested with moral evaluations. There are also conflicting demands placed on doctors in terms of their requirement to act in the best interests of their patients and their duty to serve the interests of the state. As Parsons recognized, doctors serve the state as agents of social control in their role as gatekeepers to the sick role with authority to determine who is 'healthy' and who is 'sick', but also have an obligation to act in the best interests of individual patients. When patients request, or even demand, a sick note, problems can arise for the doctor in determining whether disease exists and the designation of 'sick' and privileges of the sick role can be justified. For example, back pain is the major reason for time off work but it is often difficult to determine its cause or severity except by relying on patients' reports, which could present problems in evaluating the legitimacy of their claims to the sick role. In such situations of uncertainty, should doctors give priority to the interests of the patient, or to their societal function in ensuring that people do not malinger or occupy the sick role inappropriately? Similarly, should doctors inform the licensing authority if they are aware that a patient diagnosed with epilepsy is driving a car and thus contravening the state's regulations, even if they know how important it is for the patient to drive, and should doctors inform patients who are thinking of being tested for human immunodeficiency virus (HIV) of the potential problems of being diagnosed as a carrier for insurance premiums when this might discourage testing?

A further source of conflict for doctors arises from the competing interests of individual patients and the wider patient population. For example, doctors are often involved in rationing scarce resources of staff time, beds and medical equipment and might have to decide which patients should be given a transplant or undergo other medical procedures, as well as the priority to be assigned to treating different cases. In the absence of clear and explicit criteria, such choices rest on the judgement of individual clinicians. A recent illustration is the decision made by some consultants not to administer tests and carry out coronary artery by-pass surgery on people who continue to smoke. This is based on the argument that scarce resources should not be spent on people who smoke, as such people have longer hospital stays and less chance of recovery than non-smokers, and treating them deprives patients who have never smoked or who have stopped smoking. However, such reasoning raises questions of how far the notion of culpability and self-inflicted ill health should extend. For example, what is the situation in the prescribing of nebulizers to asthmatic smokers and the treatment of drunken victims of road accidents?

Doctors can also experience conflicts between maintaining the confidentiality of the doctor–patient relationship and disclosing information to a patient's parent or spouse. This raises the question of whether medical confidentiality is absolute or whether there are any situations when interests are best served by passing on information about a patient. For example, are there are any circumstances in which a doctor at a clinic should disclose that a patient has acquired immunodeficiency syndrome (AIDS), or is positive for HIV, when this is against the patient's wishes? Such situations frequently pose dilemmas for doctors and raise questions concerning their primary duties and responsibilities, as well as possibly presenting conflicts in relation to their own beliefs and values. However, there are powerful arguments to support the view that priority should be given to maintaining the confidentiality of the doctor–patient relationship. In particular, this has the benefit of preserving patients' trust in doctors and their willingness to consult and discuss their problems freely in the future; destroying this trust undermines the very foundation of the relationship between doctor and patient.

Psychosocial and clinical outcomes

The social interaction between individual doctors and patients is a major determinant of the success of the consultation in terms of both patients' and doctors' satisfaction with the encounter and the clinical outcomes achieved. For example, although information communicated by patients is central to diagnosis and treatment decisions, unless patients feel at ease and are encouraged to talk freely they might not disclose problems that are troubling them, or express their worries and concerns. Indeed, it is well known that some patients who feel very embarrassed or worried about a problem will initially present with a condition that does not give rise to these feelings and forms a 'ticket of entry' to the consultation. Whether such patients disclose the real problem that is troubling them, or whether this remains 'hidden', often depends on what they perceive as the general atmosphere of the consultation and the opportunities for discussion. It is also estimated that about 10% of patients do not have their prescription filled by the chemist, which suggests that the consultation might not have been successful in identifying these patients' problems or resulted in treatment that was unacceptable to the patient.

Patients' satisfaction with the consultation depends on their perception of the doctors' interpersonal and clinical skills, and might in itself have a positive effect on the pain and other symptoms experienced. For example, a longitudinal study of patients attending neurological clinics for the diagnosis and treatment of severe headache showed that, for half the patients seen, the main factor related to a reduction in symptom severity was the patients' satisfaction with the initial consultation. Of particular importance was being given information and advice they felt was relevant to their worries and which enabled them to make sense of their symptoms and achieve a sense of control over their illness (Fitzpatrick et al 1983). Similarly, a series of randomized control trials of patients with diabetes mellitus, hypertension and peptic ulcer, indicated that the amount of emotion (positive or negative) expressed by doctor or patient, and the quality of information sought by patients and given by doctors, formed important influences on patients' functional capacity and physiological measurements on follow-up, and their satisfaction with care (Kaplan et al 1989). Another beneficial effect of the social relationship between doctor and patient is what has been termed the 'placebo' effect (which literally means 'I will please'). This is calculated to account for as much as one-third of the success of any drug (Beecher 1955). To take account of this healing effect, trials of new drugs often involve the administration of an inert substance to a control group for comparison.

The social interaction between doctor and patient can also influence doctors' own feelings of satisfaction. For example, failure to elicit patients' worries and interpretation of symptoms can sometimes lead doctors to believe that patients have consulted inappropriately and that their time and skills are being wasted. This can be illustrated in relation to consultations for childhood respiratory conditions, which account for 30% of all consultations for children aged below 11 years. Many of these consultations are for a condition that is 'trivial' from a biomedical perspective. However, a study of mothers who had consulted their general practitioner for this reason revealed that their decision to consult was often due to fears that their child would experience long-term chest damage, or even die from choking in phlegm or vomit or through an asthma attack or cot death, and there was also a common belief that antibiotics were required to break up the phlegm (Cornford et al 1993). Eliciting and addressing such lay beliefs could avoid potential conflicts and enhance doctors' job satisfaction, as well as promoting the quality and effectiveness of patient care.

TYPES OF DOCTOR–PATIENT RELATIONSHIP

The significance of the social relationship between doctor and patient for the clinical, psychosocial and behavioural outcomes of the consultation has resulted in considerable attention being given to the various forms and determinants of this relationship. Whereas

53

Parsons identified the general societal expectations that guide the behaviour of doctors and patients, his portrayal of an asymmetrical relationship in which the doctor occupies the dominant position by virtue of his or her specialist knowledge and the patient merely cooperates (a 'paternalistic' relationship), is viewed as only one possible form of relationship an between individual doctor and patient. Other forms arise from differences in the relative power and control exercised by doctors and patients (Table 4.2). In reality, these different models perhaps do not exist in pure form, but nevertheless most consultations tend towards one type.

■ Models of the doctor–patient relationship

A paternalistic (or guidance–cooperation) relationship, involving high physician control and low patient control, describes Parsons' model where the doctor is dominant and acts as a 'parent' figure who decides what he or she believes to be in the patient's best interest. This form of relationship traditionally characterized medical consultations and, at some stages of illness, patients derive considerable comfort from being able to rely on the doctor in this way and being relieved of burdens of worry and decision making. However, medical consultations are now increasingly characterized by greater patient control and relationships based on mutuality.

A relationship of mutuality is characterized by the active involvement of patients as more equal partners in the consultation and has been described as a 'meeting between experts', in which both parties participate as a joint venture and engage in an exchange of ideas and sharing of belief systems. The doctor brings his or her clinical skills and knowledge to the consultation in terms of diagnostic techniques, knowledge of the causes of disease, prognosis, treatment options and preventive strategies, and patients bring their own expertise in terms of their experiences and explanations of their illness, and knowledge of their particular social circumstances, attitudes to risk, values and preferences.

A consumerist relationship describes a situation in which power relationships are reversed; with the patient taking the active role and the doctor adopting a fairly passive role, acceding to the patient's requests for a second opinion, referral to hospital, a sick note, and so on.

A relationship of default can occur if patients continue to adopt a passive role even when the doctor reduces some of his or her control, with the consultation therefore lacking sufficient direction. This can arise if patients are not aware of alternatives to a passive patient role or are timid in adopting a more participative relationship.

Different types of relationship, and particularly those characterized by paternalism and mutuality, can be viewed as appropriate to different conditions and stages of illness. For example, in emergency situations it is generally necessary for the doctor to be dominant, whereas in other situations patients can be more actively involved in treatment choices and

TABLE 4.2	Types of doctor–patient relationship	
Patient control	**Doctor control**	
	Low	**High**
Low	Default	Paternalism
High	Consumerist	Mutuality

Reprinted with permission from Sage Publications from Stewart & Roter (1989 p. 21).

54

other decisions regarding their care. However, considerable variation in the nature of the relationship between doctor and patient cannot be explained entirely in terms of the patient's medical condition, but is also influenced by the expectations of doctor and of patient and the structural context of the consultation.

Influences on the doctor–patient relationship

A major determinant of the nature of the doctor–patient relationship and the extent and forms of communication within the consultation is the doctor's clinical practice style. Two polar types of consultation style have been identified, based on video-recordings of consultations; these have been designated 'doctor-centred' and 'patient-centred' (Byrne & Long 1976).

A doctor-centred consultation is characterized by the traditional Parsonian model and paternalistic approach, based on the assumption that the doctor is the expert and the patient merely required to cooperate. Doctors adopting this approach focus on the physical aspects of the patients' disease and employ tightly controlled interviewing methods to elicit the necessary medical information. Questions were thus mainly of a 'closed' nature, such as 'how long have you had the pain?' and 'is it sharp or dull?'. These questions aim to provide information to enable the doctor to interpret the patient's illness within his or her own biomedical disease framework, while providing little opportunity for patients to express their own beliefs and concerns.

At the other end of the continuum are doctors whose consultation style conforms to a 'patient-centred' approach. These doctors adopt a much less controlling style and encourage and facilitate their patients to participate in the consultation, thus fostering a relationship of 'mutuality'. An important feature of this approach is the greater use of 'open' questions, such as 'tell me about the pain', 'how do you feel?' and 'what do you think is the cause of the problem?'. This approach also requires that doctors spend more time actively listening to patients' problems through picking up and responding to patient cues, encouraging patients to express their own ideas or feelings, clarifying and interpreting patients' statements, and generally using a more participative style with the various options presented and discussed with patients.

Studies show that individual doctors can be classified fairly consistently as holding either doctor-centred or patient-centred consultations. This suggests that doctors develop a particular consulting style and do not vary this significantly in relation to the patient's problems. However, doctors classified as having a patient-centred style tend to be the most flexible, showing the greatest ability to respond to differences in patients' needs or the circumstances of the consultation.

These differences in communication style reflect not only doctors' communication skills but also differences in their attitudes and orientations to the medical task. Doctors who hold a strictly disease-centred model talk in terms of what has been referred to as the 'voice of medicine' (Mishler 1984). They thus focus almost exclusively on the objective description of physical symptoms and the classification of these within a reductionist biomedical model, with the aim of reaching a differential diagnosis as quickly as possible and prescribing appropriate treatment. By contrast, doctors taking a more patient-centred approach aim to understand patients' own illness framework in terms of their subjective experience and meanings of illness, to identify possible psychosocial causes of illness onset and the impact of chronic and disabling illness on the patient's self concept and everyday activities, and to understand patients' beliefs, priorities and preferences for treatment (Box 4.1). This approach to the medical task requires that the doctor listens to the 'voice of the patient', and facilitates and encourages the patient's active involvement in the consultation and communication of his or her beliefs, feelings and the psychosocial context of their illness experience.

| BOX 4.1 | Key aspects of a of patient-centred consultation |

- Biopsychosocial perspective (willingness to become involved in the full range of difficulties patients bring to their doctors and not just their biomedical problems)
- Patient-as-a-person (understanding the individual's experience of his or her illness)
- Sharing power and responsibility (mutual participation of patient and doctor)
- Therapeutic alliance (creating a situation in which the patient feels able to be involved in treatment decisions)
- Doctor-as-a-person (doctor is aware of and responds to patient cues)

From Mead & Bower (2000).

56

Influence of time

General practice consultations average about 6 minutes, although this obscures wide variations, with the actual length of consultations ranging from about 2 minutes to over 20 minutes. Pressures of time encourage a more tightly controlled doctor-centred (or 'paternalistic') consultation with less attention paid to the social and psychological aspects of a patient's illness. As a result, fewer psychological problems are identified and more prescriptions are issued (Howie et al 1992). However, the doctor's own approach to medicine and practice style appears to exert a more important influence on the content of consultations than the time available. This was demonstrated by an experiment in general practice in which the time available for consultations was increased to 10 minutes (Ridsdale et al 1992). As a result, all doctors asked more questions. However, other skills, such as facilitating patients to participate and explaining the nature of their medical problem, were employed more frequently only by those doctors who already emphasized these aspects of communication. Doctors who usually employed these behaviours least frequently tended to do more of what they already did, such as asking closed questions, rather than changing their style of communication, and did not usually take advantage of the extended consultation time available. By contrast, general practitioners with a more patient-oriented approach often preferred to run over time, and possibly kept other patients waiting if they felt it was necessary to spend additional time with a particular patient. These doctors might also deliberately restrict their list size, so that they can provide what they regard as good-quality care. This suggests that the length of time available for consultations is itself partly a function of practice style, as well as the pressures of time serving to constrain the consultation. However, although a more participative, patient-centred consultation does require greater time, giving sufficient time to listen and respond to patients' worries and concerns can reduce the number of return visits and hence the total consultation time for an episode of illness.

Patient characteristics and behaviours

Although having less power than doctors in the consultation, patients can nevertheless influence the interaction by their willingness or otherwise to ask questions and assume a more participative role. It appears that younger people are more likely to expect a relationship of mutual participation than elderly people. Patients with a high social and educational level also tend to participate more in the consultation in terms of asking questions and asking for explanations and clarification than patients from a lower socioeconomic background and educational level. This possibly reflects their greater knowledge and confidence and the smaller status gap between doctor and patient. For example, a study of 1470 general practice consultations showed that only 27% of working-class patients sought clarification of what the doctor had said, compared with 45% of middle-class patients. These requests for information by patients in turn led to fuller explanations being given by doctors and a rather longer consultation (Tuckett et al 1985). However, despite these differences, patients' desire to participate in the consultation generally increases over the course of an illness as they gain more knowledge and understanding of the condition. Thus patients are often passive and unquestioning during initial hospital consultations, whereas by the second or third consultation they generally initiate questions themselves and take a more participative approach.

Interaction in the consultation and the information and explanations provided by doctors has been shown to reflect their assumptions of the interests of different patient groups (Street 1991). For example, there is some evidence that doctors volunteer more explanations to some groups of patients, including more educated patients and male patients, even when the explanation is not explicitly requested by the patient. Some patients can therefore be doubly disadvantaged; because of both their passive communication styles and the doctor's (mis-) perceptions of their informational needs and desires.

Influence of structural context

A particular feature of general practice is the opportunity for personal continuity of care, with doctors and patients often knowing each other over a long period. Consultations therefore often take place in a familiar context and can benefit from the doctor's prior awareness of the patient's social situation, past history and concerns. By contrast, patients rarely experience this personal continuity in a hospital situation. In addition, communication on the ward is frequently limited by patients feelings of a lack of privacy and difficulties of interaction can arise if the doctor or medical team stand at the end of the bed rather than coming close to and preferably sitting at the same level as the patient.

The content of consultations is also influenced at a macro level by the system of financing of health care. Consultations financed on a fee-for-service basis generally occupy a longer time and doctors' practice style is more patient-oriented than when they are paid on a per capita or salaried basis. This is because a fee-for-service payment is often associated with a greater availability of resources, there is less institutional pressure to achieve a high patient throughput, and doctors feel a greater need to achieve a high level of patient satisfaction. Patients who are paying on a fee-for-service basis also tend to expect a longer consultation and a full discussion with the doctor and are frequently more active in asking questions.

PARTNERSHIPS IN TREATMENT DECISION MAKING

Models of decision making

One aspect of the doctor–patient relationship that is now receiving particular attention is the roles of doctors and patients in treatment decisions. Three main models of medical decision-making – paternalist, shared and informed decision-making – correspond with the three main types of doctor–patient relationship (Table 4.3). The traditional paternalist model regards the doctor, as medical expert, as solely responsible for treatment decisions with the patient expected merely to cooperate with advice and treatment. By contrast, relationships of mutuality regard shared decision-making as the ideal. This requires that both parties are involved in the decision-making process, share information, take steps to build a consensus about the preferred treatment and reach agreement (consensus) on the treatment to implement (Box 4.2).

TABLE 4.3 Models of treatment decision-making in a doctor–patient dyad

Analytical stages		Paternalistic (intermediate)	Shared (intermediate)	Informed
Information exchange	Flow	One way (largely)	Two way	One way (largely)
	Direction	Doctor → patient	Doctor ↔ patient	Doctor → patient
	Type	Medical	Medical and personal	Medical
	Amount[a]	Minimum legally required	All relevant for decision-making	All relevant for decision-making
Deliberation		Doctor alone or with other doctors	Doctor and patient (plus potential others)	Patient (plus potential others)
Deciding on treatment to implement		Doctors	Doctor and patient	Patient

[a] Minimum required.

BOX 4.2 Four Requirements for Shared Decision making

1. Both doctor and patient are involved in the decision-making process
2. Both parties share information
3. Both parties take steps to build a consensus about the preferred treatment
4. An agreement (consensus) is reached on the treatment to implement

Based on Charles et al (1999)

A third model, the informed model, involves a partnership between doctor and patient based on a division of labour. Initially, the doctor communicates to the patient information on all relevant options, and their benefits and risks, so as to enable the patient to make an informed treatment decision. Information transfer is therefore seen as the key responsibility and only legitimate contribution of the doctor to the decision-making process, with the deliberation and decision-making being the sole prerogative of the patient. This model thus forms the extreme opposite of the paternalist model and, in some cases, patients might have decided on a broad course of action before entering the surgery and press the doctor to cooperate.

In practice, the three models of treatment decision-making described by Charles et al (1999) often do not exist in pure form and they therefore allow for intermediate approaches. For example, a variant of the traditional paternalist model, sometimes referred to as the 'professional as agent' model, describes a situation where the doctor continues to assume responsibility for directing the healthcare utilization of the patient but makes the treatment decision, assuming either that he or she knows or has elicited the patient's preferences for future health states, life choices, and so on. In addition, it is acknowledged that a clinical encounter can often involve a hybrid of elements of more than one model. For example, a consultation might initially be characterized by a two-way information exchange between doctor and patient but, if problems arise in achieving a shared decision, the clinician might then use the power imbalance in the relationship to persuade the patient to follow his or her advice, often with a promise of a subsequent review of the situation. This is illustrated by

Waissman (1990), who describes the initial process of negotiating to reconcile doctors' and patients' choices regarding the use of home or hospital dialysis for children with renal disease, and also shows how the doctor's decision and choice of home dialysis was later renegotiated by parents and other arrangements made if they continued to have difficulty in managing the dialysis at home. Another mixed scenario occurs where a doctor who favours a shared decision-making model thinks, as the interaction proceeds, that the patient has gained enough confidence and gathered enough information to make the decision on his or her own. At this point, the process might shift from a shared to an informed model as a result of the learning that has occurred during the interaction itself.

Shared decision making and treatment choices

The rights of patients to be involved in making informed choices about their health care, including the requirement that informed consent should include a discussion of treatment options, has been endorsed by the NHS reforms of 1991 and the Patient Partnership strategy (NHS Executive 1996). This endorsement of shared decision-making in medical care has been encouraged by the interaction of a number of social and medical factors. One influence has been patients' increased medical knowledge, which has been made possible by the greater access to medical information through the media, internet and other sources. In addition, prevailing social values endorse individual autonomy and responsibility, with younger patients thus having a greater desire to take personal control, although a consumerist ideology also engenders more critical attitudes to medical and other services (Coulter 1997).

Another impetus for shared decision making comes from the increasing prevalence of chronic illness in the population. This means that patients are often required to manage their illness on a long-term basis, taking responsibility for monitoring symptoms and adjusting their treatments, with this being facilitated by a more equal partnership with doctors in the management of the illness. In addition, for many conditions it is necessary to make choices between treatment options and to balance the various risks and benefits (both short- and long-term), often in situations of considerable medical uncertainty (Logan & Scott 1996). This has been associated with considerable variations in professional decision making and supports the view that patients should contribute their preferences and priorities directly to this process. Moreover, there is evidence that doctors frequently make inaccurate guesses about patients' concerns, and that doctors' and patients' preferences and treatment choices often differ, although the direction of these differences varies for different conditions. For example, studies of cardiovascular conditions suggest that patients are more averse to drug treatment than health professionals and would prefer higher thresholds for beginning antihypertensive treatment, because they value the benefits of this treatment less than doctors do and are more distressed about side-effects. By contrast, patients often wish to receive prescriptions for upper respiratory tract infections in situations where doctors regard this as inappropriate (Montgomery & Fahey 2001). Similarly, studies conducted in the USA, where surgical rates are relatively high, indicate that some informed patients with mild symptoms resist prostatectomy and hysterectomy in situations where these procedures are advocated by specialists. A greater patient voice and shared decision making does not, therefore, necessarily increase demands on services and could ensure that resources are employed more appropriately and increase the effectiveness of care.

Shared decision making has received particular emphasis in relation to the prescribing of drug treatments. Traditionally, studies have identified that about 50% of patients with chronic conditions do not take their treatment as prescribed, with major reasons being

59

because they do not share the doctors' view of the appropriateness of the drugs prescribed, or are worried about immediate side-effects or possible long-term harmful effects of the drugs. The aim is to explore these issues by adopting a shared decision-making approach and to reach a 'concordance' between doctor and patient (Box 4.3). Achieving concordance does not necessarily mean that both parties are convinced that a particular drug or other course of action is the best possible treatment for the patient. In some situations, where both parties have differing preferences and views, they might achieve concordance and endorse a particular treatment as part of a negotiated agreement. In particular, this could occur when there is not a true situation of equipoise (equipoise occurs where options really are options) as for example in the demand for antibiotics to treat viral infections. In this case, although a 'shared decision' is reached, it could more accurately be described as an informed decision that reflects the doctor's preference (Gwyn & Elwyn 1999). However, in such situations the concordat reached can then be reviewed at subsequent consultations and changes agreed. What is important is that both parties participate in communicating their views, concerns and preferences and share responsibility for the final decision. The aim of concordance in relation to prescribing decisions is thus to achieve the best use of medicines compatible with what the patient desires and is capable of achieving, rather than the traditional approach of imposing a medical decision that the patient can challenge only through non-compliance after they leave the consultation.

Patients' preferences for participation

The emphasis on shared decision-making model raises questions of whether and when patients desire to be involved in this way. This has been found to depend partly on a patient's state of health; patients in crisis situations or who feel weak or distressed might prefer to have decisions made for them rather than being more actively involved. Differences in the desire for involvement also reflect the complexity of treatment choices. For example, studies of patients with breast cancer and with colorectal cancer identified 20% of the former and 4% of the latter preferring an active role in terms of making their own treatment decisions, with 17% of patients with colorectal cancer and 28% of patients with breast cancer preferring to share responsibility with the doctor for deciding which treatment was best for them. However, 78% of patients with colorectal cancer and 52% with breast cancer preferred to leave the decision to the doctor, although generally wanting the doctor to consider their opinion (Beaver et al 1999). The higher proportion of patients with breast cancer wishing to be actively involved in decision-making might reflect the clear treatment choices with little impact on survival, as well as the younger age of these patients. These differing desires for involvement identify a key challenge for health professionals: to be sensitive to individual patients' needs. However, most patients desire information about their condition and treatment, even if not wishing to actively participate in treatment decisions.

BOX 4.3	Concordance

'Concordance is based on the notion that the work of the prescriber and patient in the consultation is a negotiation between equals and that the aim is a therapeutic alliance between them. This alliance may, in the end, include an agreement to differ. Its strength lies in a new assumption of respect for the patient's agenda and the creation of openness in the relationship, so that both doctor and patient together can proceed on the basis of reality and not of misunderstanding, distrust or concealment.' (Marinker 1997, p 8)

DOCTORS' COMMUNICATION SKILLS

Doctors frequently overestimate the amount of information they have provided to patients, and also believe that patients are satisfied with the communication they received during a consultation, as it is difficult for patients to convey dissatisfaction in the consultation. However, the most common complaints about doctors by patients and the public relate to communication, and particularly that doctors do not listen, will not give information and show a lack of concern or lack of respect for the patient. As a result, large numbers of patients leave the consultation without asking questions about things that are troubling them or do not receive what they regard as a satisfactory response. A recent qualitative study based on 35 patients aged 18 years and over consulting 20 general practitioners, found that only four of the 35 patients voiced all their concerns during the consultation (Barry et al 2000). The most common voiced concerns related to symptoms, requests for diagnoses and prescriptions. The most common unvoiced concerns were worries about possible diagnosis and what the future holds, ideas about what is wrong, side-effects, not wanting a prescription, and information relating to social context such as housing, work or social networks. Concerns that were not raised often led to specific problem outcomes, such as major misunderstandings, unwanted prescriptions, non-use of prescriptions and non-adherence to treatment.

Content and process skills

Patients' perceptions of inadequacies of communication arise partly from *what* doctors communicate (content skills). This refers to the substance of questions and the information gathered, including the emphasis given by doctors to understanding the patient's perspective (ideas, concerns, expectations, impact of condition on everyday life, etc.), and the treatments they discuss. The content of communication is influenced by a number of practical and situational factors (time available, initial or subsequent visit, NHS or private patient) but most importantly by how doctors perceive the nature of the medical task and their relationship with patients.

There are also questions of *how* doctors communicate (process skills). This refers to how they discover the history or provide information, the verbal and non-verbal skills they use, how they develop a relationship with the patient, and the way they organize and structure the communication, including the emphasis given to actively listening to patients, facilitating and encouraging their questions, and discussion of worries and concerns. Process skills relate to five stages and tasks of the consultation (Box 4.4). The skills required to achieve each of these stages are now taught in specialist communication courses and involve both verbal and non-verbal behaviours.

BOX 4.4   Communication Skills and Steps to be Achieved in the Consultation

1. Initiating the session (establishing the initial rapport and identifying the reason(s) for the consultation)
2. Gathering information (exploring the problem, understanding the patients' perspective, providing structure to the consultation)
3. Building the relationship (developing rapport and involving the patient)
4. Explanation and planning (providing the appropriate amount and type of information, aiding accurate recall and understanding, achieving a shared understanding and planning)
5. Closing the session

From Silverman et al (1998).

Patients are regarded as particularly sensitive to and observant of the non-verbal communications conveyed by their doctors, because illness usually involves emotions such as fear, anxiety and emotional uncertainty. Patients therefore often look for clues to assess the situation. By maintaining eye contact, looking attentive, nodding encouragingly and using other gestures, the doctor can provide positive feedback to the patient and facilitate his or her participation. By contrast, continued riffling through notes, twiddling with a pen or failing to look directly at the patient convey disinterest and result in patients failing to describe their problems or to seek information and explanation. Similarly, the patient's body language and eye contact can convey whether he or she is feeling tense, anxious, angry or upset (Lloyd & Bor 1996). Indeed, it is estimated that in a normal two-person conversation the verbal component carries less than 35% of the social meaning of the situation, and that 65% or more is carried by the non-verbal components such as eye contact, gaze, facial expression and posture. Physical proximity and the relative positions of doctor and patient in the consulting room also influence interaction. Seating of equal height and the lack of a physical barrier between participants encourage communication. This was demonstrated by an experiment in which a cardiologist removed the desk from his clinic on alternate days. When the desk was removed, 50% of the patients sat back in their chair and in at-ease positions, whereas only 10% did so when he was sitting behind his desk, with a corresponding decline in the amount of communication by patients (Pietroni 1976).

The current emphasis on shared decision making places particular demands on doctors' communication skills, because it is necessary for doctors to transfer technical information to patients about treatment options, risks and their probable benefits in as unbiased, clear and simple way as possible. This is a particular challenge in situations where the availability of reliable evidence is limited, or when decisions need to be made within the time constraints of a normal consultation. In addition, doctors might need to help the patient to conceptualize and weigh the risks versus the benefits, to share their treatment recommendations with the patient and/or affirm the patient's treatment preference, while being careful not to impose their own values about the best treatment onto the patient. Specialist training programmes are therefore being introduced to assist doctors in assimilating the philosophy and skills required for involving patients in decision making. In addition, direct doctor–patient communication is increasingly complemented by decision-boards, audiotapes, linear videotapes and computer programmes. These help to overcome the constraints of time and the demands of providing complex information in non-technical language, and might help facilitate treatment choices.

Special situations and groups

Particular challenges of communication and demands on doctors arise in disclosing a diagnosis of cancer and giving other 'sad or bad' news. Traditionally, doctors withheld such information for as long as possible. This was often justified as being in the patient's own interest, although maintaining a patient's uncertainty once the diagnosis was firmly based might also have been functional for doctors in protecting them from the stress associated with such disclosures. A more open approach is now generally adopted, supported by patients' desire to be informed and the effects that this can have in reducing uncertainty and promoting positive coping. For example, Jenkins et al (2001) found that 87% of hospitalized cancer patients interviewed desired all the information about their disease, good and bad, and 98% preferred to know whether or not their illness was cancer. The 13% who stated that in general they preferred to leave disclosure of details up to the doctor tended to be older patients (over 70 years of age) but they still wanted to know certain specific details. However, although the vast majority of patients with cancer want a great deal of very specific information concerning their condition and treatment, such information must, of course, be handled sensitively and might involve eliciting and responding to patients' personal worries, such as the pain they might experience, the side-effects of treatment, how they will feel and what they will be able to do. However, the difficulties experienced by doctors in coping with patients' emotional responses mean that they often develop routinized forms of disclosure to inform patients about the diagnosis of a terminal condition, rather than responding to an individual patient's needs.

Doctor–patient communication can also present particular challenges in relation to recent immigrants and refugee groups if their command of English is poor or if they are not familiar with the organization of health care and the expectations of service providers in the NHS. In addition, doctors' lack of familiarity with different cultural beliefs regarding the causes or meanings of illness, and different beliefs about appropriate treatments, can form barriers to doctor–patient communication (see Chapter 10).

Doctors who become patients are also a group who can experience particular problems in the doctor–patient relationship. A study of recently sick doctors found that some doctor-patients complained that they were not given information about their illness or were not counselled appropriately because it was assumed that they were already adequately informed, whereas they felt a need to occupy a more usual patient role and for the treating doctor to provide relevant clinical information and discuss their illness as they would with any other patient (McKevitt & Morgan 1997). Other doctor-patients thought they were too involved in the decision making and management of their illness because the treating doctor was unable to take control of the consultation. Some also commented that their doctor seemed embarrassed to treat them, with these problems being most common where the treating doctor was of a lower grade or younger than the patient. Most doctors commented that they found it instructive to experience the doctor–patient encounter from the patient's perspective and some suggested that this transformed their professional sympathy into empathy.

CHANGES IN THE DOCTOR–PATIENT RELATIONSHIP

The increasing size of general practices, together with the greater involvement of nurses, health visitors, counsellors and other health professionals in the provision of primary care, means that continuity in terms of the relationship between an individual general practitioner and patient is increasingly replaced by relationships with different members of the primary care team. This identifies a challenge of achieving good interprofessional communication and continuity of care among members of the team to maintain the quality of interaction and provision of individualized patient care.

The philosophy of patient-centred care and the shift towards shared treatment decisions also require new methods of involving consumers in the initial development of clinical guidelines that provide a framework for practice (Wersch & Eccles 2001). Shared decision making is also being facilitated by new courses and educational interventions to enhance these skills and competencies among health professionals. Interactive and multimedia systems are also being developed to provide patients with the information they want to receive at a pace acceptable to them, and to support an individual's treatment choices with individualized data. More generally, greater access to high quality medical information on the internet will increase the numbers of 'information-rich' patients who can bring detailed and often complex questions to their doctor and desire to participate in decisions regarding their care.

A technological development with implications for the doctor–patient relationship is the widespread use of computers in the consultation. This can have a significant impact on communication, and especially on the information disclosed by patients. However, the effects of computers have been found to be influenced by whether patients are seated in a position to have access to the computer screen, and on the doctors' ability to maintain their personal touch in terms of their verbal skills and eye contact with patients (Ridsdale & Hudd 1994). Also of increasing importance with greater computerization is the need to assure the confidentiality of patient data, thus maintaining the essential trust between doctor and patient.

A further development is the expanding use of telemedicine as a means of delivering health care. This gives rise to the increasing possibility of patients engaging in teleconsulting, often from their own homes, thus expanding access to care. However, it will also present new challenges in establishing a relationship between individual patients and healthcare providers, and facilitating their communication.

64

References

Barry CA et al 2000 Patients' unvoiced agendas in general practice consultations: qualitative study. British Medical Journal 320:1245–50

Beaver K, Bogg J, Luker KA 1999 Decision-making role preferences and information needs: a comparison of colorectal and breast cancer. Health Expectations 2:266–276

Beecher R 1955 The powerful placebo. Journal of the American Medical Association 159:602–606

Byrne PS, Long BL 1976 Doctors talking to patients. HMSO, London

Charles C, Whelan T, Gafni A 1999 What do we mean by partnership in making decisions about treatment? British Medical Journal 319:780–782

Cornford C, Morgan M, Risdale L 1993 Why do mothers consult when their children cough? Family Practice 10:193–196

Coulter A 1997 Partnerships with patients: the pros and cons of shared clinical decision-making. Journal of Health Service Research Policy 2:112–121

Fitzpatrick RM, Hopkins AP, Howard-Watts O 1983 Social dimensions of healing. Social Science and Medicine 17:501–510

Gwyn R, Elwyn G 1999 When is a shared decision not (quite) a shared decision? Negotiating preferences in a general practice encounter. Social Science and Medicine 49:437–447

Howie JGR et al 1992 Attitudes to medical care, the organisation of work, and work stress among general practitioners. British Journal of General Practice 42:181–185

Jenkins V, Fallowfield L, Saul J 2001 Information needs of patients with cancer: results from a large study in UK cancer centers. British Journal of Cancer 84(1):48–51

Kaplan SH, Greenfield S, Ware JE 1989 Assessing the effects of patient–physician interactions on the outcomes of chronic disease. Medical Care 27:S110–127

Lloyd M, Bor R 1996 Communication skills for medicine. Churchill Livingstone, London

Logan RL, Scott PJ 1996 Uncertainty in clinical practice: implications for quality and costs of health care. Lancet 347:595–598

Marinker M (Chairman of Working Party) 1997 From compliance to concordance: achieving shared goals in medicine taking. Royal Pharmaceutical Society of Great Britain, London

McKevitt C, Morgan M 1997 Anomalous patients: experiences of doctors with an illness. Sociology of Health and Illness 19(5):644–667

Mead N, Bower P 2000 Patient-centredness: a conceptual framework and review of the empirical literature. Social Science and Medicine 51:1087–1010

Mishler EG 1984 The discourse of medicine, dialectics of medical interviews. Ablex Publishing Corporation, Norwood, NJ

Montgomery AA, Fahey T 2001 How do patients' treatment preferences compare with those of clinicians? Quality and Safety in Health Care 10:39–43

NHS Executive 1996 Patient partnership: building a collaborative strategy. Department of Health, Leeds

Parsons T 1951 The social system. Free Press, Glencoe, IL

Pietroni P 1976 Language and communication in general practice. In: Tanner B (ed) Communication in the general practice surgery. Hodder & Stoughton, London

Ridsdale C, Hudd S 1994 Computers in the consultation: the patient's view. British Journal of General Practice 44:367–369

Ridsdale L, Morgan M, Morris R 1992 Doctors' interviewing technique and its response to different booking time. Family Practice 9:57–60

Silverman J, Kurtz S, Draper J 1998 Skills for communicating with patients. Radcliffe Press, Oxford

Stewart M, Roter D (eds) 1989 Communicating with medical patients. Sage, London

Street R 1991 Information-giving in medical consultations: the influence of patients' communicative styles and personal characteristics. Social Science and Medicine 32:541–548

Tuckett D, Boulton M, Oban C, Williams A 1985 Meetings between experts: an approach to sharing ideas in medical consultations. Tavistock Publications, London

Waissman R 1990 An analysis of doctor–patient interactions in the case of paediatric renal failure: the choice of home dialysis. Sociology of Health and Illness 4:432–451

Wersch van A, Eccles M 2001 Involvement of consumers in the development of evidence based clinical guidelines: practical experiences from the North of England evidence based guideline development programme. Quality and Safety in Health Care 10:10–16

Hospitals and Patient Care

Myfanwy Morgan

Hospitals employed 54 400 medical staff (whole-time equivalents) in England in 1998, with a further 29 700 doctors working in primary care. Many hospitals not only engage in patient care but also serve as centres of education and training for doctors, nurses and other health workers, and provide a setting for research. A patient admitted to hospital thus enters a complex organization with a variety of goals, and with a well-developed system of rules and procedures for coordinating the different activities and the large numbers and categories of staff. This chapter examines the changing patterns of hospital use and patients' experiences of hospital care. It also considers the importance of staff attitudes, and describes the social categorization and labelling of patients by doctors and nurses, and the ways in which nurses' perceptions of their role influences the process and outcomes of care.

PATTERNS OF HOSPITAL USE

■ Changing patterns of hospital use

There has been a steady reduction in the total number of hospital beds since the early 1960s. This trend has continued, with a decline from 297 000 beds for all specialties in England in 1987–8 to 194 000 beds in 1997–8 (a 34% reduction). This decline in the numbers of hospital beds has occurred across all specialties and has been associated with increasing outpatient attendances and inpatient admissions (Table 5.1). The latter has been made possible by substantial reductions in length of stay, which have occurred for all specialities, age groups and diagnoses. For example, in the 1940s patients admitted to hospital for myocardial infarction had a length of stay of 5–7 weeks, compared with 5–7 days today.

TABLE 5.1	Hospital beds (thousands) and activity in England 1997-8 and percentage change since 1987-8	
	1997/8 (thousands)	**Change since 1987-8 (%)**
Beds available		
All specialties	194	-35
Acute	108	-16
Geriatric	30	-43
Mental Illness	37	-45
Learning disability	8	-76
Maternity	11	-31
Finished consultant episodes[a]		
All specialties	11530	+19
Acute[b]	9016	+24
Mental illness[b]	534	+128
Outpatient attendances		
All specialties	41635	+17
Acute	36887	+17
Mental illness	2126	+32

From Department of Health (1999) Tables B11, B16 and B18.
These figures exclude medical and surgical beds in the independent sector, which increased from 7035 beds in 1981 to 11 681 in 1995.
[a] Refers to a period of healthcare under one consultant in one hospital provider. This underestimates the number of patients treated, as one patient could have more than one episode of care within the data year.
[b] Figures for 1997-8 for acute specialties and mental illness compared with 1992-3.

67

Similarly, groin hernia repair required a length of stay of about 6 weeks in the 1940s; this reduced to an average of 4.9 days in 1985, and today involves either one night in hospital or is performed as day surgery. Indeed, rates of day surgery increased from 1355 operations in 1984 to 2439 in 1994 (an 80% increase), and accounted for over half of all elective operations by 1994 (Department of Health 1996). Changes in psychiatric care show a similar pattern; whereas patients admitted in the 1940s and early 1950s often spent many years in hospital, they are now generally discharged within 1 month, and many patients are admitted for much shorter periods.

Explaining patterns of hospital use

General hospital patients

The substantial reduction in lengths of hospital stay has occurred partly as a result of changes in medical views regarding recovery following surgery or major illness. For example, long periods of bed rest used to be regarded as therapeutic, whereas mobilization as soon as possible following surgery is now viewed as beneficial. In addition, shorter stays and the use of outpatient or day surgery as an alternative to inpatient care is now regarded as advantageous in reducing the stress of hospitalization, especially for young children.

Patients' needs for long periods in hospital have reduced as a result of clinical developments. These include more effective pain control, the availability of new diagnostic tests that reduce the need for long periods of observation and the development of less invasive medical technologies and surgical procedures, such as laparoscopic techniques and the use of lasers and lithotripsy to replace conventional open surgery.

New ways of financing hospital services have provided powerful economic incentives to reduce lengths of stay and increase the throughput of patients. NHS hospitals used to receive a global budget to cover their activity. This was based on the size and composition of their catchment population and rates of hospital use. Hospitals therefore had little incentive to increase patient admissions and throughput. Indeed, a large number of patients could lead to risks for hospitals (or particular units) of having a budget overspend; a situation referred to as the 'efficiency trap'. However, new methods of funding means that the revenue received by a hospital or unit is now related to the number of cases treated. As a result, reduced lengths of stay and higher levels of throughput increase a hospital's revenue. This in turn has encouraged new measures to further reduce lengths of stay. These include the greater availability of portable technologies (e.g. home dialysis) and other innovations in service delivery, such as hospital at home schemes, in which care that has traditionally been provided in hospital is provided at home, either as an alternative to inpatient admission or to allow early discharge with rehabilitation provided at home (Iliffe 1998).

Although reductions in available beds have been accompanied by both higher rates of admission and a greater emphasis on primary and community-based care, there are concerns about the adequacy of current levels of funding and service provision. In particular, large numbers of emergency admissions, especially by elderly people in winter months, leads to problems of cancelled operations and people waiting on trolleys for admission to a bed. Pressure on beds can also, in some situations, result in lengths of stay being inappropriately short, leading to greater risks of clinical complications and readmissions, and can lead to difficulties for patients and relatives in coping following discharge unless accompanied by appropriate discharge planning. More generally, there are problems of long waiting times for outpatient appointments and elective surgery. This reflects both the increasing demands for care and the limited resources (beds, staff, etc.) that exist in many NHS hospitals, as well as the effects of organizational and behavioural factors, including consultants' own priorities and the way that waiting lists are managed, which often involves patients being selected from the list rather than forming an orderly queue (Morgan 1992). There are currently particular concerns that long waiting times for hospital treatment in England and Wales contribute to the lower relative survival rates for cancers compared with the rest of Western Europe. A retrospective survey of all new patients attending acute hospital trusts in England with a cancer diagnosed and confirmed during October 1997, showed that patients with an urgent referral for breast cancer waited a median of 9 days from referral to the first outpatient appointment and a median of 27 days to first definitive treatment. The figures were 19 and 53 days respectively for urgent referrals for prostate cancer (Spurgeon et al 2000). The government has responded to this situation by setting a target of 2 weeks from referral by a general practitioner to first hospital outpatient appointment for all suspected cases of cancer. Other approaches to the waiting list problem have included funding patients to be treated in the private sector and financial initiatives that provide earmarked money for additional operations to reduce waiting lists. Increasing numbers of people also pay privately for elective surgical procedures rather than wait in a queue for admission to a NHS bed.

Psychiatric patients

A major change in the provision of care for psychiatric patients has been the process of deinstitutionalization. This has involved the gradual closure of large Victorian psychiatric hospitals that provided long-term custodial type care for up to 1000 patients at any one time. This process began in the 1950s with the adoption of a policy of 'community care', and increased in momentum during the 1980s. As a result, care for psychiatric patients now occurs outside the hospital, with short periods of admission to psychiatric wards in general hospitals if required for diagnosis and treatment, followed by discharge back to the 'community' to live in their own homes, in hostels or other supported accommodation, or with relatives. This marked shift in the pattern of psychiatric care has occurred in most countries and has been attributed to the interaction of a number of attitudinal, clinical and economic factors, although views differ of their relative importance.

Some regard the introduction of the major tranquillizers in the mid-1950s as the key factor making community care possible, by enabling people to be treated and aggressive behaviour controlled outside the hospital setting. Others argue that this exaggerates the therapeutic achievement these drugs represent and identify several hospitals that adopted the policy of early discharge well before the new drugs were introduced. They suggest that a more important factor was the prior change in ideas regarding mentally ill people, who were no longer viewed as violent and dangerous and requiring long-term custody and care but could be treated and returned to the community. Prior (1991) further suggests that changes in the location of care were associated with changes in psychiatric knowledge and practice, which increasingly emphasized the observation, assessment and rectification of patient behaviours and ability to perform Activities of Daily Living (ADLs), which could best be assessed and developed within a normal setting.

A third explanation of the new emphasis on community care was the increasing humanitarian concerns about the harmful effects of long periods spent in large psychiatric hospitals. Particularly influential was a book ('Asylums') by Erving Goffman (1961), based on his own observational study of a large psychiatric hospital in the USA. Goffman identified these hospitals as performing a disabling function and causing 'institutionaliza-tion' among patients. This condition is characterized at a psychological level by patients' lack of interest in leaving the institution, and their general apathy and lack of concern about what is going on around them. Institutionalized patients also demonstrate disturbed and regressive behaviour, including an inability to make choices and decisions, to plan activities or to undertake simple everyday tasks. They can also lose interest in and neglect their own appearance and develop mumbled speech and a characteristic shuffling gait. Goffman (1961) attributed this condition to organizational processes within the institution, especially the high level of depersonalization that occurred in the interests of organizational efficiency. For example, patients were subjected to what he described as 'batch processing', which refers to a situation where individuals were all treated alike and performed activities such as getting up, bathing and eating according to an institutional schedule with little scope for individual choices, preferences and decision-making. Personal possessions were also kept to a minimum to make it easier for staff to cope with large numbers of patients, and there was often little regard for privacy. As a result, patients frequently lost their self-identity, took on a passive role and became dependent on the institution, with institutional pressures being particularly strong for patients who experienced long lengths of stay and had little contact with the outside world. Recognition of the harmful effects of the institutional environment, together with a number of scandals regarding the neglect and ill treatment of patients in psychiatric hospitals and other long-stay institutions provided an important pressure towards a policy of deinstitutionalization on humanitarian grounds.

Economic factors were identified as playing a significant role in promoting the policy of community care (Scull 1984). This centred on the need to renovate the large psychiatric institutions built in the Victorian era and their considerable running costs, with a policy of community care being seen as reducing costs to the health service. However, the overall

69

costs of community care depends on the level of service, and can be more expensive than institutional care if there is considerable provision of small residential units and high levels of domiciliary services (see Chapter 16).

Deinstitutionalization has been of benefit to large numbers of psychiatric patients who previously would have spent many years in a custodial style of care. A recent follow-up study of long-stay psychiatric patients resettled in the community shows that, when carefully planned and adequately resourced, community care is beneficial to most individuals and has minimal detrimental effects on society (Trieman et al 1999). However, the reduction in hospital beds has not been accompanied by a corresponding increase in residential places in other settings and there are concerns about whether the needs of some groups are being met adequately in the community. This is highlighted by media reports of instances of violent and aggressive behaviour among psychiatric patients living in the community and of high levels of homelessness among people with mental illnesses. In addition, the shift to community care can place a considerable burden of care on informal carers, which forms a largely hidden cost of care (Chapter 16). Patients' actual experience of psychiatric wards is also variable and is affected by pressures on the service. This tends to be particularly great in inner London and can lead to high thresholds for admission and a concentration on acute wards of the most 'difficult' and disruptive patients (especially young men with schizophrenia). In this situation there are also frequently problems of a lack of easy access to beds for short-term management of crises or for respite care (Quirk & Lelliott 2001).

STAFF ATTITUDES AND PATIENT CARE

The provision of a rehabilitative environment within hospitals is particularly important on wards for elderly people and those with mental illness problems. However, achieving this approach to care depends on both the availability of sufficient staff and on favourable staff orientations and approaches to care. The effects of staff attitudes and goals were demonstrated by an observational study of stroke patients cared for on a specialist stroke unit (SU), an elderly care unit (ECU) and a general medical ward (GMW) (Pound & Ebrahim 2000). There was no difference in staffing levels between the SU and ECU but the typical interaction between nurses and patients differed between these sites (Table 5.2). What the researchers referred to as 'emotional labour' consisted of interactions that were gentle, warm, respectful and attentive and which involved a personal rather than a standardized response. This occurred most frequently in ECUs. ECUs were also characterized by greater frequency of 'rehabilitation nursing', which meant that nurses encouraged patients to

TABLE 5.2	Summary of typical interaction between nurses and stroke patients			
Setting (patients per nurse)	Emotional labour observed	Failures of emotional labour observed	Standardized interaction observed	Rehabilitation nursing observed
SU (1.8)	Occasionally	Nearly always	Rarely	Rarely
ECU (1.7)	Nearly always	Rarely	Occasionally	Always
GMW (2.9)	Rarely	Rarely	Nearly always	Never

From Pound & Ebrahim (2000).
SU, stroke unit; ECU, elderly care unit; GMW, general medical ward.

wash, dress and go to the toilet independently where possible and spent the extra time with patients that this necessitated. By contrast, nurses on SUs were more likely to perform these tasks for patients and, although kindly in their approach, were often observed to treat patients as non-persons to whom things were done. The ECU was also characterized by greater communication and involvement of nurses in working with physiotherapists to carryover patients' physiotherapy activity to the wards and emphasize a holistic approach to care. A key factor contributing to these different patterns of care was identified as the greater formal training in rehabilitation among nurses in ECUs, which encouraged a rehabilitation philosophy and approach in the unit. Nurses working in ECUs also appeared to have accepted their low status and to regard emotional labour as an important aspect of their nursing role. By contrast, nurses working on SUs were concerned to enhance their professional status by undertaking an extended clinical/technological role. They therefore focused on functional and technical aspects of care that were regarded as enhancing their status, such as testing for swallow reflexes, inserting nasogastric tubes and so on. The findings of this research suggest that a greater emphasis on rehabilitation nursing in stroke units might enhance the positive effects of the specialized medical treatment provided by these units. However, achieving this depends on the attitude of members of staff and their perception of their role, with caring and emotional work with patients generally being less valued than technological skills on most wards within the acute hospital, although highly valued in hospice settings and wards where the primary goal is that of palliative and supportive care.

The notion of emotional labour described by Pound & Ebrahim (2000) forms one aspect of what Strauss et al (1982) described as the 'sentimental' work undertaken by health professionals. This comprises different forms of interaction that together comprise a patient-centred approach to care. Strauss et al identified seven types of sentimental work based on observations they conducted in six hospitals over a period of 2 years (Box 5.1). Aspects of sentimental work include:

● a style of communication that seeks to create a partnership with patients in the medical task (interactional work)

● the provision of emotional support to patients through their hospital experience to promote patients' well-being and facilitate the conduct of medical procedures (trust work, composure work and biographical work)

● maintaining patients' sense of identity in the face of illness and experience of impersonal care (identity work, rectification work).

Strauss and colleagues note that sentimental work occurs mainly at the margins of the main line (medical-nursing, technical) of action in acute hospital settings and, although assisting the achievement of these tasks, is often not recorded. However, if the ideology of the ward or unit emphasizes sentimental work, interaction involving caring and emotional labour is accorded greater value and priority by staff, rather than being excluded or devalued in professional–patient interactions.

Increasing emphasis is now given in medical and nurse training to patient partnership, empowerment and choice, and thus to implementing the various dimensions of sentimental work. However, this approach to care is by no means universal, even within settings that are formally concerned with rehabilitation and care. For example, a study of five hospital wards caring for older people identified staff as often performing nursing tasks on patients without asking their permission rather than promoting patients' independence and feeling of being in control of their own lives. They also often failed to encourage patients to make choices and to participate actively in their own care, or to provide patients (and their relatives) with

---

BOX 5.1   Typology of Types of Sentimental Work Undertaken Among Hospital Patients

1. **Interactional work and moral rules**: following taken-for-granted rules regarding behaviour (e.g. listening carefully, not breaking in abruptly on the speaker, not shouting, not being brusque or breaking in on privacy). Orienting and preparing the person you are working 'on', explaining the options, decisions or overall work, and getting consent to doing anything to their body and pacing work in relation to patients energy and their capacity for enduring pain
2. **Trust work**: establishing trust through demonstrating competence and showing concern for patients' physical, interactional and personal sensibilities through talk, reassuring touching, subtle gestures, etc.
3. **Composure work**: giving reassuring words and gestures to help patients through a painful or frightening experience
4. **Biographical work**: eliciting information about the patients' social circumstances, support and lifestyle to aid medical diagnosis and decisions such as the pacing of prescribed therapy, as well as facilitating relationships between nurses and patients
5. **Identity work**: an extension of biographical work that involves helping patients maintain and improve a sense of identity in the face of illness. This includes long conversations with terminally ill patients to keep spirits up and further a patient's closure on his or her life, or to prepare people for their post-hospital lives
6. **Awareness of context work**: this refers to staff withholding information that they believe patients will find difficult to handle. However, the practice is now of greater disclosure and recognition that non-disclosure is an unstable situation because patients move to suspicion or full awareness of the situation
7. **Rectification work**: this occurs when patients express aggrievement or a sense of insult during or following the flouting of interactional rules, or when their composure has been shattered. It involves 'picking up the pieces' and reassuring patients that they really are people despite being treated as a non-person (e.g. following some visits to machined sites for diagnosis or therapy or following some ward rounds).

From Strauss et al (1982).

---

information about future care options and answer their questions clearly, with the least empowering ward being an elderly care rehabilitation ward (Faulkner 2001). Achieving personalized care and a rehabilitative environment for chronically ill patients takes time and training. It also requires sufficient numbers of qualified staff and the valuing by staff of these aspects of care.

◼ Social evaluation of patients

Staff views

A further aspect of professional–patient relationships is the tendency in some situations for staff to evaluate patients in both social and medical terms. In particular, the considerable range of patients attending Accident and Emergency (A&E) departments, and their varying medical needs, provides considerable opportunity for such evaluation. A classic study that was conducted in three A&E departments (Jeffrey 1979) identified a group of patients depicted by junior doctors as 'good' patients in terms of their medical condition. These patients presented with conditions that allowed junior A&E staff to practise and develop the clinical skills necessary to pass professional examinations or to practise their chosen specialty, or were acutely ill patients (e.g. head injuries, cardiac arrests, road traffic accidents) who tested the general competence and maturity of staff in coping with their rapid early treatment.

At the other end of the continuum were patients described in negative social terms and categorized as 'rubbish' (dross, etc.). These consisted of four main groups of patients – people presenting with 'trivia', drunks, regular overdoses and tramps. Each of these groups was regarded as having broken the unwritten rules of appropriate patient behaviour.

Patients presenting with medical 'trivia' were viewed as having a condition that is neither due to trauma nor is urgent and therefore not a legitimate demand on an A&E service.

Normal overdoses were regarded as calls for attention for which there was no therapy to correct the state, and some ambivalence was expressed about whether drunks and tramps were 'really ill' or required other types of assistance. Most patients presenting with overdoses were not regarded as adhering to the expectation of illness as an undesirable state because their condition was often viewed as self-inflicted to put pressure on someone or get attention. Similarly, tramps were often regarded by staff as wanting to be treated as ill to gain the secondary benefits of warm accommodation and meals.

There is an expectation that patients should cooperate with competent authorities in trying to get well, but drunks and overdoses were often non-cooperative in their receipt of medical care, and were also regarded by staff as living their lives in such a way as to sustain the same injuries in the future. Negatively labelled patients were frequently observed to be 'punished' by being afforded low priority and experienced an increased wait before completing treatment. They might also receive a less sympathetic and more punitive approach to care.

The social evaluation and labelling of patients by staff has been studied mainly in A&E settings, which form an open access service. However, this social evaluation also occurs on hospital wards. Patients labelled by nurses as 'popular' ('good') are seen as polite, stoical and often entertaining, and as trying to help themselves and to cooperate with staff. By contrast, 'unpopular' ('bad') patients are regarded as too demanding, a label that includes asking too many questions, complaining, being irritable, being attention-seeking or not being cooperative or helping themselves (Johnson & Webb 1995). However, evaluations were found to be complex and could occur at more than one level. For example, patients could be unpopular physically because of the difficulties involved in performing their care, but liked at an interpersonal level perhaps because they were stoical or humorous. These evaluations are not necessarily fixed but can change over time as nurses gain more information about patients or there is a change in the context of care. As Johnson & Webb (1995) noted, qualified nurses might experience feelings of dissonance and guilt because they are aware of the 'professional' way of working in which personal preferences and views should not intrude, but also of their departures from this in terms of their social evaluations and designations.

Another area in which social and moral evaluations play an important role is in relation to clinical decision making and the need for doctors to make choices and implicit rationing decisions. For example, judgements of whether to take cardiac patients on for surgery or angioplasty often involve both a technical discourse relating to the coronary anatomy and feasibility of surgery and also a social discourse, which refers to age, lifestyle (weight and smoking) and various structural factors (i.e. gender, class and ethnicity) and draws on notions of 'deservingness' in using scarce health service resources and 'risk' in relation to likely outcomes (Hughes & Griffiths 1996).

Patient views

Recent studies have complemented research on staff attitudes and practises by examining patients' own perspectives and responses to staff evaluations. This work has identified the reasons why patients attend A&E departments for what is deemed medical 'trivia',

73

suggesting that this often occurs because individuals feel unable to evaluate the medical seriousness of the condition, especially in relation to the illness of a very young child (Kai 1996). The choice of A&E attendance rather than primary care usually occurs for practical reasons, as a result of the more immediate access (i.e. lack of a booked appointment system) and provision of an out-of-hours service. Whereas previously the aim was to change the behaviours of those designated as inappropriate attenders at A&E departments, recent policies aim to respond to patient patterns of A&E attendance through the establishment of minor injuries units and general practitioner and nurse specialists within A&E departments to respond to medically trivial conditions. In addition, a national nurse-led telephone advice system has been set up (NHS Direct) to provide information and advice as to whether medical care is necessary. This illustrates the way in which behaviours can be constructed as inappropriate or appropriate, depending on prevailing assumptions, views and forms of provision.

There are also questions over the perceptions and experiences of patients who are regarded as possessing medically or socially undesirable characteristics (e.g. tramps, drug addicts, HIV-positive patients). For HIV-positive patients this potentially stigmatizing information is noted in patients' files, with healthcare workers therefore being privy to potentially discrediting information and among the very few, or only, people who know of their stigmatizing illness (see Chapter 13). This raises important issues of confidentiality. In addition, a health professional's reaction to the patient forms an important aspect of the patient's social experience of illness. Negative reactions or tactless comments by health professionals have been identified as an important source of trauma for patients with stigmatizing conditions, and people who are HIV positive might encounter a refusal to treat and stereotyped attitudes. As a result, the specialist centres for people who are HIV positive are often viewed very positively by patients in terms of the attitudes of staff and care provided (Green & Platt 1997).

PATIENTS' EXPERIENCE OF HOSPITAL CARE

Stress and anxiety in hospital patients

Admission to hospital is routine for hospital staff but forms a major event in people's lives and is often a source of considerable anxiety and stress. Currently, about 8% of men and 12% of women in the population are admitted to hospital each year. For these people, the fact that 'something is wrong,' requiring diagnosis, treatment or both, often forms a source of anxiety in itself. For some patients there are further uncertainties about whether they will be cured, left with a physical disability or faced with an early death. Patients are also frequently apprehensive about the discomfort and pain they might experience in undergoing diagnostic or operative procedures, and often worry about having an anaesthetic. In addition, the actual experience of being a patient in hospital is often stressful. Particular sources of stress include a lack of privacy, lack of familiarity with the different categories of staff and with the general routines of the ward, problems of being disturbed on the ward and not being able to sleep, and not being given sufficient information about their medical condition or treatment. Patients about to be discharged might also worry about how they will manage at home. For young children, admission to hospital and separation from their parents and familiar surroundings can be particularly traumatic. As a result, there is now greater emphasis and provision for parents to spend long periods of time on the ward and in some cases to participate in their child's care.

Recognition of the high level of stress that is often experienced by hospital patients has led to a greater emphasis on preparing patients (and children) for hospital admission through written information and personal communication to explain their treatment and hospital stay. This patient preparation has been demonstrated to have positive effects on measures of anxiety, pain and satisfaction among patients undergoing surgery or treatments such as radiotherapy (Shuldham 1999). It is also of particular importance for day surgery, as this requires that patients are admitted and discharged on the same day and manage their recovery at home. Increasing use is now made of audio tapes and cassettes to provide patients with information about their condition and treatment options, and to ensuring that information is 'patient-centred', and thus reflects the priorities and needs of patients rather than those of the health professionals (Meredith et al 1995). The sick person's reaction to being in hospital in terms of anxiety, worry, fear and depression, also draws attention to the importance of 'emotional labour' by hospital staff, which acknowledges that the object of medical work is alive, sentient and reacting. Work done or with or on human beings needs to take into account their response to that work and provide information, support and comfort that responds to individual patients needs.

Patient participation and empowerment

A major shift in health policy has been occurring since the early 1980s: from patients as passive recipients of care to patients as consumers who make demands and have needs that the health service must strive to meet. This is illustrated by the government's strategy for the health service as set out in 'The NHS plan' (Department of Health 2000), which requires that Hospital Trusts and other parts of the NHS take account of the public's and users' views in developing the service, and that patients are fully involved in decisions about their own care as active partners with professionals and have information about their health and health care to make informed decisions about it if they wish.

The incorporation of a public/user voice is seen as an essential element at every level of the service, acting as a lever for change. This is being implemented through a variety of fora set up to elicit the views of local groups and communities, including the appointment of patient/user/public representatives to key committees concerned with the quality and development services (at both national and local levels) and supporting them in this process. It is also proposed that different sectors of the service have clear statements and commitment to user and public involvement.

These various initiatives are giving rise to new ways of organizing aspects of the service through involving staff at all levels and patients in redesigning processes in clinics to increase their efficiency and acceptability, and developing rapid access and integrated care schemes. At an individual level, emphasis is given in professional training and assessment to communication and patient partnership skills. There has also been an increase in patient information materials (leaflets, booklets, videos, etc.) that aim to respond to patients' own questions and concerns and help patients with a specific condition to understand what the disease is, and its parameters, stages of treatment, what is likely to happen to them and the options available. Patients admitted to NHS hospitals are also now accorded greater rights, including the right of access to their health records, participation in treatment decisions and full disclosure of treatment options as part of informed consent. These measures taken together aim to address a major cause of dissatisfaction among hospital patients regarding communication about their condition and treatment, as well as a perceived lack of information about the hospital and its routine which contribute to patients' feelings of stress (Bruster et al 1994).

There is evidence that patient involvement in decisions regarding their hospital treatment increases satisfaction with care and reduces psychological morbidity (Mahler & Kulik 1990). However, people have differing desires for involvement in treatment decisions, and individual preferences might also vary in relation to the type of treatment. For example, a study of women with breast cancer, for which treatment options mainly relate to type of surgery and are fairly well defined, found that 20% of women wished to have an active role in making the final decision, 28% preferred a shared role in treatment decision making and 52% wished to leave the final decision to the doctor. By contrast, among patients with colorectal cancer (for which the management, options and outcomes are less clearly defined), only 4% preferred an active role, 17% preferred shared decision-making and 78% preferred to leave the final decision to the doctor. However, although patients differed in their desire for involvement in treatment decisions, all groups of patients were keen to have information about their condition and thought that treatment choices should be discussed (Beaver et al 1999).

THE CHANGING ORGANIZATION OF THE HOSPITAL

Hospitals were founded as institutions for the care of the sick poor, who were removed from the community because of infectious disease. However, they became the major site of clinical practice and the location of technologies for diagnosis and treatment. Like any large organizations, hospitals are in a continuous process of evolution and change. Recent changes include a different staff–patient ratio, as the reduction in lengths of stay has meant that throughput has increased and patients receive more active intervention and care throughout their hospital stay and are then discharged for convalescent care. There has also been greater emphasis on pooled resources as a means of achieving greater efficiency. Thus, whereas hospital beds were formerly designated as the responsibility and resource of individual consultants, they are now generally controlled by a bed manager or senior nurse. This allows greater flexibility and avoids situations in which consultants might retain patients until they were ready for a new admission to their 'firm's' beds; equally, it avoids the need for junior doctors to spend considerable time locating beds (Green & Armstrong 1993). In addition, there is a greater emphasis on hospitals meeting targets in terms of waiting times, reducing cancelled operations and the time for admission through A&E, and so on.

A second change relates to the increased blurring of professional roles. This includes changes in the roles of healthcare assistants and nursing and therapy assistants to respond to the shortage of qualified nursing staff, as well as to the new roles being taken on by qualified nurses. One type of role is the enhanced nursing role, which requires qualified nurses to develop their skills in the social and rehabilitative dimensions of nursing, so that they can work autonomously in planning, implementing care and discharging patients in nurse-led intermediate care units. These units provide care for patients (usually elderly) who are referred from medical wards, are past the acute phase of illness but are not ready to return home. These units and an enhanced nursing role more generally are likely to become increasingly important with the growing numbers of very elderly people and the greater emphasis on a patient-centred approach and the social and emotional dimensions of care. However, another trend is towards nurses taking on an extended clinical role as clinical nurse specialists to fill the gap left by the reduction in junior doctors' hours of work, and undertaking such tasks as preoperative assessment in elective surgery, intravenous antibiotic administration, electrocardiograms and suturing minor wounds. This clinical role might also become further extended with the introduction of limited nurse prescribing and test ordering, as well as with the gradual move towards multiprofessional education.

A third change is the current trend for care to move outside the hospital. This is exemplified by the expansion in minor surgery undertaken by general practitioners, the availability of home dialysis and fetal monitoring, and developments in specialist clinics in primary care and consultant outreach sessions, the substantial increases in day surgery, and the emphasis on treating chronic conditions in the community. These changes have been accompanied by increasing numbers of nurses, physiotherapists, midwives and other health professionals working in the community, with some hospital consultants holding specialist outreach sessions for diabetes, ophthalmology and other conditions. In addition, developments in telemedicine mean that, in future, there will be less need to bring patients into specialist units, with the diagnosis made or tests ordered and treatment begun following a telemedicine consultation for patients attending at a primary care site.

The future evolution of the hospital is unclear. However, current trends suggest that the hospital will become the centre of a vertically integrated system in which acute beds play only a modest role. This change in function and blurring of the primary/secondary interface has implications for clinical training and medical work, as well as for patients' experiences of medical care. In particular, it emphasizes the importance of good coordination between primary and secondary services, and communication between staff and between staff and patients. It is also important that the increasing introduction of new treatments and technological developments within the hospital does not detract from the qualitative aspects of care and communication that have beneficial effects for both patients' experience of hospital and the outcomes achieved.

References

Beaver K, Bogg J, Luker KA 1999 Decision-making role preference and information needs: a comparison of colorectal and breast cancer. Health Expectations 2:266–276

Bruster S et al 1994 National survey of hospital patients. British Medical Journal 309:1542–1546

Department of Health (DoH) 1996 Health and personal social services statistics for England. HMSO, London

Department of Health (DoH) 1999 Health and personal social services statistics for England. HMSO, London

Department of Health (DoH) 2000 The NHS plan: a plan for investment, a plan for reform. Cmnd 4818-1. HMSO, London

Faulkner M 2001 A measure of patient empowerment in hospital environments catering for older people. Journal of Advanced Nursing 34(5):676–686

Goffman E 1961 Asylums. Doubleday, New York

Green J, Armstrong D 1993 Controlling the 'bed state': negotiating hospital organisation. Sociology of Health and Illness 15:337–352

Green G, Platt S 1997 Fear and loathing in health care settings reported by people with HIV. Sociology of Health and Illness 19(1):70–92

Hughes D, Griffiths L 1996 'But if you look at the coronary anatomy...': risk and rationing in cardiac surgery. Sociology of Health and Illness 18(2):172–197

Iliffe S 1998 Hospital at home: from red to amber? British Medical Journal 316:1761–1762

Jeffrey R 1979 Normal rubbish: deviant patients in casualty departments. Sociology of Health and Illness 1(1):90–107

Johnson M, Webb C 1995 Rediscovering unpopular patients: the concept of social judgement. Journal of Advanced Nursing 21:466–475

Kai J 1996 What worries parents when their pre-school children are acutely ill, and why: a qualitative study. British Medical Journal 313:983–986

Mahler HI, Kulik J 1990 Preferences for health care involvement, perceived control and surgical recovery: a prospective study. Social Science and Medicine 31(7):743–751

Meredith P, Emberton M, Wood C 1995 New directions in information for patients. British Medical Journal 311:4–5

Morgan M 1992 Waiting lists. In Beck E, Lonsdale S, Newman S, Patterson D (eds) The status and future of health care in the UK. Chapman and Hall, London

Pound P, Ebrahim S 2000 Rhetoric and reality in stroke patient care. Social Science and Medicine 51 1437–1446

Prior L 1991 Community versus hospital care: the crisis in psychiatric provision. Social Science and Medicine 32(4):483–489

Quirk A, Lelliott P 2001 What do we know about life on acute psychiatric wards in the UK? A review of the research evidence. Social Science and Medicine 53:1565–1574

Scull AT 1984 Decarceration: community treatment and the deviant – a radical view, 2nd edn. Polity Press, Cambridge

Shuldham C 1999 A review of the impact of pre-operative education on recovery from surgery. International Journal of Nursing Studies 36:171–177

Spurgeon P, Barwell F, Kerr D 2000 Waiting times for cancer patients in England after general practitioners' referrals: retrospective national survey. British Medical Journal 320:838–839

Strauss A et al 1982 Sentimental work in the technological hospital. Sociology of Health and Illness 4(3):254–278

Trieman N, Leff J, Glover G 1999 Outcome of long stay psychiatric patients resettled in the community: prospective cohort study. British Medical Journal 319:13–16

David Locker

Since the early 1970s, sociologists have increasingly turned their attention to the issues and challenges involved in chronic illness and disability. Studies of people with disabilities were undertaken before this time but were concerned largely with psychological factors and their role in the rehabilitation process.

During the 1970s, considerable effort was invested in developing appropriate measures of chronic illness and disability, estimating the prevalence and severity of disability, assessing the needs of people with disabilities and identifying gaps in service provision for these individuals and the families who cared for them. In the 1980s, more attention was paid to the experience of living with chronic illness and disability (Anderson & Bury 1988, Conrad 1987). A growing number of studies have begun to describe in some detail what it is like for individuals and families to live with a long-term, disabling disorder. The rationale underlying this work is that 'a sound, effective and ethical approach to chronic illness must lie in awareness of and attention to the experiences, values, priorities and expectations of (these people) and their families' (Anderson & Bury 1988). This means that a detailed understanding of the impact of chronic illness and disability on daily life is necessary for the providers of medical and social services to offer appropriate care and support.

This recent emphasis on chronic illness reflects the fact that chronic disabling disorders, rather than acute infectious diseases, are the major cause of mortality in industrial societies and present a significant challenge to the medical-care system (see Chapter 1). Even where chronic conditions are not fatal, they are major sources of suffering for individuals and families. As Verbrugge & Jette (1994) indicate, people mostly live with rather than die from chronic conditions. Given that the populations of western societies are ageing (see Chapter 11), it is predicted that the proportion of consultations in medical practice devoted to the psychosocial and other problems of daily living associated with chronic illness will increase. As a result, there will be a fundamental shift in medical practice from 'cure' to 'care' (Williams 1989).

The emergence of an interest in chronic illness also coincided with an increase in government provision for people with disabling disorders. In the UK, 1970 saw the passing of the Chronically Sick and Disabled Persons Act, which made it mandatory for local authorities to identify people with disabilities, to determine their needs and to provide services to meet those needs (Topliss 1979). In 1974, a Minister for the Disabled was appointed with specific responsibilities for the group. These developments led to an increase in services and financial benefits for people with disabilities and those who cared for them, although these were somewhat eroded during the late 1980s.

A further development that stimulated a greater awareness of the needs and priorities of people living with chronic illness was the emergence of the 'disability movement' (Conrad 1987). This consisted of groups dedicated to self-help and political action. The former offered help and support through the sharing of individual experience; the latter used the political process to secure fundamental rights and to promote independent living. The aim here was to ensure that people with chronic disabling disorders would themselves define their needs and the most appropriate way of providing for them, rather than having these imposed by putative 'experts' and professionals.

CHARACTERISTICS OF CHRONIC ILLNESS

The term 'chronic illness' encompasses a wide range of conditions affecting almost all body systems. Cancer, stroke, end-stage renal disease, poliomyelitis, multiple sclerosis, rheumatoid arthritis, psoriasis, epilepsy and chronic obstructive airways disease are common examples. The most fundamental characteristic of chronic illnesses is that they are long term and have a profound influence on the lives of sufferers. Some are fatal and some are not; some are stable with a certain prognosis, others might show great variation in terms of their day-to-day manifestations and their long-term course and outcome. In the majority of cases, medical intervention is palliative; it seeks to control symptoms but cannot offer a cure. Consequently, maximizing the welfare of these individuals and their families means maintaining or improving the quality of daily life rather than attempting to eradicate the disease process itself.

Some of the problems encountered by people with a chronic disabling disorder stem directly from the symptomatic character of their illness. In this respect, every chronic condition is somewhat distinct. For example, the person with rheumatoid arthritis must cope with chronic pain, the person with respiratory disease must live with breathlessness and an inadequate oxygen supply, and the person with end-stage renal failure must cope with the demands of a dialysis machine. In other respects, the problems faced by people with chronic illness might be common to all, irrespective of the nature of their condition. Many such individuals experience unemployment or reduced career prospects, social isolation and estrangement from family and friends, loss of important roles, changed physical appearance and problems with self-esteem and identity. Another fundamental characteristic of chronic conditions is that these assaults on the body, daily activities (encompassing home, work and leisure) and social relationships (including relationships with self and others) must be managed in the course of everyday life. When chronic illness becomes severe, daily life can be entirely consumed in coping with its symptoms, the medical regimens intended to control it and its social consequences (Locker 1983).

Prevalence of chronic illness and disability

A number of surveys of national and local populations have been undertaken in order to estimate the prevalence of disability. These have produced somewhat different results, largely because different definitions and measures of disability have been employed. The most recent study in the UK, the Survey of Disability in Great Britain undertaken in 1985 by the Office of Population Censuses and Surveys (OPCS), found that 14.2% of the adult population were disabled (OPCS 1988). Rates increased substantially with age and were higher among women than men. Other studies have reported that the most common causes of significant disability are neurological, musculoskeletal and respiratory diseases such as stroke, multiple sclerosis, Parkinson's disease and rheumatoid arthritis. Similarly, it has been estimated that about 35 million Americans, or one in seven, have disabling conditions sufficiently severe to interfere with daily life. One factor increasing the prevalence of some types of disability is medicine's increasing success at averting the death of many people with developmental abnormalities such as spina bifida and the consequences of accidents such as spinal cord resection. HIV/AIDS has also been transformed from an invariably fatal condition into a chronic illness by the advent of therapies that control the replication of the virus responsible for the disease.

Studies of disability probably underestimate the prevalence of chronic illness. Conditions such as diabetes, psoriasis and epilepsy might not be identified by conventional measures of disability. Consequently, the percentage of the population living with a chronic condition is likely to be higher than the 14.2% identified by the OPCS survey. One estimate derived from work by the Royal College of Physicians suggested that just over one-fifth of the population was subject to some type of chronic illness.

More recent surveys have provided data on the prevalence of specific conditions among specific age groups. These confirm the difference between estimates of the prevalence of chronic conditions and estimates of the prevalence of disability. For example, a survey of a sample of the population aged 45 years and over living in the north of England found a prevalence of stroke of 17.5 persons per 1000. However, the prevalence of stroke-related dependence was lower, at 11.7 persons per 1000 (O'Mahoney et al 1999). Similarly, projections based on national data collected in 1997 suggest that, by 2020, 60 million persons in the USA will be affected by arthritis, with 11.6 million being limited by this condition (Morbidity and Mortality Weekly Report 2001). These data also indicated that the prevalence of persons with arthritis had increased by approximately 750 000 persons per year since 1990. Other evidence from the USA suggests that, from 1982 to 1999, there was an overall reduction in the prevalence of disability among elderly people (Manton & Gu 2001) and European data indicate a reduction in the prevalence of disability in more recent cohorts of elderly women (Winblad et al 2001). Nevertheless, the ageing of the population will probably mean an increase in the numbers of people living with a disabling condition, even though the prevalence is falling.

Impairment, disability and handicap

A systematic approach to thinking about chronic illness is to be found in the International Classification of Impairments, Disabilities or Handicaps (ICIDH), a manual that classifies the consequences of disease (Badley 1993, Wood 1980). To better understand these consequences, it offers three concepts: impairment, disability and handicap. Impairment is concerned with abnormalities in the structure or functioning of the body or its parts, disability with the performance of activities, and handicap with the broader social and psychological consequences of living with impairment and disability. Because it is dependent on the social context in which it occurs, handicap can best be understood by sociological enquiry. Formal definitions of these terms are given in Box 6.1.

The three concepts are also organized into a model or theoretical framework, which relates these dimensions of experience to each other (Fig. 6.1).

This model has caused some confusion, especially if the arrows are interpreted to indicate time; so that an individual with a chronic condition moves along the sequence and inevitably becomes handicapped. In fact, the arrows mean 'may or may not lead to'. Disability might result from impairment and handicap might result from disability, but this is not necessarily so. The examples given in Box 6.2 illustrate this point. Moreover, there is no necessary relationship between the severity of impairment and the severity of disability and/or handicap that results. For example, a study of people with multiple sclerosis found that the psychosocial handicaps they suffered were not related to the severity of the underlying disease (Harper et al 1986). Similarly, a study of individuals with chronic respiratory disease found that clinical measures of lung function were not good predictors of disability, and there was considerable variability in the extent of handicap associated with a given level of disability (Williams & Bury unpublished and 1989).

Although the ICIDH scheme has been widely used it has been subject to some criticism, particularly in the USA, where alternative schemes have been developed and adopted (Nagi 1991, Verbrugge & Jette 1994). At the heart of the problem is the use of the term 'handicap' and the way in which is has been defined. In the USA the term 'handicapped' has been used to describe people in a pejorative way and is now generally avoided. In addition, the term carries the implication that the problems people experience are intrinsic, that is, the product of personal deficiencies and failings. Finally, because the definition of handicap

---

BOX 6.1 ICIDH Definitions

- **Impairment**: any loss or abnormality of psychological, physiological or anatomical structure or function
- **Disability**: a restriction or lack (resulting from an impairment) of ability to perform an activity in a manner or within the range considered normal for a human being
- **Handicap**: a disadvantage for a given individual, resulting from an impairment or a disability, that limits or prevents the fulfilment of a role that is normal (depending on age, sex and social and cultural factors) for that individual

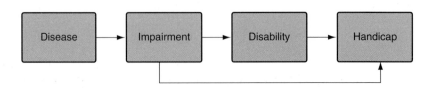

Fig. 6.1 Linear model of disease and its consequences.

BOX 6.2 Interrelations of Impairment, Disability and Handicap

- An individual with arthritis (disease) will have pain and swelling in involved joints, which will be stiff and limited in their range of motion (impairment). Consequently, there might be difficulty in carrying out activities such as walking or climbing stairs (disability). This could disadvantage the individual in terms of mobility around the community or finding a job, which in turn could lead to social isolation or relative poverty (handicap)
- People with extreme short sight or diabetes are impaired but, because these conditions can be corrected with devices or drugs, they would not necessarily be disabled in terms of any limitations in the activities they perform. However, in certain circumstances they may be handicapped by their conditions. For example, short sight might prevent access to certain occupations and diabetes could impose a burden on the individual because of dietary restrictions and the need for regular insulin injections
- A person with a severe facial disfigurement that has been present since birth or the result of an accident, would be impaired. The person would not experience any limitations in the tasks or activities of daily life and would not be disabled. However, he or she could be handicapped in the sense that social attitudes towards physical attractiveness could lead to low self-esteem and difficulty in forming romantic relationships
- A person with cerebral palsy might have a range of impairments, including problems with speech or use of the limbs. These could lead to disabilities in many activities, including mobility around the community, difficulties with self-care and difficulties with communication. As a result, the individual could be handicapped in a number of areas of life. Alternatively, recognition of the person's intellectual abilities could open opportunities for a high status professional career with a high income. In turn, this would facilitate autonomy and choice.

Adapted from Badley (1995).

---

uses the word 'role', which generally refers to activities and tasks, some have found the distinction between disability and handicap unclear.

One way around these difficulties is to think of handicap in terms of disadvantage and deprivation. For example, an individual who uses a wheelchair might be at a disadvantage in seeking work compared to the able-bodied simply because many workplaces have steps, stairs and wash-rooms or other facilities inaccessible to a wheelchair. As a consequence, individuals might be deprived of jobs commensurate with their education and skills, or could become unemployed and deprived of the income, social contacts and other benefits that accrue from work. Even less tangible problems, such as the mental burden and low self-esteem that can accompany chronic illness, can be understood in these terms: the individual is deprived of peace of mind and a sense of self-worth.

This example highlights a crucial aspect of handicap. It does not stem from the individual but from the environments in which he or she must live. An alternative definition, which makes this explicit, states that handicap consists of 'the opportunities that a person has missed because of barriers in the environment' (Halbertsma 1989). In fact, a review of recent definitions of handicap found that they all contained reference to the environment (Badley 1995). In this context, environment refers not only to the physical environment, but also to material, social and attitudinal environments.

Medical and social models of disability

The above comments regarding the concept of handicap are intended to highlight the difference between medical and social models of disability. This distinction arose out of criticisms of the ICIDH model by people who were active in organizations and movements that aimed to secure basic civil rights for people with disabilities. In the medical model, disability is defined as a deviation from biomedical norms of structure and function and the disadvantages that disabled people experience are seen as the direct and inevitable consequence of their impairments and disabilities (Bickenbach et al 1999). Consequently, disability is a problem of a person best addressed by medical intervention to cure the disease or help the person adjust to their limitations. The social model sees the problems experienced by people with disabilities as being the direct product of the physical, social and attitudinal environments referred to above. The problem is not that disabled people cannot meet the demands of everyday life; rather, the problem is a failure of the environment to adjust to the needs and desires of people with disabilities. Political action and social change are necessary to ensure the full participation of people with disabilities in all areas of social life (WHO 1999).

Although the ICIDH model attempted to offer a non-medical account of disablement, the language it used to describe the links between impairment, disability and handicap, its description of the nature of handicap and its failure to focus on the key role played by the environment meant that it embodied many of the features of the medical model (Bickenbach et al 1999).

A revised model: functioning, disability and health

An early modification to the ICIDH model emphasized the need to view handicap as emerging out of external factors that interact with disease/impairment/disability. One attempt to describe these factors made reference to the physical environment, the social situation of the person and the resources available to them (Badley 1987). In a more recent contribution, Verbrugge & Jette (1994) provided a more elaborate classification, including both personal and environmental factors in the process that links impairment/disability and their outcomes (Box 6.3). The importance of these factors is that they provide avenues for interventions that aim to improve the quality of life of persons so affected.

In response to criticisms of the original ICIDH model, a more comprehensive modification has recently been developed by the World Health Organization (Halbertsma et al 2000). This is called the International Classification of Functioning, Disability and Health known as ICF (WHO 1999). This has moved away from being a 'consequences of disease' model, to a 'components of health' model. Its key components are:

- body structures and functions, and impairments in structure or function

- activities, which are tasks or activities undertaken by a person, and difficulties or limitations an individual might have in executing those activities

- participation, which consists of involvement in life situations in the context of where an individual lives. Participation restrictions are problems a person might experience with respect to involvement in life situations.

Each of these components, and the relationships between them, are influenced by contextual factors, that is, personal and environmental factors of the kind described in Box 6.3. This scheme attempts to integrate the medical and social models of disability into a broader biopsychosocial model that gives due recognition to the significance of the environment in influencing functioning and overall health and well-being.

THE MEANING OF CHRONIC ILLNESS

From a sociological point of view and from the point of view of those living with a chronic illness, the disadvantage and deprivation they experience is, perhaps, the important

BOX 6.3	Factors Influencing the Disablement Process

Extra-individual factors
- Medical care and rehabilitation (surgery, physical therapy, speech therapy, counselling, health education, job retraining, etc.)
- Medication and other therapeutic regimens (drugs, recreational therapy, aquatic exercise, biofeedback meditation, rest/energy conservation, etc.)
- External supports (personal assistance, special equipment and devices, day care, respite care, meals-on-wheels, etc.)
- Buildings, physical and social environment (structural modifications at home/job, access to buildings and public transport, health insurance and access to medical care, laws and regulations, employment legislation, social attitudes, etc.)

Intra-individual factors
- Lifestyle and behaviour changes (overt changes to alter disease activity and impact)
- Psychosocial attributes and coping (positive affect, emotional vigour, locus of control, cognitive adaptation to disability, personal support, peer support groups, etc.)
- Activity accommodations (changes in kinds of activities, ways of doing them, frequency or length of time doing them)

Reprinted with kind permission from Elsevier Science Ltd from Verbrugge & Jette (1994).

85

consideration. This is because such experiences are closely allied with the quality of life. Arguably, within the right environments, the quality of life of many people with impairments and disabilities would not be much different from that of those without.

Because of its significance, two issues concerning disadvantage and deprivation warrant further attention: first, their multidimensional character; and second, the significance of material and social resources in managing the problems created by chronic illness. As mentioned above, many of these problems have their origins in the interaction of individuals with their environments.

Dimensions of disadvantage and deprivation

Whereas early sociological approaches to chronic illness and disability drew on the theory of the sick role (Parsons 1951) (see Chapter 4), labelling theory (Lemert 1967) and Goffman's analysis of stigma (Goffman 1963) (see Chapter 13), more contemporary approaches have used detailed case studies to understand what it means to live with a chronic disabling disorder. This 'experience of illness' perspective is to be found in numerous books and scholarly papers published over the last 20 years and all have disadvantage, deprivation and quality of life as their central concern.

Stated simply, the meaning of chronic illness is to be found in its practical and symbolic consequences (Blaxter 1976, Bury 1988). These consequences take the form of problems that people with chronic disabling conditions and their families must solve if they are to attain a quality of life of minimal tolerability.

For example, one study of people with rheumatoid arthritis found that all faced the following (Locker 1983):

- problems managing the symptoms of the disease and the medical treatments designed to control them
- problems with the practical matters of everyday living, such as self-care, household management and mobility around the home and community

- problems with respect to finding work or maintaining a meaningful role in the work-force
- economic problems following unemployment
- problems in social relationships and family life.

The emotional burden of being chronically ill, its psychological consequences in the form of depression and frustration and feelings of vulnerability were prominent among this group of people, as was the necessity of adapting to a more limited life. The participants in this study also encountered what might be termed cognitive problems. That is, they were faced with the task of making sense of the onset of chronic illness and sought answers to the unanswerable question 'Why me?'. In addition, they were constantly engaged in efforts to make sense of the day-to-day variation in levels of pain and stiffness in an attempt to establish order in their world and render their unpredictable existence predictable. As many studies have revealed, a significant aspect of being or caring for a person with a disability is the 'daily grind'; the never-ending and unrewarded practical and psychological work involved in coping with these problems on a daily basis. A more detailed account of some of these issues is presented below.

The significance of resources

A crucial factor that has an influence on how, and the extent to which, the problems associated with chronic illness and disability are managed, is the resources to which individuals have access. These resources take many forms: time, energy, money, social support, appropriate housing, formal services that foster independence rather than exacerbate dependence, and knowledge and information are perhaps the most important. Psychological resources and dispositions are also important. The magnitude and range of resources available to individuals and families, and the coping strategies of which they form a part, influence how well the consequences of chronic conditions are managed.

In a sense, the fact that personal and social resources must be allocated to solving mundane practical matters is part of the handicap that flows from chronic illness. Money might have to be used to pay someone to clean the house and do the shopping rather than to make life more enjoyable. As chronic illness progresses, it is sometimes the case that available resources shrink. Physical resources can decline as a result of the worsening of the disease, money might decline when the individual becomes unemployed and his or her spouse gives up work to adopt a full-time caring role, and social support can be eroded as friendship networks or families collapse under the strain of chronic illness. In these instances, life becomes nothing more than the work and effort of solving illness-related problems and getting through the day.

The concept of resources is a crucial one. On the one hand, it provides one of the mechanisms that link disability, disadvantage and deprivation, whereas on the other, it draws attention to the unequal distribution of resources in society and the ability/inability of individuals from different socioeconomic groups to maintain a satisfactory existence in the face of chronic illness. In this way, it links personal concerns with wider social and political issues. People from working-class backgrounds, women, ethnic minorities and those who live in deprived urban communities are likely to be the most vulnerable in the face of chronic illness.

It is also the case that the illness experience can vary with historical period and culture. As Bury (1988) has indicated, chronic illness has two levels of meaning. One is to be found in the kinds of problems described above. The other is to be found in the significance or connotations that particular conditions carry, and the extent to which a given condition renders an individual culturally incompetent, that is, unable to perform ordinary activities in socially appropriate ways. The extent to which an individual is devalued by chronic illness will also be influenced by what the illness means in its particular cultural environment. For example, chronic obstructive airways disease is 'linked in the public mind to smoking (so) that the image of a wheezing, coughing, breathless old man is often greeted with little sympathy' (Williams & Bury 1989, p 609). This lack of sympathy can reflect a lack of attention to, and resources invested in, those suffering from the disease. Similarly, AIDS is closely allied in public thinking to devalued and socially stigmatized groups such as male homosexuals and intravenous drug users, and behaviours that predispose the person to disease transmission. In this sense, AIDS constitutes a major assault on privacy. To reveal AIDS does not just reveal the presence of a disease, it reveals much more about identity and lifestyle. In this way, the handicapping nature of chronic illness flows also directly from social and cultural values.

MAJOR THEMES IN RESEARCH ON THE EXPERIENCE OF ILLNESS

It is not possible to convey the realities of living with chronic illness within the confines of a short chapter such as this. However, some impression can be gained of its pervasive effects by a brief discussion of some of the major themes evident in research on the experience of illness. Conrad (1987) has identified a number of such themes. Five are mentioned here; another – stigma – is the subject of Chapter 13.

Uncertainty

Many chronic conditions are surrounded by uncertainty. This can begin at the time when the individual first notices that something is wrong and might continue throughout the entire course of the illness. Many chronic illnesses have a slow and insidious onset and emerge in the form of vague symptoms that persist for years before diagnosis (prediagnostic uncertainty). With multiple sclerosis, the delay between appearance of symptoms and diagnosis can be as long as 15 years (Robinson 1988). During this time, sufferers are convinced that something is wrong but often find their complaints dismissed by medical practitioners as trivial or as evidence of malingering or hypochondria. This can be a very trying time for the individual and his or her family. When a diagnosis is finally obtained, it often comes as a relief; it legitimates the person's complaints and experiences and brings to an end conflicts with others over the reality of the symptoms (Robinson 1988).

However, uncertainty can follow the diagnosis itself. This is often so with respect to predicting the course and outcome of the disease (trajectory uncertainty). Coupled with the uncertainty that can surround day-to-day fluctuations in symptoms (symptomatic uncertainty), this can severely disrupt family life. It makes both short- and long-term planning impossible and often means that living arrangements have to be revised constantly. Managing this uncertainty by whatever means available can become a major component of daily life.

A good example of uncertainty is provided by rheumatoid arthritis. The symptoms of this disease, joint pain and stiffness, are highly unpredictable. The location and severity of the pain varies from day to day, and can even change during the course of a day. What seems to be a 'good day' in the morning can become a 'bad day' by the afternoon. This variability and unpredictability means that people with rheumatoid arthritis find it difficult to make sense of their symptoms and to contain them within acceptable boundaries. Many attempt to impose a degree of certainty on their existence by trying to identify events that precede acute phases or particularly painful days. Cold or damp weather and physical and emotional stress are frequently seen as the cause of pain and avoided as far as possible. However, a 'bad day' for which no apparent reason can be found leaves sufferers confused and adds to their distress (Locker 1983).

Family relations

There is clear evidence that chronic illness can place intolerable strains on families. This can arise because of the necessity to provide high levels of care and support, the emotional connotations of giving and receiving help and changes in family roles and relationships. Even where families are able and willing to provide help, the person with a chronic disabling condition might feel that he or she is a burden and refuses the assistance that is needed. It is also the case that particularly distressing symptoms, such as chronic pain, can lead the individual to withdraw from family life altogether. In some instances, both individual and family become isolated from the wider world. Marital breakdown is not uncommon in these instances.

MacDonald (1988) provides insights into the effects of chronic illness on marital and family relationships in her study of people living with the sequelae of rectal cancer. Two-thirds of the people she interviewed had a colostomy, with the remainder having been treated by excision of the cancer and anastomosis. Most of the individuals reported a loss of sexual capacity and a decline in the quality of the marital relationship. This was partly due to the physical effects of surgery and partly due to feelings of shame and embarrassment. These feelings of stigma were most marked among younger men, who reported that the consequences of surgery and fears for the future had created a barrier between them and their wives.

The consequences of surgery also had a profound effect on social relationships in general. Again, shame and embarrassment about noise and odours from the stoma, worries about offending others and feelings of self-disgust caused many to avoid social contacts and to lead a far more restricted life.

Biographical work and the reconstitution of self

All chronic disabling conditions pose a threat to identity and self-concept. One of the reasons for this is that the onset of chronic illness constitutes a 'biographical disruption' (Bury 1982) and calls into question both past and future. It necessitates a fundamental rethinking of both biography and self-concept. Williams (1984) argues that people with chronic illness must indulge in a process he calls 'narrative reconstruction', in which the individual's biography is reorganized to account for the onset of illness. This identification of cause, which draws on lay theories concerning the aetiology of illness, is part of the process of coming to terms with chronic illness. It gives meaning and order to the individual's world.

Charmaz (1987) has described how chronically sick people are involved in a constant struggle to lead valued lives and maintain definitions of self that are positive and worthwhile. This can be difficult; cultural definitions of disability devalue the individual and interactions with others can constantly undermine the individual's sense of self-worth. Charmaz (1987) considers the 'loss of self' to be a powerful form of suffering experienced by the chronically ill.

Managing medical regimens

People with chronic disabling disorders must learn to manage their symptoms and manifestations during everyday life. The person with rheumatoid arthritis, for example, learns rapidly how much activity is possible before pain rises to intolerable levels. Daily life is then planned and organized in ways that allow the individual to accomplish a few valued activities before pain intercedes and he or she is forced to rest. The individual must also learn to manage the medical regimens prescribed to control symptoms. These can include diet, drugs or the use of advanced technologies such as a dialysis machine. In some instances, the treatment can be as bad as the disease, consuming time, energy and financial resources and requiring hard work (Jobling 1988). The whole life of the chronically sick person can become organized around treatment.

An illuminating example is provided by a study of people with post-polio respiratory impairment, whose capacity to breathe had deteriorated to such an extent that permanent connection to a positive-pressure ventilator by means of a tracheostomy became necessary (Locker & Kaufert 1988). This highly efficient form of mechanical ventilation substantially improved physical and psychological health, allowed for far greater mobility than older technologies and transformed the quality of everyday life. However, the use of this machine meant that the individual concerned, and those providing care and support, had to learn a wide range of skills in order to manage the machine, including recharging batteries, suctioning tubing and maintaining the humidification system. Because this machinery often malfunctioned, usually without warning, it had to be monitored carefully and strategies had to be developed to cope with sudden failure. The potential for respiratory crises left both sufferers and family members feeling vulnerable and insecure. As a consequence, the machine, and tending to the needs of the machine, became a central focus of everyday life.

A less dramatic example is provided by a study of people with psoriasis, a disfiguring skin disease (Jobling 1988). 'Treatment' involves strict conformity over weeks, months or even years, to a programme of repetitive daily bathing, rubbing and scrubbing. This is followed by anointment with oils, creams, pastes or ointments, some of which might involve a noxious smell. Regular exposure to the sun's rays, or at least an equivalent produced by a machine, is another component. All of this can take several hours a day.

It is often the case that any prescribed regimen is substantially altered by the person concerned. This allows them to exert control over their illness and to maximize their well-being by avoiding some of the negative aspects of medical treatments.

Information, awareness and sharing

For the person with a chronic illness, information is a significant resource for managing daily life. It reduces uncertainty, helps the individual to come to terms with the illness and allows for the development of strategies for managing the illness in everyday life. Nevertheless, many people with chronic conditions express dissatisfaction with the amount of information they are able to obtain about their disorder. Difficulty with communication is a major problem in the relationships between people with chronic illnesses and their doctors. Many patients with rectal cancer who were interviewed by MacDonald (1988) were dissatisfied with what they were told about their operation, and some felt inadequately prepared for dealing with the colostomy and its effects. Some reported not knowing what a colostomy was, even at the time of surgery, and many complained of inadequate follow-up care from their family doctor.

Given these problems in communication, information might be culled from a variety of sources: from books and publications, from self-help groups or from others with the same or similar illnesses. This information provides the basis for action and the feeling that it is possible to do something about and have some control over the illness.

THE DOCTOR–PATIENT RELATIONSHIP IN CHRONIC ILLNESS

Patients with chronic disabling disorders can be difficult for a medical practitioner to treat. This is only partly due to the fact that medicine has relatively few interventions that make a real difference to the patient's condition. It also arises because the medical gaze is frequently a narrow one, concerned predominantly with disease to the exclusion of its social and emotional consequences for patients and families. Moreover, the complexity of many chronic conditions, a lack of knowledge on the part of the physician concerning the individual's illness and the fact that hospitals are largely organized around the care of acute rather than chronic diseases make it difficult for the individual to obtain care and support appropriate to their needs (Albrecht 2001, Bury 1997).

Anderson & Bury (1988) indicate the need for 'a reorientation of the focus for care from repairing damage caused by disease to education and understanding for living with chronic illness'. In this sense, information, advice and support are among the most important interventions a doctor has to offer, their goal being to help the patient live as normal and satisfying a life as possible within family and community. Such help needs to be approached with care and sensitivity; patients need to be offered choices, not have them made by others on their behalf. This means ensuring that individuals are helped to be independent and not encouraged into dependency.

By giving due attention to the particular problems associated with a chronic condition, the care that is offered to both the sufferer and the family can be made more appropriate and relevant to their social and emotional concerns. This presupposes that the professional is fully aware of the many meanings of chronic illness, the burdens carried by the individual and those who provide informal support, and the contextual factors that shape these meanings and burdens. This, in turn, highlights the issues of communication and information (see Chapter 4) and the importance of a free exchange of information between doctors and those with a chronic illness. Each has much to teach the other in working together to maximize the individual's quality of life.

References

Albrecht G 2001 Rationing care to disabled people. Sociology Health and Illness 23:654–677

Anderson R, Bury M (eds) 1988 Living with chronic illness: the experiences of patients and their families. Hyman Unwin, London

Badley E 1987 The ICIDH: format, application in different settings, and distinction between disability and handicap. International Disability Studies 9:122–128

Badley E 1993 An introduction to the concepts and classifications of the international classification of impairments, disabilities and handicaps. Disability and Rehabilitation 15:161–178

Badley E 1995 The genesis of handicap: definition, models of disablement and role of external factors. Disability and Rehabilitation 15:53–62

Bickenbach J, Chatterji S, Badley E, Ustun T 1999 Models of disablement, universalism and the classification of impairments, disabilities and handicaps. Social Science and Medicine 48:1171–1187

Blaxter M 1976 The meaning of disability. Heinemann, London

Bury M 1982 Chronic illness as biographical disruption. Sociology Health and Illness 4:167–182

Bury M 1988 Meanings at risk: the experience of arthritis. In: Anderson R, Bury M. (eds) Living with chronic illness: the experiences of patients and their families. Hyman Unwin, London

Bury M 1997 Health and illness in a changing society. Routledge, London, p 110–140

Charmaz K 1987 Struggling for a self: identity levels of the chronically ill. Research in the Sociology of Health Care 6:283–321

Conrad P 1987 The experience of illness: recent and new directions. Research in the Sociology of Health Care 6:1–31

Goffman E 1963 Stigma. Prentice Hall, Englewood Cliffs, NJ

Halbertsma J 1989 The ICIDH: a study of how it is used and evaluated. A review of the application of a classification relating to the consequences of disease. WCC Standing Committee on Classification and Terminology of the National Council of Public Health, Zoetermeer, The Netherlands

Halbertsma J et al 2000 Towards a new ICIDH. Disability and Rehabilitation 22:144–156

Harper A et al 1986 An epidemiological description of physical, social and psychological problems in multiple sclerosis. Journal of Chronic Diseases 39:305–310

Jobling R 1988 The experience of psoriasis under treatment. In: Anderson R, Bury M. (eds) Living with chronic illness: the experiences of patients and their families. Hyman Unwin, London

Lemert E 1967 Human deviance, social problems and social control. Prentice-Hall, Englewood Cliffs, NJ

Locker D 1983 Disability and disadvantage: the consequences of chronic illness. Tavistock, London

Locker D, Kaufert J 1988 The breath of life: medical technology and the careers of people with post respiratory poliomyelitis. Sociology, Health and Illness 10:24–40

MacDonald L 1988 The experience of stigma: living with rectal cancer. In: Anderson R, Bury M. (eds) Living with chronic illness: the experiences of patients and their families. Hyman Unwin, London

Manton K, Gu X 2001 Changes in the prevalence of chronic disability in the United States black and non-black population above age 65 from 1982 to 1999. Proceedings of the National Academy of Science USA 98: 6354–6359

Morbidity and Mortality Weekly Report (MMWR) 2001 Prevalence of arthritis – United States, 1997. Morbidity and Mortality Weekly Report 50:334–336

Nagi S 1991 Disability concepts revisited: implications for prevention. In: Pope A, Tarlov A (eds) Disability in America: toward a national agenda for prevention. National Academy Press, Washington DC

Office of Population Censuses and Surveys 1988 OPCS Surveys of disability in Great Britain: the prevalence of disability among adults. HMSO, London

O'Mahoney P, Thomson R, Rodgers H, James O 1999 The prevalence of stroke and associated disability. Journal of Public Health Medicine 21:166–171

Parsons T 1951 The social system. Free Press, New York

Robinson I 1988 Reconstructing lives: negotiating the meaning of multiple sclerosis. In: Anderson R, Bury M. (eds) Living with chronic illness: the experiences of patients and their families. Hyman Unwin, London

Topliss E 1979 Provision for the disabled. Martin Robertson, London

Verbrugge L, Jette A 1994 The disablement process. Social Science and Medicine 38:1–14

WHO 1999 ICIDH-2: International classification of functioning and disability. Beta-2 draft, short version. World Health Organization, Geneva

Williams G 1984 The genesis of chronic illness: narrative reconstruction. Society, Health and Illness 6:175–200

Williams S 1989 Chronic respiratory illness and disability: a critical review of the psychosocial literature. Social Science and Medicine 28 791–803

Williams S, Bury M 1989 Impairment, disability and handicap in chronic respiratory illness. Social Science and Medicine 29:609–616

Winblad I et al 2001 Prevalence of disability in three birth cohorts at old age over time spans of 10 and 20 years. Journal of Clinical Epidemiology 54:1019–1024

Wood P 1980 The language of disablement: a glossary relating to disease and its consequences. International Rehabilitation Medicine 2:86–92

7

Dying, Death and Bereavement

Graham Scambler

The facts and circumstances of death have varied historically and geographically. Before concentrating on contemporary Britain, it is worth putting recent British experience into a broader global perspective. In 1955, the average life expectancy at birth worldwide was 48 years; by 1995 it had risen to 65 years. The World Health Organization (WHO 1998a) predicts that it will rise to 73 years by 2025, by which date it is also anticipated that no country will have an average life expectancy of less than 50 years. Reductions in infant mortality and in early childhood deaths are primarily responsible for this (see Chapter 1). However, a marked diversity remains between continents and countries. Table 7.1 documents the age structures of populations and life expectancy at birth globally.

Some 16 countries actually experienced a decline in life expectancy at birth between 1975 and 1995 (WHO 1998a). This applies to a number of Eastern European countries: for example, in the Russian Federation life expectancy for males fell dramatically from 64 in 1985–1990 to 57 in 1994; for females the fall was from 74 and 71. These declines appear to reflect increases in particular causes of death, influenced by deteriorating public service provision as well as by falling material standards of living. Middle-aged men have suffered the most severe decline, with increases in deaths from cardiovascular disease, accidental poisonings, suicide and, most strikingly, homicide (so that by 1993–4 Russia surpassed the USA as the country with the highest homicide rate). In Uganda, where AIDS is the leading cause of death for young adults, life expectancy at birth declined from a peak of 56 to 41 in 1995–2000 (Seale 2000).

TALKING ABOUT DEATH

The inescapable fact of death provides one of the principal parameters of the human condition. As Lofland (1978) writes, 'it can neither be "believed" nor "magicked" nor

TABLE 7.1	Age structures of populations and life expectancy globally			
	Distribution (%) by age group (1996)			Life expectancy at birth (1995–2000)
	0–14 years	15–64 years	65+ years	
Africa	43.7	53.2	3.2	53.8
America	28.8	63.2	8.0	72.4
Asia	31.5	63.1	5.4	66.2
Europe	18.9	67.1	14.0	72.6
Oceania	25.9	64.5	9.6	73.9
World	31.1	62.3	6.6	65.6

Adapted from WHO (1998b).

"scienced" away'. Increasingly, through the twentieth century to the present, physicians and other healthcare workers in countries like Britain have been called upon to give often prolonged treatment and support to the terminally ill and their families. A higher proportion of people than ever before experience 'slow' as opposed to 'quick' dying, that is, dying has typically become a more protracted process. The reasons for this have been well documented and are summarized in Box 7.1. For obvious reasons, this change has enhanced the salience of communication around death. It is ironic, therefore, that many historians have maintained that death over the last century or so has become more and more 'unmentionable'. Aries (1983) characterizes modern – demythologized and secularized – death as invisible death: 'we ignore the existence of a scandal that we have been unable to prevent; we act as if it did not exist, and thus mercilessly force the bereaved to say nothing. A heavy silence has fallen over the subject of death'. According to Aries, death has grown fearful again, imbued with all its 'old savagery'.

Countering this view that the denial of death is now ubiquitous, however, Seale (1995) has pointed to evidence that 'scripts' for proclaiming 'heroic self-identity in the face of

BOX 7.1	Conditions Facilitating 'Quick Dying' in the Pre-Modern Era and 'Slow Dying' in the Modern Era
Conditions facilitating quick dying	Conditions facilitating slow dying
Low level of medical technology	High level of medical technology
Late detection of disease (or fatality)producing conditions	Early detection of disease (or fatality) producing conditions
Simple definition of death (e.g. cessation of heart beat)	Complex definition of death (e.g. irreversible cessation of higher brain activity)
High incidence of mortality from acute disease	High incidence of mortality from chronic or degenerative disease
High incidence of fatality-producing injuries	Low incidence of fatality-producing injuries
Customary killing or suicide of, or fatal passivity towards, the person once he or she has entered the 'dying' category	Customary curative and activist orientation toward the dying with a high value placed on the prolongation of life

Reproduced with permission of Sage Publications Inc. from Lofland (1978).

death' are currently being promoted by many professional 'experts' and appropriated by growing numbers of lay people. His contention is that these scripts, less 'masculine' and more 'feminine' in orientation than their predecessors, redefine 'heroic death' as involving a struggle to gain knowledge, opportunities to demonstrate courage, and a state of emotional calm or equilibrium in which dying people and carers alike participate. The emphasis is on care, concern and emotional expression. Some deaths, Seale admits, cannot be written into such scripts; for example, those of the very old, the mentally confused and sudden unexpected deaths. And there are rival scripts: there are those, for example, who prefer the benefits of continuing the everyday project of the self oblivious of oncoming death, with others sharing the burden of awareness in an attempt to protect the dying person from the strain of knowing. But Seale conjectures that what he terms 'scripts of heroic death' are gaining ground.

Independently of differences between writers like Aries and Seale, it is not surprising that deciding whether to tell someone he or she is dying continues to be regarded as problematic for health workers. When asked, most people anticipate that they would want to be told if they were dying; physicians are themselves unexceptional in this respect. But how much credibility should be attached to such responses? Can young, healthy individuals accurately predict how they will feel as death approaches?

Cartwright et al (1973), who interviewed relatives of a national sample of people who had died in the preceding year in Britain, were told by relatives that 37% of those dying knew as much, and a further 20% 'half knew'. Nearly three-quarters of the relatives felt they had themselves known. It was also apparent from this study that the relatives received more information from all sources than did the people who were dying. Less information was forthcoming if death occurred in a hospital than if it occurred at home; in both contexts, however, the general practitioner was the key informant. Herd (1990), in a study of terminal care in a semirural part of Britain, also found principal lay carers to be less aware and knowledgeable about what was happening if death took place in hospital than if it took place in the home. A more recent study by Seale & Cartwright (1994), however, suggests a changing picture. In 250 accounts from lay relatives, friends and others who knew people in a random national sample of adult deaths, 54% reported that both parties had been aware that the person was dying. In 36% of situations the respondent knew, but the dying person did not; in 8% neither knew; and in 1% the respondent did not know, although the deceased did.

Awareness of dying

Glaser & Strauss (1965) found there to be four common types of 'awareness context' in relation to the dying. They define 'awareness context' as: 'what each interacting person knows of the patient's defined status, along with his recognition of others' awareness of his own definition'. The four types are summarized in Box 7.2. Some commentators have assumed that 'closed', 'suspected' and 'mutual pretence' awareness contexts are intrinsically undesirable and that health workers, especially physicians, are exclusively to blame for the fact that they frequently exist. As a study by McIntosh (1977) suggests, however, such assumptions can be naive and misleading. McIntosh interviewed both patients and physicians. Most patients he spoke to suspected malignancy. The majority sought information from members of the hospital team but, according to McIntosh's estimate, two out of every three did not 'really' want their diagnostic suspicions confirmed and fewer still 'really' wanted to know their prognosis. They sought exclusively information that would reinforce an optimistic conception of their condition: uncertainty afforded hope. Most patients also felt – somewhat unrealistically, given McIntosh's documentation of physicians' predisposition not to disclose – that they would be told everything if they asked.

BOX 7.2 'Awareness Contexts' in Relation to Dying

1. **Closed awareness**: the patient does not recognize his or her impending death, although everyone else does
2. **Suspected awareness**: the patient suspects what others know and attempts either to confirm or to invalidate these suspicions
3. **Mutual pretence awareness**: each party defines the patient as dying but each 'pretends' that the other has not done so
4. **Open awareness**: health workers and patient are each aware that the latter is dying, and they act on this awareness fairly openly

Reproduced with permission of Aldine Press from Glaser & Strauss (1965).

95

Timmermans (1994) has suggested that Glaser and Strauss's 'open awareness context' requires refinement 'to include the diversity of viewpoints of family members and patients'. He delineates three types of open awareness. The context of 'suspended open awareness' occurs when patients and their relatives simply ignore or 'deny' the information. This can arise in three sets of circumstances. First, it can be a transitory feature after the disclosure of the terminal condition and prognosis. Disbelief here is an initial reaction to cope with the shock of disclosure – 'the open awareness context is nascent: the news has been given but its radical consequences have not been fully assimilated'. Second, disbelief can become a permanent and preferred state, with even the reality of the underlying condition being called into question. And third, patients can come to question or doubt the outcomes of their conditions in situations of unexpected deterioration or improvement. The context of 'uncertain open awareness' occurs when patients and relatives do not dismiss the possibility of death but 'prefer the uncertainty of not understanding exactly what is going on'. The context of 'active open awareness' occurs when hope for recovery is abandoned and patients and their families understand the full ramifications of the impending death and try to find ways of coming to terms with it.

Mamo (1999) suggests that the analyses of both Glaser & Strauss and of Timmermans disregard the importance of emotions, arguing that they fail to address 'the complexity of emotional management and the existence of emotional surges in the context of dying'. She maintains that cognitions and emotions are in fact intertwined: 'awareness emerges and subsides in a complex web of emotions and cognition'. She commends further study, in particular of the multiple ways in which emotional work is performed by dying patients and their families.

As McIntosh found, physicians are not always ready to communicate openly. In a Canadian study of 118 encounters during which 17 male surgeons disclosed the results of biopsies to women with breast cancer, Taylor (1988) found that each surgeon appeared to have adopted a favoured 'strategy' that he used routinely, thus 'bypassing the individuality of each case'. Four techniques were discerned. The first – communication – was deployed by some surgeons when they were in a position to make a reasonable and definite prognosis of the condition in terms comprehensible to the patient. Many surgeons claimed to use this technique, but in fact few did. Only 10% of the 118 disclosures were of this type. The second – admission of uncertainty – was used by a small minority of surgeons when no clinical prognosis was justified; 15% of the disclosures took this form. The third technique – dissimulation, or the pronouncement of a prognosis that could not be clinically substantiated – occurred when surgeons were reluctant to share the extent of their uncertainty with their patients; 30% of the disclosures fell into this category. The final technique – evasion – or 'the failure to communicate a clinically substantiated prognosis', was used by a number of surgeons who preferred not to respond directly to patients' questions. 'For those surgeons whose patients asked direct questions to which the appropriate technical response might reveal a low chance of long-term survival, repressing information was a favoured policy.' Not infrequently, replies to specific questions drew on general statistics not easily applicable to the individual case. In 45% of disclosures surgeons used evasion as a means of coping with direct questions posed by women.

If one thing is clear it is that there is no easy, general answer to the question 'To tell or not to tell?'. Hinton (1967) offers physicians the following counsel:

> Although it is not an infallible guide as to how much the dying patient should be told, his apparent wishes and questions do point the way. This means that the manner in which he puts his views should be closely attended to – the intonations and the exact wording may be very revealing. It also means that he must be given ample opportunity to express his ideas and ask his questions. If the questions are sincere, however, then why not give quite straight answers to the patient's questions about his illness and the outcome? It makes for beneficial trust.

A study by Hinton (1980) highlights the importance of giving dying patients the opportunity to talk. He interviewed 80 patients with terminal cancer at a mean of 10 weeks before death; 66% told him that they recognized they might or would soon die, 8% were non-committal, and 26% spoke only of improvement. Some patients spoke of dying to either their spouse or the staff and not to the interviewer, but they tended to say less to their spouse than to the interviewer and less still to members of the staff. This tendency is illustrated in Fig. 7.1. Hinton concludes that people are often ready to share their awareness if someone is prepared to listen.

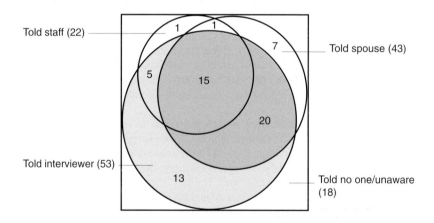

Fig. 7.1 Awareness of the possibility of dying as shown by different people by 80 patients with terminal cancer. The square represents the 80 patients and the three shaded circles their communicated awareness to staff, spouse and interviewer.
(*Reproduced with permission from Hinton 1980*).

Stages of dying

How people come to terms with the prospect of imminent death depends on many factors (Hinton 1984). Of obvious importance is the nature of the physical and mental distress experienced. A number of national surveys have been conducted, relying on data from surviving relatives or others. Table 7.2 lists the main symptoms experienced by people dying from cancer, heart disease and stroke from a large national study in Britain in 1990. Pain, nausea and vomiting, difficulty swallowing, constipation and pressure sores seem more prevalent for people dying of cancer. Breathlessness is a particular problem for people with heart disease. Mental confusion and incontinence affect more people dying from strokes. In general, cancer caused a large number of symptoms and a larger proportion of these were defined as 'very distressing' for the dying person; but the duration of symptoms for cancer was less than for other conditions (Addington-Hall et al 1998). It has regularly been found that, when compared with lay carers, health workers tend to underestimate patients' symptoms and to overestimate the success of treatment (Herd 1990).

97

Among the many factors that can influence how individuals cope with terminal illness are age, family intimacy and support, and religious convictions. There is enormous individual variation and hence unpredictability in any given case. Kubler-Ross (1970) has claimed, however, that people who know they are dying typically pass through five 'stages' (Box 7.3).

Several writers have criticized Kubler-Ross's specification of discrete stages of dying, usually on the grounds that it represents an overgeneralization based on subjective data. Certainly Kubler-Ross's stages should not be regarded either as unidirectional or as sequential.

PLACE OF DEATH

Those, like Aries, who argue that death has become increasingly invisible during the twentieth century attach considerable significance to the fact that, since the 1930s and 1940s, death has been substantially removed from the community or 'hospitalized'. In the hospital, according to this thesis, death is no longer an occasion of ritual ceremony over

TABLE 7.2	Symptoms experienced in the last year of life in Britain (1990)		
	Cancer %	Heart disease %	Stroke %
Pain	88	77	66
Breathlessness	54	60	37
Nausea and vomiting	59	32	23
Difficulty swallowing	41	16	23
Constipation	63	38	45
Mental confusion	41	32	50
Pressure sores	28	11	20
Urinary incontinence	40	30	56
Bowel incontinence	32	17	37
N =	2063	683	229

From Addington-Hall (1996).

BOX 7.3   Stages of Dying

First stage: denial and isolation

Many people, on being told they are dying, experience a temporary state of shock. When the numbness disappears, a common response is: 'No, it can't be me'. One's own death is all but inconceivable. 'Denial' is usually a temporary defence but some take it further, perhaps 'shopping around' for a more amenable clinical opinion (only three of the 200 patients in Kubler-Ross' study attempted to deny the approach of death to the very end). A deep feeling of 'isolation' is normal at this stage.

Second stage: anger

When the initial stage of denial can no longer be maintained, it is often replaced by feelings of anger, rage, envy and resentment. The question 'Why me?' is posed. The anger can be displaced and at times projected onto the environment almost at random (although it can, of course, be justified as well as unjustified). The hospital team, especially the nursing staff, frequently bear the brunt of these outbursts.

Third stage: bargaining

The third stage of 'bargaining', Kubler-Ross argues, has only rarely been acknowledged. The point is that terminally ill people will sometimes negotiate – openly with health workers or secretly with God – to postpone death: postponement will be the reward for a promise of good behaviour. For example, many patients in the study promised to donate parts of their bodies to medical science if the physicians undertook to use their knowledge of science to extend their lives.

Fourth stage: depression

When terminally ill patients can no longer deny their illness, when they are compelled to endure more surgery, when they grow weaker, the numbness or stoicism or anger gives way to a sense of great loss. This 'depression' can be reactive, for example, a woman with cancer of the uterus might feel she is no longer a woman, or what Kubler-Ross calls preparatory, that is, based on impending losses associated with death itself.

Fifth stage: acceptance

The final stage of 'acceptance' is one in which dying patients commonly find a sort of peace, a peace that is largely a function of weakness and a diminished interest in the world. 'It is as if the pain has gone, the struggle is over...'. Kubler-Ross adds that this is also the time during which the family usually needs more help, understanding and support than the patient.

Reproduced with permission of Tavistock Publications from Kubler-Ross (1970).

---

which the dying person and his or her kin and friends hold sway. The physicians and hospital team are the new 'masters of death', of its moment as well as its circumstances. This interpretation of changing events is once again open to criticism. Seymour (1999) has shown, for example, that the common representation of the medicalized, hospitalized death as antithetical to an idealized 'natural death' is simplistic. She found that the next of kin tended to see death as 'natural' when medical technology delivered outcomes they expected, appeared amenable to human manipulation and intention, was accessible to their understanding, and seemed to 'fit' with the wider context of the dying person's life. There is no doubt, however, that the hospitalization of death has continued: two-thirds of deaths in Britain now occur in hospitals, compared with only a half in 1960 (Seale 2000).

There is a growing feeling that the hospital is too frequently an inappropriate place in which to die. In his essay on 'The Loneliness of Dying', Elias (1985), who is fully aware of how emotionally taxing, as well as rewarding, a death in the family home can be, nevertheless stresses that in modern hospitals 'dying people can be cared for in accordance with the latest biophysical specialist knowledge, but often neutrally as regards feeling; they may die in total isolation'. Most hospitals are designed to provide for acute illness, and terminally ill people in acute wards can both disturb other patients and members of ward staff and be disturbed by them; most hospitals do not set aside a whole or part of a ward for dying patients because they are anxious to avoid the stigma of a 'death ward'. Several alternative locations exist in Britain, including special units within conventional hospitals, but the most discussed are the home and the hospice.

The home

For many health workers and lay persons alike, despite the statistical trend to hospitalization, the home remains the 'natural' and 'proper' place in which to die. As Bowling & Cartwright (1982) discovered, however, the care of dying people at home imposes severe physical, financial and psychological strains on relatives. In Herd's (1990) study, 74% of lay carers (four out of every five of them female relatives) mentioned 'emotional strain' as a problem, and 51% mentioned 'physical strain'. Table 7.3 ranks those aspects of home care that Herd's lay carers defined as 'worrying'. Lay carers are also likely to find their own activities restricted: Bowling & Cartwright report 26% describing their activities as 'severely restricted' and a further 19% as 'fairly restricted'. The extent to which professional and other support is at hand is likely to be contingent upon *ad hoc* factors affecting local planning and provision. Currently, hospitalization in Britain is a function of the absence of local planning and provision. There are shortages of helpers ranging from Macmillan nurses to home helps and providers of meals-on-wheels.

The hospice

The hospice movement was founded in the mid-nineteenth century and was largely pioneered in Britain, although inpatient hospices still deal with only 4% of dying people, and generally with those dying from cancer. The favoured pattern in Britain is to build small units in the grounds of general hospitals, using their facilities but remaining administratively independent. The range of care provided in a hospice is intermediate between that of a long-stay hospital and that of an acute hospital. The staffing ratios are similar to those of an acute hospital, but the call for diagnostic and other 'support' services is much less. The average length of stay is also closer to that of patients in an acute hospital than that of patients in a long-stay hospital, and costs are in keeping with this.

TABLE 7.3	Worrying aspects of home care identified by lay carers
	Number (%) of respondents
Anxiety about medication	26 (49)
Inability to leave patient unattended	22 (42)
Not knowing what to expect	18 (34)
Inability to help	15 (28)
Fear of being alone when death took place	11 (21)
Anxiety about what to do when death took place	5 (9)
Anxiety about calling the doctor	3 (6)
Other	5 (9)

Reproduced with permission from Herd (1990).

Central to the philosophy of the hospice is the view that the whole professional caring team should work in unison to develop the skills the dying person needs. Dramatic improvements in care originated in hospices in the last quarter of the twentieth century, for example, in standards of palliative medicine; hospice teams have reduced levels of uncontrolled pain to 8% and less (Parkes 1984). It should not be assumed, however, that, given the choice, everybody would opt for death in a hospice. In one study, which compared the care given in four radiotherapy wards of an acute hospital, in a Foundation Home visited by two general practitioners and in a hospice (Hinton 1979), little difference was found between the acute hospital and the Foundation Home, but there was some evidence that patients were less depressed and anxious in the hospice and preferred the more frank communication available there. It was also found, however, that patients gave most praise to the outpatient system of care, despite experiencing more anxiety or irritability at home. The author concluded: 'treatment cannot be judged solely by the mental quiet it brings; freedom or hope may be preferred even if they bring worry'. It has been found that home-centred patients tend to experience more pain than hospital-centred patients, and their relatives more stress; but it does not follow that, even knowing this, patients and their relatives would necessarily choose to leave home. It should not be concluded that because adequate support for home care is rarely available the hospitalization of death should be accelerated.

Figure 7.2 summarizes the sources of help available to people who are dying in Britain.

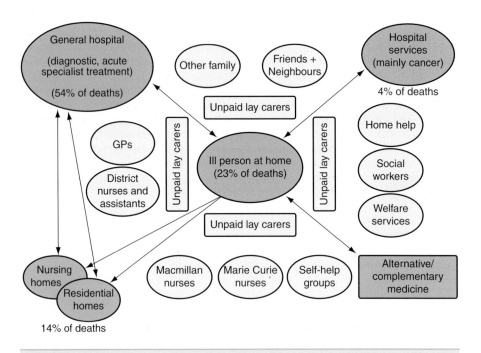

Fig. 7.2 Sources of help for people who are dying.
(*Reproduced with permission of Open University Press from Field & James 1993*).

PATTERNS OF DEATH AND BEREAVEMENT

Sudnow (1967) has drawn a distinction between biological and social death. The problem of how to define biological death has been resolved by the medical profession for the time being in favour of the irreversible cessation of higher brain activity. Sudnow uses the term 'social death' in a general sense to refer to how organizations deal with different modes of dying and death. More specifically, social death is marked, within the hospital setting, by that point at which a patient is treated essentially as a corpse, although still perhaps biologically alive. He gives an example of social death preceding biological death. A nurse on duty with a woman she explained was 'dying' was observed to spend 2 or 3 minutes trying to close the woman's eyelids. After several unsuccessful attempts she managed to shut them and said, with a sigh of relief, 'Now they're right'. When questioned, she said that a patient's eyes must be closed after death, so that the body will resemble a sleeping person. It was more difficult to accomplish this, she explained, after the muscles and skin had begun to stiffen. She always tried to close them before death. This made for greater efficiency when the time came for ward personnel to wrap the body. It was a matter of consideration toward those workers who preferred to handle dead bodies as little as possible.

101

Mulkay (1993) interprets the concept of social death more broadly. Social death might precede biological death, as in Sudnow's example, or, alternatively, social existence might continue long after death, 'for example, when distraught parents visit the grave of a dead child and talk and write to that child about their previous life together and about the reunion to come' (Clegg 1988). The defining feature of social death, then, is the cessation of the individual person as an active agent in others' lives. Mulkay argues that the profile of social death has changed considerably over the last century as a result of people's collective responses to changes in the social distribution of biological death, changes in the social setting of death, and changes in the clinical nature of death. Consider the elderly, for example. Mulkay suggests that the start of the 'death sequence' in our society occurs, particularly for men, at the time of retirement from work. This is a key transition, when people's participation in social life significantly diminishes – independently of personal variations in state of health – owing to the socially recognized approach of death. From retirement on, elderly people in Britain are typically channelled away from the principal arenas of social activity and their ties with the wider society progressively weakened in anticipation of their biological end (Williams 1990). With admission to a hospital or, increasingly, a residential or nursing home, where the bureaucratic 'neglect of the patient as a person' (Field 1989) converges with the physical, emotional and communicative withdrawal of the living from those on the death sequence, the death sequence of society at large is repeated in microcosm.

Trajectories of dying

Glaser & Strauss (1968) distinguish seven 'critical junctures' in what is sometimes called the 'career' of the dying patient:

1. the definition of the patient as dying

2. staff and family then make their preparations for the patient's death, as the patient might do if he or she knows that death is near

3. at some point there seems to be 'nothing more to do' to prevent death

4. the final descent, which can take weeks, days or merely hours

5. the 'last hours'

6. the death watch

7. death itself.

When these critical junctures occur as expected – as it were, on schedule – then all those involved, including sometimes the patient, are prepared for them. When, however, critical junctures occur unexpectedly, hospital staff and the patient's family alike can be unprepared. If a patient is expected to die quite soon, for example, but vacillates sufficiently often, then both staff and family are likely to find the experience stressful.

Predictability, then, makes the work of hospital teams easier. Miscalculations in forecasting can play havoc with the organization of work. When crises do occur, the staff attempt to regain control as quickly as possible, but sometimes the disruption of work is accompanied by a shattering of what Glaser & Strauss (1965) have called a ward's characteristic 'sentimental mood' or order. They cite an example:

> In an intensive care unit where cardiac patients die frequently, the mood is relatively unaffected by one more speedy expected death; but if a hopeless patient lingers on and on, or if his wife, perhaps, refuses to accept his dying and causes 'scenes', then both mood and work itself are profoundly affected.

Glaser & Strauss (1968) differentiate between a number of patterns of death, 'dying trajectories', paying special attention to the distinction noted earlier between 'quick' and 'slow' dying. Quick dying, they claim, can take three forms: 'the expected quick death'; 'unexpected quick dying, but expected to die'; and 'unexpected quick dying, not expected to die'. They report that, in general, unexpected quick deaths are more disturbing for staff and families than expected quick deaths. Even expected quick deaths, however, can give rise to distinctive difficulties. Glaser and Strauss focus on staff–family interaction and note, for example, that the likely presence of the family at the bedside when death occurs requires careful handling by the staff, because a 'scene' will disrupt ward order and worry other patients. Slow dying 'is fraught with both hazard and opportunity'. On the one hand, the dying could take 'too long', be unexpectedly painful or unpleasant, and so on; on the other hand, a slow decline can allow time for wills to be made or families to come together, and can provide the setting for quiet and dignified endings. All these consequences are less likely to occur with quick dying.

Bereavement and mourning

Just as experiences of impending death vary from person to person, so does the experience of losing a relative or friend. Much depends on the nature of the relationship. However, a sudden, unexpected death is often harder to get over than one where there was time to grieve before the occurrence of death: this is known as 'anticipatory' or 'prebereavement mourning'.

In his anthropological study of death in Britain, Gorer (1965) argues that mourners typically pass through three stages:

1. a short period of shock, usually lasting from death until the disposal of the body

2. a period of intense mourning, accompanied by withdrawal of attention and affect from the external world and by physiological changes like disturbed sleep, vivid dreams, failure of appetite and loss of weight

3. a final period of re-established social and physical homeostasis, with sleep and weight stabilized and interest again directed outwards.

Gorer's principal thesis is that, in an increasingly secular Britain, only the first of these three periods is socially acknowledged and surrounded by ceremony and ritual. After the funeral or postfuneral meal, mourners are frequently abandoned to cope alone. To counter this social isolation during a time of continuing need for succour and support (periods 2 and 3), he advocates the creation of new secular rituals to replace now defunct religious ones.

Kamerman (1988) suggests that this twentieth-century process of 'deritualization' has been accompanied by a process of 'rationalization'. By this he means that death has increasingly come to be subsumed under conventions or routines that render it nonintrusive. Responses to death have become more 'business-like'. Both deritualization and rationalization are epitomized by the growing preference for cremation over burial. Approximately two-thirds of bodies are now cremated in Britain.

As if in affirmation of the need for continuing support after the funeral, several studies have shown elevated rates of morbidity and mortality and of visits to general practitioners among samples of recently bereaved persons.

It remains the case that many health students and workers receive minimal preparation for coping with terminal care and bereavement. Glaser and Strauss argue that much non-technical conduct in relation to the dying and bereaved is influenced by common-sense assumptions, 'essentially untouched by professional considerations or by current knowledge from the behavioural sciences'. The argument for the provision of a good grounding in those aspects of care – psychological, social, organizational and ethical – is a strong one. MacLeod's (2001) small ethnographic study of 10 doctors' reflections on learning to care for people who are dying suggests that medical training is still often inadequate and that in practice learning frequently occurs as a result of retrospectively identified 'turning points' or specific encounters with dying patients.

References

Addington-Hall J 1996 Heart disease and stroke: lessons from cancer care. In: Ford G, Lewin I (eds) Managing terminal illness. Royal College of Physicians, London

Addington-Hall J, Altmann D, McCarthy M 1998 Variations by age in symptoms and dependency levels experienced by people in the last year of life, as reported by surviving family, friends and officials. Age and Ageing 27:129–136

Aries P 1983 The hour of our death. Penguin, London

Bowling A, Cartwright A 1982 Life after death: a study of the elderly widowed. Tavistock, London

Cartwright A, Hockey L, Anderson J 1973 Life before death. Routledge & Kegan Paul, London

Clegg F 1988 Decisions at a time of grief. Cambridge University Press, Cambridge

Elias N 1985 The loneliness of dying. Basil Blackwell, Oxford

Field D 1989 Nursing the dying. Tavistock/Routledge, London

Field D, James N 1993 Where and how people die. In: Clark D (ed) The future for palliative care. Open University Press, Buckingham

Glaser B, Strauss A 1965 Awareness of dying. Aldine, Chicago, IL

Glaser B, Strauss A 1968 Time for dying. Aldine, Chicago, IL

Gorer G 1965 Death, grief and mourning in contemporary Britain. Cresset Press, London

Herd E 1990 Terminal care in a semi-rural area. British Journal of General Practice. 40:248–251

Hinton J 1967 Dying. Penguin, London

Hinton J 1979 Comparison of places and policies for terminal care. Lancet ii:29–32

Hinton J 1980 Whom do dying patients tell? British Medical Journal 281:1328–1330

Hinton J 1984 Coping with terminal illness. In: Fitzpatrick R et al (eds) The experience of illness. Tavistock, London

Kamerman J 1988 Death in the midst of life: social and cultural influences on death, grief and mourning. Prentice Hall, Englewood Cliffs, NJ

Kubler-Ross E 1970 On death and dying. Tavistock, London

Lofland L 1978 The craft of dying: the modern face of death. Sage Publications, Beverly Hills, CA

McIntosh J 1977 Communication and awareness in a cancer ward. Croom Helm, London

MacLeod R 2001 On reflection: doctors learning to care for people who are dying. Social Science & Medicine 52:1719–1727

Mamo L 1999 Death and dying: confluences of emotion and awareness. Sociology of Health & Illness 21:13–36

Mulkay M 1993 Social death in Britain. In: Clark D (ed) The sociology of death. Blackwell, Oxford

Parkes C 1984 'Hospice' versus 'hospital' care: a re-evaluation after 10 years as seen by surviving spouses. Postgraduate Medical Journal 50:120–124

Seale C 1995 Heroic death. Sociology, Health and Illness 29:597–613

Seale C 2000 Changing patterns of death and dying. Social Science and Medicine 51:917–930

Seale C, Cartwright A 1994 The year before death. Averbery, Aldershot

Seymour J 1999 Revisiting medicalization and 'natural' death. Social Science and Medicine 49:691–704

Sudnow D 1967 Passing on: the social organization of dying. Prentice Hall, New York

Taylor K 1988 'Telling bad news': physicians and the disclosure of undesirable information. Sociology, Health and Illness 10:109–132

Timmermans S 1994 Dying of awareness: the theory awareness contexts revisited. Sociology, Health and Illness 16:322–339

Williams R 1990 A protestant legacy: attitudes to death and illness among older Aberdonians. Clarendon Press, Oxford

World Health Organization (WHO) 1998a World Health Report. WHO, Geneva

World Health Organization (WHO) 1998b World Health Statistics. WHO, Geneva

Social Structure and Health

8 Inequality and Social Class

Graham Scambler and David Blane

In Bethnal Green in the year 1839 the average age of death in the different social classes was as follows: 'Gentlemen and persons engaged in professions, and their families ... 45 years; tradesmen and their families ... 26 years; Mechanics, servants and labourers, and their families ... 16 years' (Chadwick 1842). The average age of deaths in these social classes was found to vary somewhat from area to area, but similar differences between the classes were found in all areas of Britain.

Although 'the average age of death' would be criticized today as a measure that is oversensitive to high childhood mortality, Chadwick's study provided some of the first evidence that health varies with social class. The population's general level of health has improved dramatically since the first half of the nineteenth century, but subsequent investigations have shown that a relationship between mortality rates and social class remains. This has been repeatedly confirmed and shown to apply equally to morbidity (DHSS 1980). It is important, therefore, to understand both what is meant by 'social class' and why it should be related to health indicators of many kinds. With this in mind, this chapter starts with details of some modern inequalities and of different ways of accounting for them, the most influential of which draws on concepts of social class. It then goes on to examine the relationship between social class and health.

SOME DIMENSIONS OF INEQUALITY IN THE UK

Wealth and income

Wealth, defined in terms of marketable assets, is very unequally distributed. In 1998 the richest 1% of the population aged 18 or over owned 23% of the country's total personal wealth, and the richest 10% over half. The poorest 75% of the population owned approximately the same as the richest 1%. If the value of housing is omitted from estimates of marketable assets, then the resulting distribution is even more skewed, with the richest 1% owning 26% and the poorest 75% a mere 14%. In 1998–9, one-half of all households in the UK reported having less than £1500 in savings, with 28% reporting no savings at all (National Statistics 2001). It can be argued that the wealth that is owned by the majority of the population is used in an attempt to guarantee the necessities of life, whereas the wealth of the rich also brings with it social power, in the sense of ownership of land and voting rights in the decisions of financial and industrial corporations.

Income, which consists mainly of earnings from employment but also includes investment income and the various state benefits, is more equally distributed than wealth. During the 1970s there was relatively little change in the distribution of income among households, but the 1980s were characterized by a substantial increase in inequality: between 1981 and 1989, whereas average income rose by 27% when adjusted for inflation, the income of the top 10% rose by 38% and that of the bottom 10% by only 7%. Income distribution seemed to stabilize during the first half of the 1990s but in the most recent period for which data are available there appears to have been a further increase in inequality (National Statistics 2001). Access to state facilities such as the education system and health service can also be seen as part of income, as can benefits in kind, which are received on top of earnings from employment. Although those on low incomes derive marginally greater benefit from the former, benefits in kind go disproportionately to those with high incomes and tend to be greatest for those with the highest salaries. Thus, large inequalities in income remain despite the redistribution achieved by mechanisms such as income tax, state benefits and access to state facilities.

Working conditions

An individual's income is strongly tied to the nature of his or her work. For a number of reasons, the difference in total weekly pay is not as great as the difference in the hourly rate. Manual workers work a greater number of hours per week than non-manual workers, and are more likely to work overtime: in 1998, 14% of the average gross weekly earnings of £327 paid to manual workers came in the form of overtime, compared with 3% of the average gross weekly earnings of £505 paid to non-manual workers (National Statistics 2000). Manual workers are also more likely to work shifts, which attract additional payment, and to be paid some form of production bonus. As these additional sources of income are likely to vary from week to week, it is more difficult for manual workers and their families to make financially sound plans, a disadvantage that is reinforced by manual workers' greater likelihood of being made redundant. Of considerable financial importance after retirement, manual workers are less likely to be members of an occupational pension scheme than non-manual workers.

Manual work is usually more physically demanding, noisier and more dangerous than non-manual work (Hunter 1975), as well as being more likely to involve the physical and social disruption of shift work. Despite its more hazardous nature, manual work lasts longer than non-manual work. Manual workers enter the workforce at an earlier age and, as has been noted, their basic working week is likely to be longer and they are more likely to work overtime. In addition, their holidays are shorter, with non-manual workers being more likely to receive in excess of 5 weeks holiday per year. Manual work is also more likely to be repetitive than the work of professionals and managers, to offer little autonomy and to be experienced as boring. Perhaps as a result, manual workers are subject to closer supervision and tighter discipline; most have to clock-in at work, automatically lose money when late for work, face dismissal if continually late, and many need a supervisor's permission to use the lavatory or obtain a drink outside the set work-breaks.

POVERTY

The inequalities so far documented have been illustrated in terms of manual compared with non-manual, professional compared with unskilled, and so on. Such comparisons are useful because they indicate the direction and size of the general trends, but they can create the misleading impression that the workforce is divided into homogeneous blocks whose members share the same income and living and working conditions and that these, in turn, are clearly higher or lower than those of the next block. In reality, there is considerable variation in income and conditions within each block and considerable overlap between them. As a result, there is always room for debate about where it is appropriate to draw lines on this continuous distribution to identify specific groups. This problem complicates the definition of poverty and attempts to identify those who are exposed to poverty first need to be clear about the sense in which the term is being used.

The term 'poverty' has been used in two ways. Absolute poverty refers to a standard of living that cannot sustain life. When the term is used in this sense it could describe, for example, destitute people in the drought-stricken areas of the Sahel. One problem with this definition, however, is its failure to specify how long people can live before their standard of living is judged incapable of sustaining life. As the experience of hunger strikers demonstrates, no standard of living is so low as to kill instantaneously, and low-grade malnutrition might influence mortality only after many years. In addition, because very few people in the rich countries of the world are starving, using the term poverty in its absolute sense fails to address the hardships that are endured by many members of these societies.

'Relative poverty' refers to a standard of living below that which is considered normal or acceptable by the members of a particular society: 'The resources [of those in relative poverty] are so seriously below those commanded by the average individual or family that they are, in effect, excluded from ordinary living patterns, customs and activities' (Townsend 1979). Using the term in this relative sense allows the concept of poverty to be applied to rich societies such as Britain, although for research purposes it does pose the problem of how to establish empirically what is considered normal or acceptable in a particular society. This relative 'poverty line' can be established by means of surveys. A less expensive method, which is frequently used in research, is to equate relative poverty with an income below the level of eligibility for the various state benefits.

Townsend's classic study of poverty in the UK found that 7% of households, containing 3.3 million people, received an income below the state benefits level, and that a further 24% of households, which contained 11.9 million people, were on the margins of poverty, defined as an income less than 40% above the state benefits level. When those in poverty were analysed according to their labour market, personal and other characteristics, the three largest groups were those employed on low wages or in casual work, the disabled and long-term sick and the elderly retired, with the unemployed and one-parent families being the next largest groups (Townsend 1979).

The threshold now generally adopted to define low income in Britain is 60% of median equivalized household disposable income (equivalization here denotes adjustment for size and composition of the household). In fact, this threshold is one of those used in the government's antipoverty strategy. In 1998–9, 18% of the British population lived in households with incomes below this level. This proportion was fairly static during the 1960s, 1970s and early 1980s, fluctuating between 10 and 15%, but it rose steeply from 1985 to peak at 21% in 1992. Children are disproportionately present in low-income households: in 1998–9, 24% of children, or 3.1 million, were living in such households in Britain. There is a clear relationship between work and income. In 1998–9, only 2% of those living in households where all adults were in full-time work were in low-income households, compared with 64% of those in households where the head or spouse were unemployed; 26% of those in households where the head or spouse was aged 60 or over lived in low-income households (National Statistics 2001).

Low income can lead to material and other forms of deprivation. Compared with that of the better paid, for example, the diet of the low paid contains far less fresh fruit, significantly less fresh vegetables, fresh fish and cheese, and more white bread, potatoes, sugar, lard and margarine (MAFF 1989). The Poverty and Social Exclusion Survey commissioned by the Joseph Rowntree Foundation sought to identify the items that a majority of the public perceive to be 'necessities', that is, which all adults should be able to afford and that they should not have to do without. About 28% of people in 1999 said they were unable to afford two or more of these items; 25% were unable to have 'regular savings of £10 a month for rainy days or retirement'; and nearly one-fifth could not afford a 'holiday away from home once a year not staying with relatives'. Other 'one-off' larger items of expenditure that more than 10% could not afford were 'replace or repair broken electrical goods', 'replace worn-out furniture', and 'money to keep home in a decent state of decoration'.

A potential shortcoming of such cross-sectional data is the extent to which they obscure the association between poverty and certain phases of the lifecycle. In societies where incomes are derived primarily from the labour market and where human reproduction predominantly occurs within nuclear families, there is an in-built tendency for an individual's standard of living to be lowest during childhood, active parenthood and old age, and to be highest during the intervening phases. This longitudinal approach has certain advantages: it draws attention to the association between poverty and childhood; it reminds us that those who are not currently living in poverty might have experienced it in the past or might realistically expect to experience it in the future; and it enables us to see that it is often the same individuals whose standard of living will dip below the poverty line during the low phases of the lifecycle. Thus, the child reared in poverty is educationally handicapped and is likely to be an early entrant to the unskilled sector of the labour market, where low wages and insecure employment will make family formation financially difficult and where the lack of an occupational pension scheme will predispose to poverty after retirement. Some idea of the proportion of the population that is likely to experience relative poverty at some stage during their lives is given by combining those who were found to be in poverty with those who were on its margins in the study quoted earlier; that is, 31% of households or 15 million people. Rather than being a marginal problem, therefore, poverty, or the realistic fear of it, is a fact of life for a substantial proportion of the population.

There is a considerable overlap between medical problems and poverty or the phases of the lifecycle where the standard of living tends to dip. The size of this overlap is illustrated by the 75% of prescriptions that are exempt from charges, a figure that can rise to 90% in some areas. The medical consequences of poverty start before birth, with poor maternal nutrition contributing to prematurity and low birth weight. During childhood, poor nutrition inhibits normal growth and development; lack of hygienic facilities predisposes to infestations with scabies, head lice and intestinal worms; damp housing increases the incidence of upper-respiratory-tract infections, which can lead to chronic ear disease, partial deafness and a poor educational record; and lack of play facilities hinders psychological development and increases the risk of accidents.

During active parenthood the health hazards stem from attempts to maximize income. Men might seek the premiums attached to shift work, or the 'danger money' associated with hazardous jobs, as well as working overtime, taking a second part-time job on top of their main employment or working in the informal economy where poor health-and-safety conditions predominate. Such strategies increase income, but at the cost of physical exhaustion, risk of accidents, disrupted family life and increased vulnerability to depression in the mothers alone at home with their young children. Other, psychological, effects include exhaustion by the ceaseless struggle to 'make ends meet' and low self-esteem because of failure in this struggle, shame because one's children cannot have the same things as other children and fear lest the furniture is repossessed, the gas or electricity is cut off or one is made homeless because of insufficient money to pay hire purchase instalments, energy bills and rent.

During old age, the health effects of poverty reflect both immediate problems and the accumulation of past effects. Malnutrition ('tea and toast syndrome') and hypothermia are obvious examples, although the large increase in mortality during the winter compared with the summer months is probably a more important effect.

In summary, relative poverty affects a sizeable proportion of the British population. Because of the relationship between poverty and ill health, an even larger proportion of the patients whom doctors treat are likely to be affected in some way by its associated problems.

SOCIAL STRATIFICATION

Many other aspects of inequality could have been examined, in addition to those already discussed, including education, career prospects and leisure activities (Reid 1989). These inequalities tend to go together, so that an individual who is disadvantaged in one area of life is likely to be disadvantaged in others. In the same way, someone who is advantaged in one area of life is likely to be similarly advantaged in others. The term 'social stratification' generally refers to this kind of socially structured inequality, and the concept of social class describes the form that social stratification takes in societies such as contemporary Britain. Most societies to date have been hierarchically structured in some way. Historical forms of stratification have included, for example, the Hindu caste system and the various estates of feudal society. Some social theorists, drawing on the work of the early German sociologist Max Weber, consider that the stratification of modern industrial societies involves three main dimensions: social class, social status or honour, and the political power of organized groups. Although class, status and power are usually related, so that, for example, unskilled labourers generally have low social status and little political influence, they are analytically distinct and can vary independently of one another. Although it is generally agreed that social class is the most fundamental dimension of stratification, sociologists often differ in their precise definition and treatment of class and there are a number of competing theories.

The theory most widely used in the general population divides society into two stereotyped groups of roughly equal size. The 'middle class' consists of people who earn monthly salaries in non-manual jobs, borrow money to buy their own homes and encourage their children to get as much formal education as possible. The 'working-class', by contrast, consists of people who earn weekly wages in manual jobs, rent their homes, mainly from a local authority, and try to get their children started in a good job as soon as they are allowed to leave school. Most of the population appear to have little difficulty in placing themselves in one or other of these two classes. One study that included an unprompted question about self-rated social class found that 40% of the population spontaneously described themselves as middle class and 48% as working class. The study's subjects were found to have made this distinction chiefly on differences in lifestyle, but they were also influenced by considerations of family background, occupation and wealth (Townsend 1979). Recent social changes might have blurred this distinction somewhat: the downward spread of home ownership, foreign holidays and wine consumption and the upward spread of job insecurity and trade unionism have all contributed to this effect.

Most academic social scientists tend to favour some version of Weber's class scheme, whereas the lay population, as we have seen, tends to use the working-class–middle-class distinction. Another approach, derived from the work of Karl Marx, is unusual in having advocates in both camps. It divides society into two main social classes on the basis of ownership and control of the land, industry and financial institutions. The 'working class' in Marx's analysis consists of the overwhelming majority of the population, who own only things they can use; and who live by selling their mental or physical labour power. Social changes since Marx's death have required considerable, and often disputed, elaboration of his original analysis.

For research purposes a more precise and detailed definition of social class is generally necessary. Many scales have been devised to meet this need, although each of these has its own particular strengths and weaknesses. The Registrar General's classification has been the most widely used in medical research. It divides the population into five social classes, I–V, with social class III being further subdivided into non-manual (IIIN) and manual (IIIM). This system of classification is based on occupation, and it groups occupations into social classes according to their skill level and general social standing in the community. Men are allocated to a social class on the basis of their own occupation, married women on the basis of their husband's occupation, children on that of their father and the retired and unemployed on that of their last significant period of employment. Single women are classified on the basis of their own occupation (OPCS 1980).

Certain characteristics of the Registrar General's classification need to be appreciated. Being based on the general social standing of different occupations, it is primarily a measure of status rather than economic class or living standards. As the earlier comments on Weber indicate, however, the link between social status and economic class is sufficiently strong for the classification to act as a reasonable indicator of lifetime earnings and conditions of life. Second, the Registrar General's social classes are not internally homogeneous. Social class II, for example, contains both tenant farmers working a few dozen acres and farmers who own thousands of acres; similarly, it contains both the corner shopkeeper and the senior manager in a multinational company. Third, the Registrar General's classification deals inadequately with women's employment, which, among other things, weakens its power as an indicator of living standards. Married women are classified by the occupation of their husband, although the standard of living of the family's members can be decisively affected by whether or not she has paid employment. It has been calculated that the number of families living in poverty would double if they were deprived of these earnings. Finally, it is possible to question the relevance of an occupationally based classification to a world of flexible labour markets, job insecurity and high unemployment rates.

Problems such as these have prompted attempts to devise a more satisfactory classification, resulting in the new National Statistics Socio-economic Classification (NS-SEC) (Rose & O'Reilly 1997). The NS-SEC assigns people to social classes based on their occupational title and responsibilities over the workforce. The basic divisions are between employers, who buy labour and exercise some degree of control and authority over it; employees, who sell labour and find themselves under the control of employers in the process; and the self-employed, who experience neither. However, employees are further differentiated according to their 'service relationship' and labour contracts. Managers and professionals have a service relationship with their employer that is characterized by a high degree of trust and delegated authority on the part of their employers. Such occupations are typically long-term and compensate for 'service' to the employer through salaries and salary arrangements (like company cars), together with salary increments, pension rights, job security and opportunities for career advancement. The labour contracts of working-class employees, on the other hand, typically specify discrete amounts of labour under close supervision in return for wages calculated on a 'piece' or time basis. Intermediate occupations are characterized by a mixed form of regulation between the service relationship and the labour contract (Chandola 2000). Table 8.1 compares the Registrar General's classification with the NS-SEC.

113

SOCIAL CLASS AND HEALTH

UK data

As the quotation from Chadwick in the opening paragraph of this chapter illustrates, it has long been recognized that the various positions in the social hierarchy are associated with different chances of premature death. Good quality data on the relationship between social class and mortality in England and Wales were published each decade for most of the twentieth century. The data reproduced in Table 8.2 are the most recent available, but the general pattern that they reveal has been a constant feature of all the earlier reports. The mortality rates increase in a step-wise fashion as one moves from the Registrar General's social class I to social class V, with the mortality rate of the latter being approximately twice that of the former. This social class gradient in total deaths due to all causes is found among both males and females and within all age groups, although the differences tend to narrow with increasing age.

Certain specific, major causes of death are listed in Table 8.3. For most causes the mortality rates increase as one moves from social class I to class V, so showing the same gradient as deaths due to all causes combined. There are exceptions, however, which show

TABLE 8.1	Registrar General's and SEC classifications of social classes	
	Registrar General	**NC-SEC**
I	Professional	1 Senior professionals/senior managers
II	Intermediate	2 Associate professionals/junior managers
IIIN	Skilled non-manual	3 Other administrative and clerical workers
IIIM	Skilled manual	4 Own account non-professional
IV	Semi-skilled manual	5 Supervisors, technicians and related workers
V	Unskilled manual	6 Intermediate workers
		7 Other workers
		8 Never worked/other inactive

N, non-manual; M, manual.

TABLE 8.2	Social class and deaths due to all causes (England and Wales, 1991–3, 1993–5)			
Social class	Still-birth rate[a]	Infant mortality rate[b]	Mortality rate (1–15 years)[c]	Standardized mortality ratio (men, 20–64 years)[d]
I	4	4	18	66
II	4	5	16	72
IIIN	5	5	16	100
IIIM	5	6	26	117
IV	6	7	22	116
V	8	8	42	189

Adapted from Drever & Whitehead (1997)
N, non-manual; M, manual.
[a] Number of deaths per 1000 live and dead births; rounded to the nearest integer, 1993–5.
[b] Number of deaths in the first year of life per 1000 live births; rounded to the nearest integer, 1993–5.
[c] Number of deaths per 100,000 population aged 1–15 years; rounded to the nearest integer, 1991–3.
[d] The ratio of the observed mortality rate in a social class to its expected rate from the total population, multiplied by 100, 1991–3.

little or no social class gradient; breast cancer in women has been the most prevalent of these, although this pattern appears to be changing. As this suggests, unlike the gradient for deaths due to all causes, the social class gradient for some causes of death has changed considerably during this century. Coronary heart disease is the most prominent of these; its mortality rate was highest in social class I and lowest in class V for the first half of the century; this gradient flattened out in the third quarter and reversed in the final quarter, so that its mortality rate is now highest in social class V and lowest in class I.

The data presented so far have been mortality rates, and their use as a measure of health has certain advantages. In the vast majority of cases, death is an unambiguous event that can be recorded with high reliability. Death is also one of the few times that an individual is legally obliged to be seen by a doctor, with the result that the recording of death is virtually complete. Mortality rates, therefore, are reliable and complete measures. Nevertheless, they are not perfect measures of health. The term 'health' implies the absence of disease as well as the absence of premature death (see Chapter 18). As a result, attempts to understand the relationship between social class and health have recently begun to examine the way in which morbidity (illness) varies with social class.

For a variety of reasons, the measurement of morbidity is more difficult than that of mortality. Consulting a doctor could be taken as a measure of morbidity. Manual workers consult doctors more frequently than non-manual workers, but it should not be assumed that this is solely because of differences in health. Differences in consultation rates result from differences in illness behaviour (Chapter 3) as well as differences in morbidity. Indeed, non-manual workers appear to be the more frequent consulters when 'use/need ratios' are used to relate consultation rates to the prevalence of illness in the various social classes. The illnesses that people report when questioned as part of a representative survey appear to avoid this problem with consultation rates, so rates of reported illness could be taken as a second measure of morbidity. Manual workers report more illnesses of all types, especially chronic and limiting long-standing illness, than non-manual workers, with the differences tending to widen in the older age groups (Drever & Whitehead 1997). All

| TABLE 8.3 | Social class and major causes of death (England and Wales; 1986–92): age-standardized mortality rates per 100 000. | | | |

Cause of death	Social class			
	I/II	IIIN	IIIM	IV/V
Males 35–64 years				
Ischaemic heart disease	160	162	231	266
Lung cancer	35	50	77	80
Cerebrovascular disease	29	27	33	40
Respiratory diseases	13	21	36	48
Females 35–64 years				
Ischaemic heart disease	29	39	59	78
Lung cancer	16	17	34	47
Cerebrovascular disease	14	22	18	34
Respiratory diseases	11	12	23	29
Breast cancer	52	49	46	54

Adapted from Drever & Whitehead (1997).
N, non-manual; M, manual.

measures of self-reported morbidity, however, involve subjective judgements about illness and its severity. The observed class differences on these measures might be due to systematic variation in these judgements. The more physically demanding nature of manual occupations, for example, might mean that illness is less easily tolerated and recognized earlier.

Some studies have used clinical measures of morbidity on samples of the whole population. These studies should provide results that are free from possible contamination by illness behaviour and systematic subjective variation. Among middle-aged men in the British Regional Heart Study, manual workers were more likely to have experienced angina than non-manual workers; similar social class differences were found in obesity and, to a lesser extent, in blood pressure (Pocock et al 1987, Shaper et al 1988, Weatherall & Shaper 1988). Among men and women of working age in the Health and Lifestyle Survey, manual workers were more likely to experience psychological malaise, to have poorer respiratory function and, to a lesser extent, higher blood pressure than non-manual workers (Cox et al 1987). Studies of this type are expensive and therefore rare. An additional disadvantage is that they usually concentrate on one specific disease, so they are unable to provide information about social class differences in overall morbidity. Like all surveys, they also suffer from non-responders, so their results are not based on the complete coverage achieved by mortality data.

In summary, for many decades reliable and complete data in Britain have shown a step-wise gradient in mortality across the social classes, with members of social class V having approximately twice the chance of dying at any particular age as members of social class I. Recently, attention has turned to morbidity, which is a more valid measure of health than mortality, but difficult to measure with comparable reliability and completeness. Social class differences have been found in various measures of morbidity. The size of these differences appears to vary considerably. The lack of a close match between social class differences in mortality and in morbidity is not surprising. Some major causes of death, such as accidents and violence, need not be preceded by illness and disease, and some common serious diseases, such as arthritis and depression, rarely cause death.

International data

British data on health inequalities are richer and longer standing those from elsewhere. In recent years, however, information on socioeconomic differences in health has become available for many other countries. In most cases, these studies have used measures of social position that differ from the Registrar General's occupational social classes. The number of years of formal education and the level of income are the most frequently used. In general, these alternative measures of socioeconomic position show the same relationship to health as the Registrar General's classes in Britain. Mortality and morbidity rates are lowest in the most advantaged group, highest in the least advantaged group and, in between, increase along a step-wise gradient. Recently, moreover, there has been a discernible tendency for studies yielding cross-country comparisons to show a widening of inequalities in health. The most dramatic widening seems to be occurring in Central and Eastern Europe, but countries with 'good health profiles', such as the Netherlands, Sweden and Denmark, are also signalling persisting or growing inequalities (Drever & Whitehead 1997).

USA

In 1990, death rates at ages 25–64 years, for males and females combined, were 471 per 100 000 for those who had received 8 years or less of formal education and 264 per 100 000 for those who had received 16 years or more (DHHS 1994). In another large-scale study, the death rates of white males showed an inverse gradient with the level of median family income. At the extremes of the income distribution, those with a median family income of less than $7500 had a death rate of 81 per 10 000 compared with 39 for those with more than $32 500 (Davey Smith et al 1992).

European Union

In the Netherlands in 1981–5, the rate of self-reported chronic illness among people aged 16 years or more was over 50% higher in those who left formal education after primary school than in those who had received a university education (Mackenbach 1993).

In Spain in 1987 the prevalence of chronic illness among women aged 20–44 years was nearly 50% higher in the poorest income group than in the highest income group (Kunst & Mackenbach 1994).

Eastern Europe

In Poland in 1988–9 the death rate among men aged 50–64 years was 22 per 1000 among those who left formal education after primary school and 10 per 1000 among those with a university education (Brajczewski & Rogucka 1993).

Among women in Russia who received primary school and university education a similar, although smaller, difference in death rates has been reported (Davis et al 1994).

Socioeconomic differences in health are therefore not confined to Britain. They have been found in every country that has examined the issue and are probably a feature of all industrialized societies. British efforts to understand this phenomenon are now part of an international endeavour.

INTERPRETATION OF THE RELATIONSHIP BETWEEN SOCIAL CLASS AND HEALTH

The association between social class and health shows that death and disease are socially structured, as opposed to randomly distributed throughout the population, and that they vary in line with the differences in living standards that were documented earlier. However, correlation does not imply causation, and the relationship needs to be examined further to establish the status and direction of causality. This can best be achieved by using the explanatory framework that was first developed by the Department of Health's Research Working Group on Inequalities in Health (DHSS 1980). This report, which has become known as the Black Report, suggested four types of explanation of social class differences in health: artefact, social selection, behavioural/cultural and materialist (Box 8.1).

Artefact

The artefact type of explanation examines the possibility that observed social class differences in mortality might be an artefact of the processes by which these two variables are measured. One example of this type of explanation is numerator–denominator bias. The Black Report relied on mortality rates that had been calculated from two sources. Death registration provided the number of deaths in each social class and the Decennial Census the number of individuals in each class. It is possible that an individual's occupation might have been described differently at these two events. Any systematic bias towards 'promoting oneself' on the census form would artefactually increase the death rates in classes IV and V.

The OPCS longitudinal study has followed a 1% sample of the 1971 census population. It eliminated any numerator–denominator bias by categorizing individuals at death according to their social class at the 1971 census. When used in this way, social class differences in mortality were found to be similar to, although smaller than, those that depend on both death registration and census information (Fox & Goldblatt 1982). Social class differences in mortality are, therefore, not an artefact of registration bias.

The relevance of artefact explanations might lie in the opposite direction. Social class differences in mortality are wider when alternative measures of social class and mortality are used. When social position is measured in terms of employment grade within particular industries, the mortality differences between the top and bottom of the social hierarchy are considerably wider than when the Registrar General's classification is used. Similarly, when death rates are measured in terms of years of potential life lost, so weighting deaths according to the age at which they occur, the resulting social class differences are wider than when standardized mortality ratios are used (Blane et al 1990).

BOX 8.1   Types of Explanation: The Black Report

1. **Artefact**: the association between social class and health is an artefact of the way these concepts are measured
2. **Social selection**: health determines social class through a process of health-related social mobility
3. **Behavioural/cultural**: social class determines health through social class differences in health-damaging or health-promoting behaviours
4. **Materialist**: social class determines health through social class differences in the material circumstances of life

Artefact explanations, in summary, do not explain social class differences in mortality, but they do suggest that the differences shown in Table 8.2 (p. 114) are conservative estimates.

Social selection

Social selection explanations argue that health determines social class through a process of health-related social mobility in which the healthy are more likely to move up the social hierarchy and the unhealthy to move down. There is little doubt that chronically sick and disabled people can be additionally disadvantaged in this way. Similarly, those who are taller than average, and in this context height is taken as an indicator of good health, have been found to have a greater than average chance of upward mobility. Health-related social mobility is therefore a real phenomenon. In theory it could explain the whole social class gradient. Whether it does so is the relevant question to ask.

The social distribution of mortality, when seen in relation to the Registrar General's classification rules, suggests that the contribution of social mobility is unlikely to be large. First, social class differences in mortality are found where health-related mobility is not possible. The social gradient in childhood mortality is similar to those among adults. The childhood gradient cannot have been created by mobility associated with child health, however, because the Registrar General's scheme classifies children according to their father's occupation. The same reasoning applies to married women. Their mortality gradient is similar to that of adult men. The married women's gradient cannot be due to mobility associated with their own health, because the Registrar General's scheme classifies them according to their husband's occupation.

Second, social class differences in mortality are found where social mobility of any type is not possible. Class gradients after retirement are similar to those during working life. The post-retirement gradients cannot be due to health-related social mobility. The Registrar General's scheme classifies retired people according to their last significant period of employment, which eliminates any subsequent social mobility.

Third, social class differences in mortality due to diseases that kill quickly, such as lung cancer, are similar to those that kill slowly, such as chronic bronchitis and emphysema. If health-related social mobility made an important contribution to social class differences in health, the gradients should be steeper for causes of death that allow time for social mobility between the onset of disease and death.

Fourth, social mobility tends to occur before the serious diseases become prevalent. Social mobility is most frequent, and movement between the working class and middle class most likely, during the early years of working life, particularly between leaving formal education and the mid-twenties age group. Serious disease, which could interfere with performance, does not become widespread until several decades later. Most social mobility takes place when the population is generally healthy and it is comparatively rare in the age groups where serious disease is prevalent.

Finally, incapacitating illness does not inevitably lead to downward mobility. The chronically sick and disabled have other options, including early retirement, unemployment and moving to a similar but less demanding job. All of these alternatives are likely to entail a reduction in income, but none of them involves downward social mobility on the Registrar General's scheme.

Research points to the same conclusion as these more general considerations. An examination of health and social mobility among men aged 45–64 years found no evidence that health-related social mobility systematically contributed to the social class differences in their mortality (Goldblatt 1989). The contribution of health to social mobility during the early years of working life is still uncertain (West 1991), but the weight of evidence indicates that its contribution is small (Power et al 1990, Wadsworth 1986). Educational achievement, the type of secondary school attended and the material and cultural resources of the family of origin, rather than health, are found to be the main influences on social mobility between formal education and the world of work (Halsey et al 1980).

Social selection explanations, in summary, are most relevant to the early years of working life and even at these ages the contribution of health-related social mobility to social class differences in health is probably small.

Behavioural/cultural and materialist

The behavioural/cultural and the materialist types of explanation both see health as determined in some way by social class, but they differ in the aspects of social class they see as responsible. Behavioural/cultural explanations involve class differences in behaviours that are health damaging or health promoting, and which, at least in principle, are subject to individual choice. Materialist explanations, by contrast, involve hazards that are inherent in the present form of social organization and to which some people have no choice but to be exposed.

Dietary choices, the consumption of drugs like tobacco and alcohol, active leisure-time pursuits and the use of preventive medical services such as immunization, contraception and antenatal surveillance are examples of behaviours that vary with social class and could account for class differences in health. Considerable weight is given to this type of explanation by the evidence that has accumulated as a result of medicine's long interest in such issues. However, the social and economic context in which these behaviours occur needs to be recognized. Diet is influenced by both cultural preferences and disposable income. The ability of nicotine to maintain a constant mood in situations of stress and monotony might predispose towards cigarette smoking in repetitive and highly supervised occupations. Other evidence cautions against a one-sided emphasis on behavioural factors. Early in the twentieth century, cigarette smoking was more prevalent among the middle class than the working class, but class gradients in mortality were similar to the present. Intervention studies have rarely produced the clear-cut improvements in health that would be predicted by the behavioural/cultural approach, despite achieving reduction in the hazardous behaviours.

The Black Report judged that materialist explanations were the most important in accounting for social class differences in health. The health-damaging effects of air pollution and occupational exposure to physicochemical hazards had already been recognized. More recently, local levels of economic and social deprivation have been identified as powerful predictors of mortality and morbidity. The health effects of income distribution and the psychosocial aspects of employment have been demonstrated. Damp housing has been shown to be associated with worse health, particularly with higher rates of respiratory disease in children. Unemployment has been associated with psychological morbidity and raised mortality among unemployed men and their spouses. Each of these factors could contribute to class differences in health because they are all more likely to be experienced by working class than middle class people.

There is thus a certain amount of evidence to support the materialist type of explanation. Nevertheless, most medical researchers would probably judge behavioural/cultural factors, and cigarette smoking in particular, to be of greater importance. The primacy assigned to materialist explanations by the Black Report can be defended on the grounds that research has so far ignored the accumulation of advantage or disadvantage that is associated with social class. As the earlier sections of this chapter have indicated, inequalities are found in many spheres of life. Social class is the concept that stresses the likelihood that advantage or disadvantage in one sphere will be associated with advantage or disadvantage in others. Those who experience occupational disadvantage are likely to be the same people who are residentially disadvantaged, and these disadvantages in their various forms are likely to accumulate through childhood and adulthood and into old age. It will not be possible to make a secure judgement about the relative importance of behavioural/cultural and materialist explanations until the effect on health of such combined and accumulating disadvantages has been established.

CONTEMPORARY DEBATES

The Black Report both offered a collation of data on health inequalities in Britain and, in identifying and assessing rival explanations, served as a catalyst for subsequent research and debate. A later influential contributor, Wilkinson (1996), drew on this accumulating research to maintain that the level of income inequality is a crucial determinant of the health of populations in more affluent societies like Britain. He argued that once certain levels of gross national product (GNP) per capita have been reached, the principal determinant of level of health status within a country is degree of income inequality. Once countries A and B have passed through what he calls the 'epidemiological transition', then the population of country A can be twice as rich as that of country B without being any healthier. In short, the populations of rich 'equal' countries have better health profiles than the populations of rich 'unequal' countries. He went on to claim that 'social cohesion' and 'trust' provide the dominant mechanisms linking a country's degree of income equality with health. He argued that there is evidence that where income inequalities are more marked, social divisions tend to be exacerbated; levels of trust and strength of community life tend to be lower; rates of social anxiety and chronic stress tend to be higher; rates of hostility, violence and murder tend to be higher; and there tends to develop a 'culture of inequality' characterized by a more hostile and less hospitable environment. Wilkinson (2000) concludes that whereas we used to assume that the direct effects of poorer material circumstances accounted for class differences in health and longevity, it might well be that a major part of the association between lower class position and diminished health status springs from the experience of low social status or subordination itself.

Wilkinson's general thesis on the nature of the epidemiological transition has been challenged on statistical grounds, and his notion of a 'psychosocial pathway' linking income inequality to health differences has been criticized by a number of commentators. Coburn (2000), for example, has argued that too many researchers have concentrated on possible social, psychological or biological mechanisms through which social factors might link with health status. This has meant they have neglected what he defines as the 'basic social causes of inequality and health'. Against Wilkinson he contends that rather than income inequality producing lower social cohesion and trust leading to lowered health status, 'neo-liberalism' (or market dominance) produces both higher income inequality and lower social cohesion and trust; as well as, it might be presumed, lowered health status. In advancing this thesis, Coburn introduces into the debate on health inequalities much wider issues of social change. Economic globalization has been underpinned, he suggests, by neo-liberalism, and neo-liberalism in turn has benefited from economic globalization. Moreover, the more neo-liberal or market-oriented a country's political regime, with the possible exception of Japan, the higher the income inequality. So in Coburn's view it is neo-liberalism that leads to income inequality and reduced social cohesion and trust, although he remains cautious about possible causal relationships between these and health inequalities.

Scambler & Higgs (2001) have taken things a stage further by adopting a concept of class that owes much to Marx's perspective mentioned earlier. According to them, the neo-liberalism to which Coburn attaches such importance should be understood as the expression of class interests. In other words, it is the changing nature of present capitalist society and of class interests that are basic to understanding the increase in income inequality and, ultimately, the 'widening gap' in health inequalities. They go on to suggest that the Labour government's philosophy of the 'third way', with its emphasis on personal responsibility, shares many properties with the Conservative government's espousal of neo-liberalism; and both must be seen as reflecting class interests. Scambler (2002) has recently expanded on this argument to put forward a 'greedy bastards hypothesis' (or GBH). This provocatively named hypothesis asserts that the well-documented growth in health inequality in Britain since the 1970s can be understood as the largely unintended consequence of the ever-adaptive behaviours of the (weakly globalized) power elite at the centre of government, which is in turn influenced, often decisively, by (strongly globalized) leading capitalists. It is this 'alliance' of the powerful and wealthy, he maintains, which plays the greatest role, although not of course the only one, in the social distribution of those factors known to bear on people's health and longevity. It is necessary to understand the rich and powerful in order to understand the poor and powerless.

Contemporary debates such as these address wider issues than were found in the Back Report in 1980 and in much subsequent research. They are valuable in that they broaden our thinking about health inequalities, but they have yet to be researched thoroughly. If Wilkinson's contribution has opened up other and more diverse areas of enquiry and debate, ways need to be found to subject these theories to proper empirical examination.

THE OVERALL PICTURE

The work of social researchers such as Chadwick and Farr made the Victorians aware of the vicious circle of 'poverty causes disease which causes poverty'. Despite the subsequent development of the welfare state, disabled people and those with chronic diseases are still at risk of relative poverty. This side of the Victorians' vicious circle, however, would now appear less important than the side that stresses the effect of material well-being, or the lack of it, on health. The health inequalities of today are primarily due to the combined effect of class differences in exposure to factors that promote health or cause disease.

This was the conclusion reached by the Department of Health Working Group that produced the Black Report. The Report went on to suggest measures for starting to eliminate health inequalities. There are 37 of these recommendations. A few were designed to ensure better information about class differences in health. Most were carefully targeted at a limited number of issues where class differences in health were thought to be widest and most likely to respond to relatively small sums of money. Disability was the subject of six recommendations designed to break its links with poverty. These covered prevention (fetal screening for neural tube defects and Down syndrome), welfare procedures (a comprehensive disablement allowance), housing (more specialist housing for disabled people) and community-care services (resources shifted towards home-help and nursing services for disabled people). This set of recommendations appears designed to prevent disability where this is presently possible (fetal screening) and, where it is not, to ensure that the lives of working-class people with disabilities are not markedly disadvantaged in terms of income (welfare procedures) and living conditions (housing and community services).

In addition to disability, equally detailed recommendations were made concerning infant and child health, cigarette smoking, occupational health and safety and local authority housing. Particular priority was given to the abolition of child poverty by means of a new

> **BOX 8.2**   Crucial Areas Identified by the Acheson Report
>
> 1. All policies likely to have an impact on health should be evaluated in terms of their impact on health inequalities
> 2. A high priority should be given to the health of families with children
> 3. Further steps should be taken to reduce income inequalities and improve the living standards of poor households

infant-care allowance, increased child benefit and the provision of free school meals. These recommendations, in common with the rest of the report, were described by the incumbent Conservative government as 'unrealistic' and the report was published 'without any commitment by the Government to its proposals'. Nevertheless, subsequent research has greatly increased our understanding of the relationship between social class and health.

When the Labour government was elected in 1997 it promptly established an 'Independent Inquiry into Inequalities in Health', (Stationary Office 1998). Even before the Acheson Report, as it was known, was published, a Green Paper entitled 'Our Healthier Nation' (DoH 1998) had stated as one of its aims improving the health of the worst off in society and narrowing what it called 'the health gap'. The Acheson Report itself noted that average mortality had fallen over the previous 50 years, but concluded that 'unacceptable inequalities in health persist' and that 'for many measures of health, inequalities have either remained the same or have widened in recent years'. This applied at all stages of the life course. The Report acknowledged that income, education and employment were fundamental determinants of ill health, as well as material environment and lifestyle. Its recommendations went well beyond the remit of the Department of Health, calling for policy development in relation to poverty, income, tax and benefits, education, employment, housing and environment, mobility, transport and pollution, and nutrition. The three main areas defined as crucial are listed in Box 8.2.

The authors of the Black Report welcomed its successor, drawing attention in particular to the recommendation relating to material factors, which specified the urgent need to reduce income inequalities and improve the living standards of households in receipt of social security benefits (Black et al 1999). However, the Acheson Report has been criticized for not prioritizing its recommendations, for being overly vague and for not costing its suggested policies, and early audits of government responses have been cautious, even pessimistic (Shaw et al 1999). It remains to be seen whether there will be a willingness to act effectively against factors, such as income inequality, which continue to underpin health inequalities in Britain.

References

Black D et al 1999 Better benefits for health: plan to implement the central recommendations of the Acheson Report. British Medical Journal 318:724–727

Blane D, Davey Smith G, Bartley M 1990 Social class differences in years of potential life lost: size, trends and principal causes. British Medical Journal 301:429–432

Brajczewski C, Rogucka E 1993 Social class differences in rates of premature mortality among adults in the city of Wroclaw. American Journal of Human Biology 5:461–471

Chadwick E 1842 Report on the sanitary condition of the labouring population of Great Britain 1842. Edinburgh University Press, Edinburgh. Reprinted 1965

Chandola T 2000 Social class differences in mortality using the new UK National Statistics Socio-Economic Classification. Social Science and Medicine 50:641–649

Coburn D 2000 Income inequality, social cohesion and the health status of populations: the role of neo-liberalism. Social Science and Medicine 51:135–146

Cox BD et al 1987 The health and lifestyle survey: preliminary report. Health Promotion Research Trust, London

Davey Smith G et al 1992 Income differentials in mortality risk among 305,099 white men. European Society of Medical Sociology Conference, Edinburgh, September 1992 (Abstract)

Davis CE et al 1994 Correlates of mortality in Russian and US women: the Lipid Research Clinics Program. American Journal of Epidemiology 139:369–379

Department of Health (DoH) 1998 Our healthier nation: a contract for health. HMSO, London

Department of Health and Human Services (DHHS) 1994 Health United States 1993. National Centre for Health Statistics, Hyattsville, MD

Department of Health and Social Security (DHSS) 1980 Inequalities in health: report of a research working group (The Black Report). HMSO, London

Drever F, Whitehead M (eds) 1997 Health inequalities. National Statistics, London

Fox AJ, Goldblatt PO 1982 Longitudinal study: socio-demographic mortality differentials. HMSO, London

Goldblatt PO 1989 Mortality by social class 1971–85. Population Trends 56:6–15

Halsey AM, Heath AF, Ridge JM 1980 Origins and destinations: family, class and education in modern Britain. Clarendon Press, Oxford

Hunter D 1975 The diseases of occupations, 5th edn. English Universities Press, London

Kunst AE, Mackenbach JP 1994 Measuring socio-economic inequalities in health. WHO Regional Office for Europe, Copenhagen

Mackenbach JP 1993 Inequalities in health in the Netherlands according to age, gender, marital status, level of education, degree of urbanisation and region. European Journal of Public Health 3:112–118

Ministry of Agriculture, Fisheries and Food (MAFF) 1989 Household food consumption and expenditure 1988. HMSO, London

National Statistics 2000 Social Trends 30. HMSO, London

National Statistics 2001 Social Trends 31. HMSO, London

Office of Population Censuses and Surveys (OPCS) 1980 Classification of occupations 1980. HMSO, London

Pocock SJ et al 1987 Social class differences in ischaemic heart disease in British men. Lancet ii:197–201

Power C, Manor O, Fox AJ 1990 Health and class: the early years. Chapman & Hall, London

Reid I 1989 Social class differences in Britain, 3rd edn. Fontana Press, London

Rose D, O'Reilly K (eds) 1997 Constructing classes: towards a new social classification for the UK. Office for National Statistics, London

Scambler G 2002 Health and social change. Open University Press, Buckingham

Scambler G, Higgs P 2001 'The dog that didn't bark': taking class seriously in the health inequalities debate. Social Science and Medicine 52:157–159

Shaper AG, Ashby D, Pocock SJ 1988 Blood pressure and hypertension in middle-aged British men. Journal of Hypertension 6:367–374

Shaw M, Dorling D, Gordon D, Davey Smith G 1999 The widening gap: health inequalities and policy in Britain. Policy Press, Bristol

Stationary Office 1998 Independent inquiry into inequalities in health (the Acheson Report). HMSO, London

Townsend P 1979 Poverty in the United Kingdom. Penguin, London:

Wadsworth MEJ 1986 Serious illness in childhood and its association with later-life achievement. In: Wilkinson RG (ed) Class and health: research and longitudinal data. Tavistock, London, p 50–74

Weatherall R, Shaper AG 1988 Overweight and obesity in middle-aged British men. Journal of Clinical Nutrition 42:221–231

West P 1991 Rethinking the health selection explanation for health inequalities. Social Science and Medicine 32:373–384

Wilkinson R 1996 Unhealthy societies: the afflictions of inequality. Routledge, London

Wilkinson R 2000 Deeper than neo-liberalism: a reply to David Coburn. Social Science and Medicine 51:997–1000

123

Annette Scambler

This chapter presents a broad sweep of health differences between the genders, starting with mortality data and life expectancy, and moving on to a general consideration of morbidity differences before detailing some issues of health of especial significance to women. A consideration of mental health and issues of masculinity and femininity connects with material on embodiment and body hatred in young women, and childbirth provides a forum for further consideration of the medicalization and control of women's bodies. To attempt to understand the relationship of gender to health it is first essential to explore the relative social positions of men and women in contemporary society.

GENDER ROLES AND WOMEN'S POSITION IN SOCIETY

A key contention is that we live in a social environment where gender plays a significant role in social status and in access to material resources, health and well-being, and where roles, responsibilities and power are not shared equally between males and females. It is tempting, when looking at gender, to focus on the enormous range of changes that undoubtedly occurred over the course of the twentieth century, and to indicate that women are now to be found in every sphere of society; that we have had a female Prime Minister and women at the head of unions and major business, leisure, academic and professional organizations. Women now comprise half the entrants to medical school and are entering the legal profession in large numbers. It would be very easy to paint a picture of women in the process of equalling or even displacing the existing male captains of industry. That would be a simplistic view. Although there have been significant shifts in gender norms in society, such changes have occurred within a complex web of power and advantage that still leaves women with a long way to go to achieve even material parity with men.

Some evidence is required here and a good place to start is with the seat of government itself. As of October 2001, after the Labour Party's second general election victory, there was a complement of 659 MPs, of whom 118 were female (two fewer than the previous parliament). That is just under 18% of the total, although over half the population is female. Contrast this, however, with the percentage of female MPs prior to Labour's 1997 victory, which was just over 9%. The doubling of the female contingent in 1997 was due largely to the introduction of women-only shortlists by the Labour Party, to counter a male bias in the selection process; this policy had to be abandoned after legal challenges under the Sex Discrimination Act. That women then lost headway at the election in 2001 has resulted in a Labour promise to reintroduce women-only shortlists via a proposed Women's Representation Act, almost 100 years after women first gained a partial vote in 1918. Despite this development, there is little evidence to suggest that the interests of women are high on the parliamentary agenda. For example, the minimum wage was delayed until the European Court became involved, despite the fact that it was estimated at the time of adoption that 80% of those to benefit would, in fact, be women. Lack of nursery education, poor childcare facilities and inflexible working hours are all examples of areas where it is suggested that more female representation might help. It would, however, be naïve to suggest that more female MPs, alone, will effect change.

◼ Changes in family size and structure

There have been significant changes in family size and structure since the 1960s. Fewer people are marrying and divorce is rising. Between 1961 and the end of the twentieth century, the percentage of households comprising 'traditional families' – composed of parents and dependent children – declined from more than one third to less than one quarter. During the same period, the proportion of households comprising lone-parent families with dependent children trebled to 7%. Now, over 30% of all dependent children live in lone-parent families, nearly 80% of them with their mothers. In 1997, the average age of first marriage had risen to 27 for women and 29 for men (a rise of 5 years over a 30-year period), and the number of divorces had doubled over the same period so that now around 40% of marriages are legally terminated (Fig. 9.1). Cohabiting now normally precedes marriage and many couples cohabit but do not marry. This trend is expected to continue (The Women's Unit 2000).

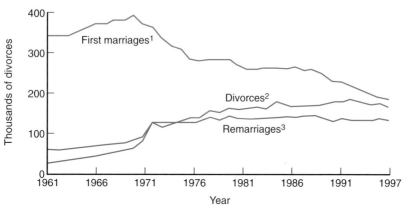

1 For both partners
2 Includes annulments
3 For one or both partners

Fig. 9.1 Marriages and divorces in the UK.

Along with changes in the structure of the family, fertility rates have also declined, with a drop from 91 births per 1000 women of childbearing age in 1961 to only 59 in 1998. Overall, women are getting married later, having their children later in life and having fewer children. Contributing factors include increased participation in higher education and employment and better contraception (72% of women were using contraception by the end of the twentieth century). At present, 40% of all live births occur to women outside marriage, but for women below 20 that figure rises to 90%. Following the Abortion Act of 1967, abortion rates rose from 3.4 per 1000 women in 1968 to 30.4 per 1000 in 1998, with the peak figures in the age group 20–24. One area of concern is the increasing trend for women to remain childless. Figure 9.2 shows the rise in female childlessness since the Second World War. Only 11% of women born in 1943 remained childless at the age of 45, but this figure has risen steadily and it is expected that nearly 25% of those born just 30 years later will never have children (The Women's Unit 2000). Some predictions are even higher than this.

Women and paid employment

It is difficult to dispute the fact that equality for the genders is still not obvious in the general area of paid work. Figures for 2002 indicate that, although there was an Equal Pay Act in 1970, the pay gap between males and females is still around 20%, despite a very small narrowing in 2001–2. This belies the varying shortfalls in different occupations. In 1996 the Equal Opportunities Commission found a 25% gap in marketing and sales, 28% in the legal profession, 35% in banking and 42% in management. Women are twice as likely to work in the public sector (32% of women workers as opposed to 15% of male workers) where pay levels do not match the private sector (Labour Force Survey 2001). Indeed, the same survey indicates that women's overall hourly pay is over £2 less then men's (£8.17 as opposed to £10.74). Women are also less than half as likely as men to reach the higher levels of management where another set of benefits kicks in (Labour Force Survey 2001). Apart from pay differentials, women are less likely to get access to company cars, private

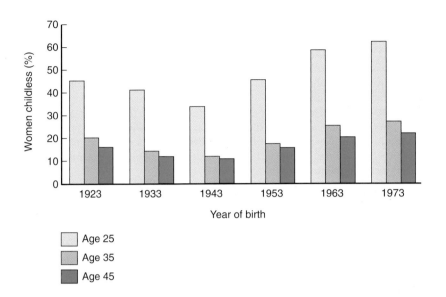

Fig. 9.2 Percentage of women childless by year of birth (England and Wales).

127

health insurance paid by the company, health screening and other forms of welfare, including access to sports clubs. They also have less access to subsidized canteens and company shares, and are less likely to get bonuses and overtime pay.

The patriarchal structure of paid employment is heavily implicated in what has undoubtedly been the 'feminization of poverty'. In relation to paid work, women's contribution has been significantly curtailed by their unpaid work in the domestic sphere of society, and still only 69% of all working age women are in work as compared to 80% of all working age men (Labour Force Survey 2001). Furthermore, in Britain, part-time working for married women and mothers became the norm after the Second World War when, unlike France (where women were called into the workforce and provided with comprehensive child-care facilities), recruitment of full-time workers was extended to the Commonwealth and women were used as cheap, part-time employees on a lower hourly pay than full-time workers and largely without benefits such as sick-pay, holiday pay, redundancy pay and so on. The pattern for women became, and still is, fragmented because of reproduction, with women moving in and out of the workforce. In 2001, figures indicated that 42% of female workers were still part-time compared with only 8% of males (Labour Force Survey 2001) and that, overall, females comprised over 80% of the part-time workforce. Part-time working is most common for mothers, with two-thirds of those with children under five in part-time employment.

This pattern of employment for women has had an enormous effect on lifetime earnings. In 2000, the Cabinet Office Women's Unit published the results of research on this issue. They found that women's lifetime earnings were substantially lower than men's and that both gender and motherhood independently affected the outcome. They concluded that there is a 'gender earnings gap' – the difference between equivalently skilled and childless males and females, and a 'mother gap' – the difference between equivalently educated females with and without children. The 'parent gap' is the difference in lifetime earnings between a mother and father in a family. As a result of the gender earnings gap, high-skilled childless women lost £143 000 over a lifetime, whereas mid-skilled childless women lost £241 000 and low-skilled childless women £197 000. The mother gap reduced the high-skill earnings by £19 000 only, but mid-skilled women lost £140 000 and low-skilled women a massive £285 000 (Davies et al 2000). Figure 9.3 shows the breakdown of the mother gap by age of mother at first birth. Data like these might well push the fertility rate even lower than it is already.

The extent of the total lost in each category gives weight to the feminization of poverty thesis as lowered lifetime earnings are reflected in substantially reduced or absent work pension funds. It is also expected that large numbers of females will become increasingly poor as the pension system continues to be privatized and individuals are made personally responsible for their maintenance.

Women are also disproportionately dependent on social security benefits as their sole or main income. As already indicated, they are more likely to be single parents, and the past 20 years have seen a doubling of the numbers in this category on income support. Additionally, the majority of families receiving the Working Families Tax Credit (formally Family Credit) are lone parents (Davies et al 2000). The sum total of all this information is that for many women, especially those at the bottom of the class structure, life can be one long slog characterized by demands on time, energy and income which cannot be met satisfactorily. The effects on women's health are examined throughout the chapter.

Two gender issues of some importance in relation to work are the ways that occupational health and work hazards research and practice have operated against the interests of women, and the effects of sexual harassment on female health. For some time now it has been pointed out that there is a male bias in occupational research. Doyal (1995), for example, discusses the problem that most research in relation to chemical risk assessment has been applied to the metabolic processes of males rather than females, and that in a wide range of occupational settings male biology is treated as the norm. She also points to the lack of attention to the size and shape of protective clothing, which often precludes women from access to certain spheres. Doyal suggests that a vicious circle exists,

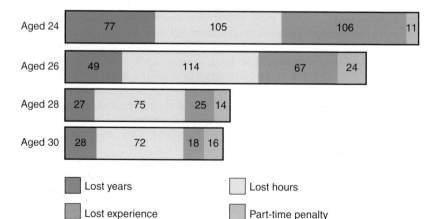

Fig. 9.3 Breakdown of the 'mother gap' in earnings for a mother of two children, by the age of the mother at the first birth: mid-skilled women.

128

where the assumption is that women's work is safe so there are no relevant guidelines, few prevention programmes and risks that remain invisible, so illness is attributed to 'hormones' or imagination, which results in claims being refused and so reinforces the prejudice that women's work is safe.

Harassment at work is also a source of much distress amongst women and can have wide-ranging effects on health. One study in the USA in the 1980s found that sexual harassment was related to deterioration in work performance and enhanced work hazard levels as concentration dipped. Common symptoms of distress included anxiety, depression, guilt and fear. Walby (1990) and Crompton (1997) both suggest that sexual harassment is a deliberate strategy used by men to exclude women from certain work contexts. Pilcher (1999) points out that this is particularly common where women have encroached on traditional male areas. She quotes one 1983 study that found that 96% of women in 'male' spheres suffered sexual harassment, and even in traditional female areas the figure was as high as 48%.

The public and private spheres

It has been suggested that society has been divided into two distinct and gendered spheres, the public and the private. The public world of paid work is deemed to have higher status than the private, and is seen as the 'real world', containing the institutions and personnel necessary to create a functioning society. It is also seen as the natural social sphere for men. Conversely, the domestic sphere is gendered female and is conceptualized as the domain of unpaid work that is performed 'for love', where the reproduction and rearing of children and the nurturing of families takes place. It is also seen as a place of leisure and a refuge from paid work, especially for men.

This ideology, although changing, still has a significant effect on male and female roles and subsequent access to material and social resources, despite the economic activity figures just quoted, and the fact that most households find it very difficult to exist on one income. Women's work in the home continues to be valued lower than paid work, and the status of 'home-worker' remains a negative one. Indeed, the current benefit structure focuses on the 'welfare to work' ideology, which clearly implies, despite rhetoric to the contrary, that society has little tolerance for women with dependent children who are dependent not on a partner's income, but on welfare. A minimal benefit level together with strict surveillance of welfare recipients and continual public pressure to seek 'proper' work outside the home are deemed to be risk factors for the well-being of such women. The expectation is that they should be able to cope both with paid work and with unpaid childcare work, despite a lack of facilities or adequate income to allow them to do so.

The low status placed on a 'woman's work' is highlighted when its lack of monetary value within the economy is addressed. An exercise performed by the Office of Statistics in 1997 looked at work done around the household. The researchers estimated that such work, valued as paid employment, would have amounted to £739 billion per annum; this would more than double the gross domestic produce (GDP). They found that women performed nearly twice as much of this work as men. Significantly, work in the home is often rendered invisible by being ignored altogether, or only recognized when there is a problem and children appear to be badly cared for or the housekeeping is deemed inadequate. Women in these circumstances might be seen as lacking in social skills (not a proper woman) and subject to public surveillance, or they could even be classified as suffering from mental illness.

The home is not necessarily a refuge for women, and there is now a catalogue of evidence delineating the problem of domestic violence and the effect it has on their mental and physical health. Although domestic violence is a significant problem in Britain, it is also a global issue and remarkably stable figures seem to exist across the world, with World Health Organization (WHO) figures indicating rates of between 20 and 30% for Western countries and those for countries in Asia, the Middle East, Central and Latin America and Africa ranging from 16 to a high of 52% in Nicaragua. The incidence in Kenya and Uganda is around 40% and several other countries show incidences approaching 40% (WHO 2000). Domestic violence includes physical, emotional, psychological and sexual violence. It ranges from slaps to murder, harassment to mental abuse, and is mainly directed towards females by males (approximately 80%). In 2000, a national snapshot study of the prevalence in Britain, conducted by the police, found acts of domestic violence committed every 6 seconds. Their research showed that 25% of all London crimes are domestic and that children witness at least 50% of such attacks. The health effects are wide-ranging, with one 1997 study of 129 abused women in Hackney finding that injuries were serious enough for 1 in 9 to need medical attention in the past year and 1 in 3 over their life-span (Camden Domestic Violence Forum 1999). A range of studies put injuries at between 30 and 70%, including bruising, broken bones, damage to the genitalia and facial injuries. Emotional distress is severe with common symptoms being depression and loss of self-esteem, sleep problems and increased risk of suicide (one US study in 1992 found that 25% of all female suicide victims had been battered women). Domestic violence is another indication that women have very different health profiles to men. It is being addressed nationally now, with publicity campaigns and Domestic Violence Forums run by local authorities, but much still needs to be done to safeguard women.

Dual roles and role conflict

Gender expectations, therefore, remain firmly entrenched around reproduction and women are finding it difficult to make significant inroads. The strain of dual roles has been a key issue in women's health research. Although there are changes in the working patterns of younger women, with the average age for childbirth now standing at 29, and many middle-class women delaying their children to the mid- or even late thirties to qualify and stabilize their careers, recent research suggests that working practice has not altered in line with these developments. There is a trend for women who have gone back to work full-time after having their first babies to give up their jobs altogether or to go part-time if they are able to. Inflexible hours of work lead to a health toll on women as they soak up the stress from trying to juggle work and home commitments. One study in Quebec in 1999 looked at the stresses of working mothers with degrees. This study found that women who juggle difficult jobs with raising a family face greater risk of stress-related illness than their husbands: 'While tension raises the blood pressure of both sexes during the day, working mothers remain stressed for longer into the evening and may increase the danger of heart disease and strokes' (Brisson 1999).

The long hours and competitive culture in Britain (which has the longest working day in Europe) also disadvantages women with home responsibilities who are unable to stay late in the evenings or get into work early, or take work home. Women in one recent study felt watched and valued less in their jobs than when they were childless, and felt let down by the system. More and more women, in the middle classes especially, are choosing to remain childless for longer periods and are assimilating into the male long-hours work culture with its heavier drinking patterns and smoking and a movement away from domesticity. Additionally, it has been noticed that young women in business are not always overtly supportive of female colleagues who are trying to juggle home and family. Many see such women as a drain on their own career progress as they see themselves 'carrying' them during periods of childhood illness or other domestic crises. What is not happening at the moment is a change in the culture of work to accommodate changing expectations of young women to their life chances.

Childbirth, therefore, still remains a barrier to the progress of women throughout society, and ironically, paid work culture also now increasingly acts as a barrier to childbirth. There has been recent concern that a whole cohort of younger women are in danger of forfeiting the opportunity to bear children because they are waiting until the middle to late thirties when the dangers of genetic abnormality and lowered fertility combine to render conception difficult and childbirth risky.

MORTALITY AND LIFE EXPECTANCY

Life expectancy

Life-expectancy rates differ globally, but in almost every country women outlive men. Part of this difference can be accounted for by an innate biological advantage, which is still not fully understood, but manifests itself in, among other things, higher male deaths *in utero* and in the early postnatal period. Recent research focuses on the immune system and suggests that the extra T cells that women possess might give them more protection against disease over the life course. It is now widely accepted, however, that any biological advantages enjoyed by women are only a small part of the overall picture, and that the social construction of gender identity and related gender roles also has a significant effect. Arber & Thomas (2001) identify four key patterns of gender differences in mortality rates and, although acknowledging the presence of a biological advantage, explain the rest of the difference socially:

- A female advantage of 5–7 years, exemplified by Western countries of the late twentieth century, but also some countries like Brazil and Korea. Length of life expected is in the 70s to low 80s. Sweden, for example, has a gap of 5 years, with males at 76.5 years and females at 81.5 years, whereas the gap in Japan is higher, at 6.6 years. In this category, the female advantage is explained through the effects caused by the gendering of social roles and lifestyles. More hazardous occupations and risk behaviours of men prescribed by the hegemonic version of masculinity are emphasized.

- A female advantage of 2–4 years, exemplified by many developing countries in Africa and Asia. This is typical of transitional societies where previously high maternal mortality has declined and the structural disadvantages of women are beginning to improve. Length of life expected for this group is in the 50s and low 60s. Examples given here are Kenya with a 3.9 years gap and figures for men and women, respectively, of 61.4 years and 57.5 years, and China with a 2.8 years gap.

- No gender difference or men outlive women, exemplified by some developing countries. Expected length of life depends on the overall economic development of the individual country and varies between the 40s, 50s and 60s. In Bangladesh, men marginally outlive women, with figures of 58.6 years and 58.2 years, respectively, and in Pakistan and India the life spans are almost equal at just under 60 years for both genders. In Algeria and Afghanistan the female excess is only 1 year. In all these countries women's status is very low, but the UN figures starkly show the effect of differing levels of economic development, with men and women in Algeria reaching the late 60s, whereas Afghani men and women can expect to die in their early to mid 40s. In these countries, women seem to have lost all their relative advantage over men through gender discrimination, which renders them especially vulnerable to violence and reduces their access to food and to health care, the latter especially important to women in such cultures where a high birth rate combines with high maternal and perinatal mortality rates.

● A female advantage of 8+ years, exemplified by countries in the former Soviet Union and in other countries of Eastern Europe. In Russia the gender gap is 13 years with men expecting to live until just over 58 and women until nearly 72. In Latvia the figures are 63.9 and 75.6 years, respectively. Startlingly, we also find that black Americans fit the same pattern, with the life expectancy of black males being 64.7 years whereas the black female figure is 73.7 years. In these countries, women's rates have improved or remained stable and men's rates have deteriorated. In the USA, recent research suggests that black men suffer a range of socioeconomic disadvantages that have enhanced alienation and risky behaviours.

132

▧ Gendered life expectancy in Britain and Europe

Life expectancy in Europe has not always favoured women. In Europe in the sixteenth and seventeenth centuries there was a big male advantage (Shorter 1982), and in the industrialized early nineteenth century male and female longevity was more or less the same. The female advantage began to appear in the second half of the nineteenth century, with the widest gender gap occurring in the twentieth century from the 1960s to 1980s. Parallel with these changes, expectation of life for both genders has almost doubled since the mid-nineteenth century (Social Trends 2001). Table 9.1 shows changes in life expectancy from 1841 to 1998. Information on 'healthy life expectancy' is also included using recent research by the Office for National Statistics (Social Trends 2001). This is defined as expected years of life in good or fairly good self-assessed general health. A gender gap remains for the years presented, but is considerably less than the general life expectancy gap. Women seem to expect to live less of their lives in a healthy state than men.

In the European Union (EU), 1995 data indicate that women in the EU live around 6.4 years longer than men. Significantly, British males rank better than British females, with men placed fifth out of the fifteen countries, whereas women could only achieve twelfth place. There were big improvements across the EU between 1970 and 1995, with women increasing by 5.5 and men by nearly 5 years.

TABLE 9.1	Life expectancy (in years) by gender								
	1841	**1901**	**1931**	**1961**	**1981**	**1986**	**1991**	**1997**	**1998**
Males									
Life expectancy	41.0	45.7	58.1	67.8	70.9	72.0	73.2	74.6	74.9
Healthy life expectancy						64.4	65.4	66.2	66.9
Females									
Life expectancy	43.0	49.6	62.1	73.7	76.8	77.7	78.8	79.6	79.8
Health life expectancy						66.7	67.6	68.6	68.7

From Government Actuary's Department, Office for National Statistics.
Data for 1841 and 1901 are for England and Wales only.

MORTALITY

As with the data for length of life, there are clear differences in mortality rates between the genders. The focus will be on Western society and this section will examine these differences, look at the main causes of death and offer some explanations for the differences.

Main causes of death by gender

At the beginning of the twentieth century the major causes of death for both males and female were infections and respiratory diseases (Social Trends 2001) (see Chapter 1). Over the course of the twentieth century, infections declined and were replaced by circulatory diseases and cancers, as the population lived longer and standards of living and health care improved. Figure 9.4 shows the changes in causes of death from 1911 to 1999 for males and females. At present, diseases of the circulatory system, the respiratory system and cancers account for approximately three-quarters of all deaths in both genders in Britain.

The figures show lower rates of all these causes of death for females and, until the 1980s, circulatory diseases were the predominant cause of death for both genders, followed by cancers and finally respiratory diseases. Diseases of the circulatory system steadily declined as the major cause of female death from the 1940s, whereas the male rate did not do so until the 1970s and then the gradient was much steeper. However, although circulatory diseases continue as the major cause of male deaths (two-fifths of deaths in males 20–64 in 1991–3), they are now closely followed by cancers (one-third of deaths in males 20–64 in 1991–3) (Drever et al 1997). In females, cancers overtook circulatory diseases as the main cause of death in 1983, and although the overall cancer rate continues to decline slowly for both genders, in females it now comprises 42% of the overall death rate in Great Britain (Social Trends 2001). The British female cancer rate compares unfavourably with other EU countries. Figure 9.5 shows the main causes of death for

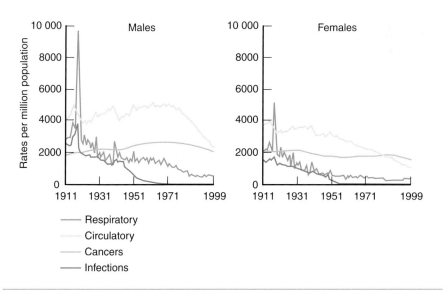

Fig. 9.4 Mortality (people aged 15–74) by gender and major cause (UK data, which have been age-standardized to the European population).

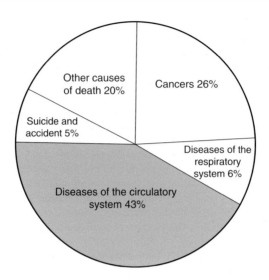

Fig. 9.5 Main causes of death of women in the fifteen European Union countries (1992).

women in the EU in 1992. For the fifteen EU countries, cancers claimed only 26% of female lives, compared with the British 42% (European Commission 1997).

Breast cancer

In the European Union in 1992, breast cancer was responsible for 21% of female deaths, and was the main cause of death in women aged 35–64 years. The incidence is rising in many EU countries and it is suspected that better screening contributes to the increase. Survival rates are also improving due to more effective treatments (European Commission 1997). However, the British mortality rate at this time for women of all ages was the second highest in the community after Denmark. The key risk factors given are age, with two-thirds of cases in women over 50, and having a mother or sister with the disease. Lesser factors appear to be early menarche before 11, late menopause after 54, childlessness and first full-term pregnancy over the age of 30 (European Commission 1997). By 2001, the Imperial Cancer Research Fund (ICRF) revealed that the rising breast cancer rate in Britain had now overtaken lung cancer as the most common form of cancer. They suggest that causal factors might include the trend for women to have babies later in life, but also increasing rates of obesity in women over 50 (ICRF 2001). By 1998, 84% of women aged 25–64 in England had been screened at least once for breast cancer in the previous 5 years compared with only 44% in 1988 when national screening began (The Women's Unit 2000). The ICRF pointed out that although 25% of women over 50 invited for screening fail to attend, improving survival rates mean that 70% of cases are now successfully treated (ICRF 2001).

Suicide

Suicide is starkly gendered in Britain with a long-established excess for males over females. In 1971 the male suicide rate was one-and-a-half times the female rate, but by 1998 the gap had widened and the male rate is now three times the female rate. For females, the rate for those aged 15–24 rose marginally in the latter years of this period whereas that for other age groups remained stable. For men the picture is very different and the trends are worrying. Suicides in those aged 15–24 increased two-and-a-half times, whereas those aged 25–44 doubled their rate in this period. Meanwhile, suicides among older men have come steadily down (Social Trends 2001).

Marital status also seems to be related to the suicide rates. The suicide rate for widowed and divorced men is double that for those who are married, and the rate for single men is slightly less than the rate for widowed and divorced but is rising steadily. Although the female rates are much lower, again it is the widowed and divorced who have the highest rates (Social Trends 2001).

EXPLAINING GENDER DIFFERENCES IN MORTALITY AND LIFE EXPECTANCY IN WESTERN COUNTRIES

With the growing interest in gender studies in Western societies, so the range of explanations relating to gender differences in mortality in such countries has increased. These include both biological explanations and a wide range of explanations based on social factors. Arber & Thomas (2001) list the following types of explanation: biological, psychosocial differences, risk behaviours, occupational and work factors, social roles and relationships, power and resources in the home and social structural differences within society.

One key factor said to be responsible for male mortality is the nature of male occupations. More occupations typically followed by men involve direct risk to life, for example through individual accidents, failure of machinery and weather and environmental hazards. Such occupations as underground and surface mining, working on the oil rigs, fishing, construction and heavy industry are typical. Additionally, it has been argued that male employment opportunities place men at higher risk of danger from the industrial process through exposure to toxic chemicals, radiation and so on, which will have a longer term reach but are implicated in a range of cancers, respiratory diseases and other conditions. What should be noted here is the connection between mortality risk and class. It is largely lower-class males who are most at risk (see Chapter 8).

Although occupations are still heavily gendered worldwide, so too is risk-taking behaviour. Masculinity, it seems, needs to be affirmed and continually renegotiated by men's participation in activities such as dangerous sports like hang-gliding, car and motorbike racing, rock-climbing and so on. Men also generally drive more than women and faster (hence the preferential insurance rates for women). Overall, males have more accidents than females and this is especially reflected in excess mortality for young men in the age group 15–25. This propensity to accidents manifests itself early in childhood in the generally more physical behaviour of young boys, leaving a question mark over the relative effects of biology and gender socialization. Boys engage in more dangerous pastimes in sport and in peer groups and take more risks than girls, but males from boyhood also engage in more physical aggression towards one another, so excess male deaths from violence and murder can be added to the equation. However, there is recent evidence that violence is growing among young women as they take on more of the behaviour patterns of young men. Recent cases of mugging and assisted rape by young women might indicate a trend here.

Another gendered form of risky behaviour is smoking. Men have always smoked more than women, and although overall trends are well down, by 1998 about one-quarter of both males and females were smoking regularly. Girls up to the age of 15 are now more likely than boys to be regular or occasional smokers (Drever et al 2000). If this trend continues, smoking-related diseases will continue to rise for women. For both males and females, heavier levels of smoking continue to be higher in lower socioeconomic classes and in single people (Rainford et al 2000), and there is some suggestion that single women working in previously male strongholds, for example City finance occupations, are increasing their levels of smoking significantly.

Male excess mortality is also linked to higher alcohol intake; but younger women have recently increased their drinking habits so gendered health patterns might be changing here as well. At the end of the 1990s, the heaviest alcohol intake for females was concentrated in those aged 16–24, with 25% drinking over 14 units per week compared to 16% 10 years previously (Davies et al 2000), whereas heavy drinking in men extended from those aged 16 to 44 (Social Trends 2001). Unlike smoking patterns, however, whereas for men higher intake still remains in the lower socioeconomic groups, for women intake is higher in the professional classes (Rainford et al 2000).

The masculine persona has also been implicated in the effect of differential health behaviour on risk of mortality. It has been contended that men more readily shrug-off the symptoms of illness in the early stages and consult later when the damage is greater. It has been argued that illness is seen as weakness and not consistent with being a 'real' man. However, an alternative view might suggest that women's closeness with their bodies through menstruation and childbirth and the long tradition of women as carers, has rendered females more aware of bodily symptoms and more socialized into the potential illness/patient role.

GENDER AND MORBIDITY – KEY DIFFERENCES

Although the explanations for gender differences in mortality are rarely disputed, morbidity differentials invite more controversy. First, there is dispute about whether, indeed, the higher morbidity traditionally attributed to women actually exists or whether it is mere artefact. Second, recent interest in men's health suggest that real changes in gendered morbidity have occurred and that men are suffering more illness and are increasing their use of the health services.

As Arber & Thomas (2001) point out, it has become an accepted fact that 'women are sicker but men die quicker'. In relation to morbidity, a major focus has been on self-reported data relating to gender differences in general health, long-standing illness, limiting long-standing illness and restricted activity 14 days prior to interview. In the mid-1990s a variety of surveys were showing small but relatively consistent female excesses in morbidity, with more females self-reporting their general health as poor or fairly poor, while longitudinal data from 1972 to 1994 showed small excesses of around 2–3% for females across that period on the other three measures (Annandale 1998, OPCS 1995). The 1998 Health Education Monitoring Survey (Rainford et al 2000) reinforces earlier results, showing 4% more females reporting both less good health and limiting long-standing illness. In the same survey 5% more women than men admitted to suffering a large amount of stress. Table 9.2, produced by the Women's Unit at the Cabinet Office, shows self-reported health problems by gender and age for 1996–7.

Other data show that women are more likely than men to consult a professional in relation to their health. In the working-age group 16–64, men average four consultations each year, whereas women average almost double this, at just over seven consultations (OPCS 1998). Studies on symptom-reporting also show significant gender differences. MacIntyre et al (1996) analysed datasets from the 1980s and found that when all reported symptoms were considered, there was a consistent and significant female excess, as there was with symptoms of 'malaise', but that the difference in physical symptom reporting, although still present, was not significant. Data also clearly indicate that gender differences

TABLE 9.2	Self-reported health problems by gender (%)				
	Age range				
Problem	**16–44**	**45–64**	**65–74**	**75 and over**	**All aged 16 and over**
Males					
Pain or discomfort	18	39	52	56	32
Mobility	6	22	36	50	18
Anxiety or depression	12	19	20	19	15
Problems performing usual activities	5	16	21	27	12
Problems with self-care	1	6	8	14	5
Females					
Pain or discomfort	20	40	51	65	34
Mobility	6	21	37	60	19
Anxiety or depression	18	24	25	30	22
Problems performing usual activities	7	17	23	40	15
Problems with self-care	2	5	9	21	6

From OPCS (2002) General Household Survey, Office for National Statistics; Continuous Household Survey, Northern Ireland Statistics and Research Agency

in health vary with age, and Arber & Thomas (2001) report that older women are more likely to suffer from chronic but non-fatal conditions and disabilities that affect their daily quality of life. Specifically, they indicate that in Britain in 1994, in those aged 65 or more, women were twice as likely as men to suffer from functional impairments needing daily support to keep them living in the community. The MacIntyre article, however, although acknowledging substantial evidence of sex differences, stresses that their direction and magnitude varies by symptom, condition and stage in life course, and that oversimplification is dangerous.

MASCULINITY, FEMININITY AND NORMALITY

Women's mental health, and the way it has been defined and treated since the earliest times within Western societies, has been one of the key concerns of the women's movement since the 1970s. Central to this whole issue has been the way in which concepts of normality in society would appear to have been constructed from a male perspective, creating the man as mentally robust and the woman as mentally fragile. Within this general model women are subordinated to a masculine construction of reality placing the male at the centre of humanity with women on the periphery. The male as a biological, social and psychological being becomes the template against which all other forms of life are compared. The male identity is superior whereas the female identity is flawed. This long-standing male/female dichotomy was strengthened when Enlightenment thinking in Europe decreed that women were not inherently logical or rational, bound as they were by their reproductive ties to nature, and so were unable to achieve cognitive skills equal to men. The essential character of womanhood was said to be constructed from common sense and intuitive understanding. With these ideas deeply embedded in social norms, the emerging concept of citizenship marginalized womanhood as 'biologically ill-equipped to exercise pure uncontaminated reason' and therefore as incapable of exercising the full rights of public citizenship. The 'normal' woman was entrenched as a semi-citizen, better suited to the private sphere of the home than the rough and tumble of the public domain, and under the 'natural authority of the male head of household' (Scambler 1998).

Connell's model (1987, 1995) describes the gender order in terms of three major social structures: how labour is organized, where power is held, and through sexual and emotional relations. These three interlinking structures interact constantly to create a gender hierarchy fundamental to which is the dominance of men over women. Connell's gender order ranks the key gender categories according to the model shown in Fig. 9.6.

At the top of the hierarchy is 'hegemonic' masculinity, focused on authority and comprising the culturally dominant ideals of paid work, physical strength and heterosexuality. This is followed by complicit masculinity. This is the level where most men live their lives, falling short of the hegemonic ideal but gaining significant social advantages from their association with it. Further down we have the subordinated masculinities, spearheaded by homosexuality, which do not fully conform to the hegemonic ideal, and where men are seen as wanting. Significantly, in Connell's model, even the lowest masculine category exceeds the feminine in the gender order, but the whole hierarchy is open to internal contestation or even crisis.

Such social constructions of masculinity and femininity, and the power relations they engender, are profoundly difficult to dislodge and structure individual and social actions deep below the surface of everyday life. Since the 1960s, the women's movement has been building-up a picture of how patriarchy functions at all its levels, and one of the most problematic relates to the construction of woman herself.

Feminists have slowly broken down the categories of male and female to expose the underlying patriarchal discourse. What has become clear is the way the social gendering of the two sexes has not just empowered men at the expense of women, but that it was the male gender that actually created this hierarchy of identity and mental well-being in the first place. Theorists from within the post-modern perspective suggest that the source of women's oppression lies in the symbolism created by masculine power structures. Irigaray (1985) cites what she calls the 'male imaginary', and asserts that men have used 'phallocentric logic' to create a symbolic order that imposes gender opposites comprising a range of dualities (rational/irrational, logical/illogical) defining women as 'other' and 'lacking', or as object in relation to the male subject (Irigaray 1985). Many feminists have additionally pointed to the fact that the traits attributed to the male are those socially valued, especially in the public domain. The female psyche, conversely, is deemed suitably placed in the devalued domestic arena.

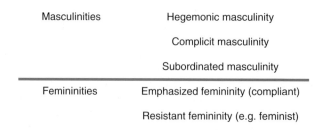

Masculinities	Hegemonic masculinity
	Complicit masculinity
	Subordinated masculinity
Femininities	Emphasized femininity (compliant)
	Resistant femininity (e.g. feminist)

Fig. 9.6 Hierarchy of gender categories (according to Connell 1987, 1995).

GENDER AND ISSUES OF MENTAL HEALTH

Others interested in the area of mental health have explored the medical treatment of women during the nineteenth and twentieth centuries and have constructed a picture of misogynistic control of women by an emerging (male) psychiatric profession. Ehrenreich & English (1979) documented the ways in which women were firstly defined as mentally fragile (they were seen as suffering from hysteria, the vapours, were too overtly sexual or were insubordinate to their husbands), and then the source of the problem was located firmly within women's reproductive systems. Women would find themselves propelled to the physician where various remedies would be applied. They could be subject to what would now be seen as sensory deprivation, confined to a darkened room and forbidden to read or exercise their minds in the interests of a cure. For cases of hysteria, slapping with wet towels was one of the techniques used to bring the woman to her senses, and for sexual proclivity the clitoris was sometimes removed.

The focus on misogynistic psychiatry gathered force, and much work was produced suggesting that patriarchal definitions of female mental health persisted throughout the twentieth century and are still apparent in the twenty-first. As Prior (1999) points out, a number of theorists have suggested that male-dominated psychiatry, heavily contaminated by patriarchal psychoanalytic theory, has tended to stereotype female behaviour within a 'catch 22' situation where women can be defined as mentally unstable if they conform to the female norm, or conversely, deviate from it. The dominant discourse of psychiatry, it is contended, incorporated the gendered dualisms outlined above, and tenets of masculinity such as rationality, competitiveness and creativity became fundamental to the notion of the mentally healthy adult, in contrast to the psychologically unhealthy 'female' characteristics of, for example, passivity, conformity and lower motivation for achievement. For a large part of the twentieth century women's mental health continued to be seen as fragile. Unhappiness, anxiety, depression and so on were regarded as a normal part of the female condition and routine treatment with drugs such as Librium, Valium and Prozac was widespread. Prescription drug dependence also became a problem as long-term prescribing became commonplace as part of what came to be seen as the 'medicalization of female unhappiness'.

What, then, of the mental health of men? How was their unhappiness or debility defined and treated? Viewed from a constructionist perspective one can suggest that the dominant masculine identity did not allow for the fragility of mental disorders deemed to be indicative of a 'weak character', such as neuroses, anxiety states and depression. These were clearly female states, or might, perhaps, emerge in males of a more artistic temperament. Thus, it has been contended, much male mental ill-health has lacked an acceptable social category and was thus rendered invisible. Doctors operating within the discourse would not define male distress as mental illness unless it appeared in a socially appropriate masculine form of deviance for men. Not permitted to express their mental debility in the same ways as females, they could, however, do so via aggressive behaviour, criminal behaviour, the use of drugs and alcohol, or in the more 'heroic' medically defined expressions of mental derange-ment such as psychotic behaviour.

This way of looking at the gendering of mental illness suggests that men suffered alongside women but that their problems were not recognized, were redefined or the unhappiness was either suppressed or channelled into alternative forms. Within the constructionist view, as Prior points out, an increase in male mental illness statistics must mean 'that the conceptualisation of mental disorder has changed so that men are now more likely to be diagnosed as having psychiatric problems' (Prior 1999). Indeed, in the late 1980s and into the 1990s studies in the USA indicated that if alcohol and drug dependence and personality disorders were included as psychiatric categories, a very large number of men would be pulled into the statistics on mental disorder, rather than boosting those on criminal justice. In positive terms this could mean a more sympathetic treatment of male unhappiness, but in negative terms it could simply imply greater medicalization of men. Prior contrasts the constructionist view with the 'social causation' perspective. From this standpoint it is contended that the actual incidence of mental problems for men is greater because their exposure to stressful life experiences has burgeoned. What becomes increasingly clear is that it is not possible to treat the issue as an either/or.

Gender differences in mental illness

Despite recent changes in male mental health behaviour, a range of data still show gender differences. MacIntyre et al's (1996) analysis presented consistent evidence of a female excess for psychological distress across the lifespan. Women were found to be significantly more likely to admit to neurotic disorders such as anxiety and depression, and to consult more for such conditions. Between 1994 and 1998, women in England and Wales were two-and-a-half times more likely to be treated for depression than men, with rates of 61 per 1000 patients. For men it was only 25 per 1000 (Social Trends 2001).

Mental illness is a difficult area to research because definitions of mental health categories are contentious and it has been suggested that prevalence statistics and those relating to medical treatment might be contaminated by under-reporting of symptoms by some sectors of society because of problems of stigma. In addition, the medical profession has had a patriarchal mind-set in relation to what constitutes mentally healthy behaviour for males and females. Busfield (2002) presents a clear and concise map of the distribution of psychiatric disorders by gender, using the data from an OPCS study of 1995, the results of which are presented below. She creates a three-fold typology of disorders, which she then relates to gender. These are disorders of thought, emotion and behaviour:

- Disorders of thought: comprising more severe conditions such as functional psychoses, including schizophrenia

- Disorders of emotion: including depression, anxiety states, phobias and neuroses

- Disorders of behaviour: including behaviour and personality disorders such as alcohol and drug dependence.

Table 9.3 gives the gender prevalence of psychiatric disorders for adults 16–64. These data were collected in the community. The data can be grouped into Busfield's three categories. She calls the first group (the neurotic disorders) disorders of emotion, and this can be seen to have a clear female excess. The second group is represented by functional psychoses and constitutes her disorders of thought; here there is no gender relationship and the balance appears to be equal. The third group is represented by alcohol and drug dependence and constitutes her disorders of behaviour; this category has a significant male excess. The findings from this survey mirror the general results from many other surveys in the community, with women predominating in the minor psychiatric morbidity category as exemplified by the disorders of emotion above.

In Britain, women make up the majority of those being admitted to psychiatric inpatient care, and have done so since the middle of the nineteenth century. There is also an abundance of research to indicate that women are much more likely to be prescribed psychoactive drugs than men, as much as double in some studies (Prior 1999). However, men are twice as likely to be sectioned as women.

What seems to be apparent is that, although women take more mental ill health to the GP and get more treatment overall, there is a gender imbalance in specialist care, with men

TABLE 9.3	Psychiatric disorders by gender (from Meltzer et al 1995)		
	Female	**Male**	**Ratio female:male**
Rates per 1000 in the past week			
Mixed anxiety and depression	99	54	1.8
Generalized anxiety disorder	34	28	1.2
Depressive episode	25	17	1.5
All phobias	14	7	2.0
Obsessive–compulsive disorder	15	9	1.7
Panic disorder	9	8	1.1
All neurotic disorders	195	123	1.6
Rates per 1000 in the past year			
Functional psychoses	4	4	0.0
Alcohol dependence	21	75	0.3
Drug dependence	15	29	0.5

getting referred on to specialists at a higher rate than women. Both Payne (2001) and Prior (1999) suggest that men pass more easily through the primary care filter, whereas women are more likely to be treated by their GPs. In addition, within specialist care, women are more likely to end up in outpatients and men more likely to be referred for inpatient treatment. Payne suggests that this reflects the gender hierarchy, with men able to command access to more resources than women. However, she sees the picture as much more complicated. The changes in mental health care enacted over the past few decades, with big reductions in psychiatric beds, the placing of psychiatric care into district hospitals and the improvement in drug treatments that reduce inpatient stay or can be offered to outpatients, might have resulted in rationing of inpatient care, which has left men more at risk than women. But why should men between 20 and 34 be so prominent in the statistics at present? Payne considers the relationship between criminal behaviour and mental ill health. Men are much more likely to be imprisoned than women (less than 5% of the prison population is female). Young men are four times less likely to be admitted to psychiatric hospital than to be imprisoned, while the reverse is true for young women (Payne 2001).

However, recent changes suggest that problematic young men are increasingly being seen as targets for the 'medical gaze' rather than just that of the criminal justice system. Young men, as has been shown, have a worryingly high and increasing suicide rate. Men, generally, are also consulting more than ever before for depressive illness. One cause might be changing norms on the acceptability of males expressing unhappiness as mental illness, as was discussed earlier, but it could also be the result of Payne's notion of 'the redundant male'. Men are now more likely to be unemployed than women, with young men especially vulnerable. Young women are more independent, have better careers and young people are in looser relationships for longer and having children later. It is suggested that young men have lost a structure to their lives and that this has resulted in a surge of unhappiness and mental illness. However, the perception is that, with young men, unhappiness results in aggressive and problematic behaviour, and Payne implies that the new psychiatric interest in this group of patients mirrors the custodial response of the criminal justice system and promotes inpatient care. The same reasoning could explain the sectioning figures; simply that men under stress are seen as much more of a public threat than women and need to be closely controlled.

FEMININITY, EMBODIMENT AND HEALTH

Another key factor deemed to have a detrimental effect on the mental well-being of women is negative body image. Frost (2001) contends that negative and frequently damaging sets of emotions focused on the body are common in females, beginning at an early age and resulting in the alienation of young women from their bodies. The range of conditions connected with what she calls 'body hatred' is disturbingly broad and affects the mental and physical well-being of a large number of females.

Eating disorders

The American psychiatric diagnostic criteria for anorexia cites disturbance in perception of body weight and shape with fear of weight gain and refusal to maintain minimal normal weight. Body image is linked to self-esteem and there is also absence of at least three consecutive menstrual cycles. Both anorexia and bulimia are female conditions, rarely affecting males, although there is some suggestion that this could be changing (present estimates are 5–10% of total), and largely absent outside Western societies. Bulimia is characterized by binge eating with loss of sense of control, compensated by behaviour to reverse the effects such as use of laxatives and self-induced vomiting. Body shape and weight are again central and bulimia can occur apart from anorexic episodes. Figures cited by Frost (2001) suggest that the full clinical condition of anorexia overwhelmingly affects adolescents and young women. Between 1 and 4% have the condition, with some American studies quoting rates up to 33% for college women. Anorexia appears to peak between ages 15 and 19, and seems to be increasing in prevalence. In Britain all ethnic groups are somewhat affected, but referrals are mainly white, middle-class women.

It would appear, therefore, that a woman's mental well-being is gendered in a complex range of ways that combine to make her especially vulnerable to lowered self-esteem, anxiety, tension and depression. Her whole being is rendered suspect from her femininity to her sexual competence, to her intellectual competence, to her capacity for paid work and physical activity and for mothering. She is unable to match social expectations in relation to her body and in Connell's hierarchy she is not just valued below hegemonic masculinity she is valued lower than the masculine underclass.

Childbirth and medicalization

Childbirth is an issue of central importance to women and is especially significant because of charges of medicalization levelled against it. It has been the subject of much debate around women's control of their own bodies and campaigns to reclaim childbirth have been prominent in the women's movement since the 1970s. In Britain, Oakley (1984) spearheaded some of the key discussions, looking especially at the way childbirth seemed to have progressed from being a normal biological and family event in women's lives to becoming a medical event, defined and ordered by medical professionals and including surveillance and control of the birth itself within hospitals. Oakley and others focused on the way in which the obstetrical profession has created a 'risk' situation out of a normal biological event by defining childbirth as potentially pathological until after a safe delivery in hospital. The woman became a patient from the moment the impending birth was confirmed by her GP, and was then subject to a range of tests and examinations throughout her pregnancy, culminating in a controlled hospital delivery. The whole process became known as 'technological childbirth', and blood and urine tests, scans and so on began to take place at intervals to maintain an ordered trajectory of the pregnancy. This plethora of tests often resulted in what came to be known as the 'cascade of intervention'. A scan might suggest a baby either growing too slowly or too quickly or a potentially small pelvic canal, for example, and early induction might ensue, culminating in an increased need for analgesics, with enhanced danger to the baby, a caesarean section or even fetal surgery. What was being suggested was that once the train of events was set in motion it was difficult to get back to a low-tech birth. Now less than 1% of British pregnant women have no prenatal tests (Graham et al 2000), and even in the mid-1990s, research showed many women did not realize that antenatal screening is optional, such are the subtle pressures on women to conform (Jackson 2001).

Between 1927 and 1997 the change from birth at home to birth in hospital was dramatic, as Table 9.4 indicates (Lloyd & Woroch 2000). Moves to promote 100% hospitalization of births, such as the Government Peel Report of 1970, made spurious connections between the reduction in perinatal mortality rates over this period and the increased hospitalization of births. Tew (1990) and others, using statistical analyses, later pointed to alternative and more significant factors in the mortality reduction, such as better nutrition and standards of living of mothers, better contraception and fewer pregnancies. Meanwhile, the average rate of caesarean sections had escalated from under 10% in the 1970s to 17% by 1997. In some hospitals this rate has touched 30%. This rise has been variously attributed to the heroic maintenance of borderline viable fetuses, medical fashion; the desire for pain-free or planned childbirth by some mothers and increased litigation threats. As an extreme example of patriarchal control in childbirth 'forced' caesarean sections are frequently cited using well-publicized enacted cases from the USA, and attempts by hospitals like St Georges in Tooting, to mirror this practice. Reasons given include lack of competence to decide her own best interests by the woman and protection of the unborn child against a non-complying mother (for a discussion, see Jackson 2001).

Various associations – the Association for Radical Midwives (ARM), The National Childbirth Trust and the Maternity Alliance – began to respond to these changes. Questioning of childbirth procedures and the whole organization of maternity care gradually came under public scrutiny. Women began to ask for women-focused birth with their needs taken into account. They began to critique the medical notion that childbirth was a "double medical emergency" for mother and baby. Some commentators saw this as a confrontation between the lay sector and the experts and evidence of the use of professional power by doctors to shroud the process of childbirth in medical mystique. ARM began to ask for more independence from the obstetrical profession and middle-class women for rights to choose the type of birth and level of technology they wanted, especially for forms of 'natural childbirth', midwife-assisted births and more recognition of the experience of childbirth as a personal and family event. Some changes were instigated as a result of

TABLE 9.4	Changes in place of birth									
	1927	1937	1946	1957	1968	1973	1984	1990	1993	1997
Hospital	15	25	54	64.6	80.7	91.4	99	99	98	97
Home/elsewhere	85	75	46	35.4	19.3	8.6	1	1	2	3

From Audit Commission (1997; figures for 1993 and 1997); Lewis (1980; figures for 1927, 1937 and 1946); Oakley (1984; figures for 1957, 1968 and 1973); OPCS (1992; figures for 1984 and 1990).
Figures are percentages of live births.
Figures for hospital include hospitals, maternity homes and poor-law institutions.

interest group action by the 1980s, with hospitals being encouraged to allow 'domino' births – birth in the hospital with a midwife and discharge into domiciliary midwife care after as little as 6 hours if no problems presented – and choices relating to pain-relief and sometimes water births and other forms of birthing techniques. By the 1990s it began to be recognized that offering choice might have political advantages (and be cheaper), and the 1993 government report, 'Changing childbirth' focused on choice for women and was proactive towards the idea of 'home birth', an issue that had suffered much negative battering from previous governments of both persuasions (DoH 1993).

CONCLUSION: DO WE NEED TO FOCUS ON MEN'S HEALTH NOW?

It would be premature to abandon a focus on women's health issues in favour of a more 'neutral' gender approach, although there is evidence that the health of males is changing and that they might be taking on some of the health profiles usually attributed to women, especially in the area of mental health, where statistical evidence supports an increase in inpatient treatment for men and more general practice consultations for depression. Other evidence also seems to suggest that men are more interested than they used to be in health matters (they are subscribing to magazines on men's health and are increasingly, especially younger men, including fitness workouts and body-building in their daily routines). However, changes in women's behaviour have also tended to move them closer to masculine norms and values, and there is evidence of younger women undertaking fitness regimes, while also taking on 'male' patterns of behaviour such as heavier drinking and smoking, more participation in contact sports and in related 'laddish' behaviour. The effect on the health of females of these changes could well be mixed. Current evidence, however, does little to suggest that there are fundamental changes taking place in the power base of society or the gender order that underpins gender health profiles.

References

Annandale E 1998 The sociology of health and medicine; a critical introduction. Polity Press in association with Blackwell Publishers, Cambridge

Annandale E, Hunt K (eds) 2000 Gender inequalities in health. Open University Press, Buckingham

Arber S, Thomas H 2001 From women's health to a gender analysis of health. In Cockerman W (ed) The Blackwell companion to medical sociology. Blackwell, Oxford

Brisson C 1999 Study on work and stress. Lavel University, Quebec

Busfield J 2002 The archaeology of psychiatric disorder: gender and disorders of thought, emotion and behaviour. In Bendelow G et al (eds). Gender, health and healing: the public/private divide. Routledge, London

Camden Domestic Violence Forum 1999 Domestic violence: a training pack for health professionals. London Borough of Camden, London

Connell R 1987 Gender and power. Polity Press, Cambridge

Connell R 1995 Masculinities. Polity Press, Cambridge

Crompton R 1997 Women and work in modern Britain. Oxford University Press, Oxford

Davies H, Joshi H, Rake K, Alami R 2000 Women's incomes over the lifetime: a report to the Women's Unit, Cabinet Office. The Stationery Office, London

Department of Health (DoH) 1993 Changing childbirth: report of the expert maternity group. HMSO, London

Doyal L 1995 What makes women sick: gender and the political economy of health. Macmillan, London

Drever F, Bunting J, Harding D 1997 Male mortality from major causes of death. In Drever F, Whitehead M (eds) Health inequalities. Office for National Statistics, London

Drever F et al 2000 Social inequalities. Office for National Statistics, London

Ehrenreich B, English D 1979 For her own good, 150 years of the experts' advice to women. Pluto Press, London

European Commission 1997 The state of women's health in the European Community. Luxembourg Office for Official Publications of the European Community, Luxembourg

Frost L 2001 Young women and the body, a feminist sociology. Palgrave, Basingstoke, UK

Graham W et al 2000 Randomised controlled trial comparing effectiveness of touch screen system with leaflet for providing women with information on prenatal tests. British Medical Journal 320:155–160

Imperial Cancer Research Fund (ICRF) 2001 November Report

Irigaray L 1985 This sex which is not one. Cornell University Press, Ithaca, NY

Jackson E 2001 Regulating reproduction. Hart Publishing, Oxford

Labour Force Survey 2001 Autumn report. The Stationery Office, London

Lloyd C, Woroch K 2000 Visions and values in health: a case-study of childbirth. Unit 5 in Visions and values in health, which forms block one of the course Working for health. Open University, Milton Keynes, UK

MacIntyre S, Hunt K, Sweeting H 1996 Gender differences in health: are things really as simple as they seem? Social Science and Medicine 42(4):617–624

Oakley A 1984 The captured womb. Blackwell, Oxford

Office of Population Censuses and Surveys (OPCS) 2002 Living in Britain. General Household Survey. HMSO, London

Office of Population Censuses and Surveys (OPCS) 1995 Living in Britain: results from the 1994 General Household Survey. HMSO, London

Office of Population Censuses and Surveys (OPCS) 1998 General Household Survey. HMSO, London

Payne S 2001 Masculinity and the redundant male: explaining the increasing incarceration of young men. In Heller T, Muston R, Sidell M, Lloyd C (eds) Working for health. Sage Publications, London

Pilcher J 1999 Women in contemporary Britain. Routledge, London

Prior P 1999 Gender and mental health. Macmillan, London

Rainford R, Mason V, Hickman M, Morgan A 2000 Health in England 1998: investigating the links between social inequalities and health. Health Education Monitoring Survey, Office for National Statistics/Health Education Authority, HMSO, London

Scambler A 1998 Gender, health and the feminist debate on postmodernism. In Scambler G, Higgs P (eds) Modernity, medicine and health. Routledge, London

Shorter E 1982 A history of women's bodies. Penguin, London

Social Trends (2001) Office for National Statistics, London, Stationery Office.

Tew M 1990 Safer childbirth? A critical history of maternity care. Chapman and Hall, London

The Women's Unit 2000 Women and men in the UK: facts and figures 2000. Cabinet Office/HMSO, London

Walby S 1990 Theorizing patriarchy. Blackwell, Oxford

World Health Organization (WHO) 2000 Violence against women. Information pack. WHO, Geneva

The Health and Health Care of Ethnic Minority Groups

Sheila Hillier

Central to the choices and constraints which structure the life chances of people in the modern world are those associated with race and ethnicity. (Mason 1996)

Everyone as a member of society is entitled to realization of the economic, social and cultural rights indispensable for dignity and the free development of personality. (General Assembly Resolution 217 A 111, Article 22. Universal Declaration of Human Rights)

Many governments are now confronting issues of multicultural diversity. There are debates about political rights, in particular what can be done to protect minority rights, devise inclusive notions of citizenship and democracy, and combat racism, both inter-personal and institutional.

The National Health Service, by its very structure and nature, is designed to be available to all citizens. This does not mean simply providing the same service to everybody – 'one size fits all' – but attempting to tailor the service to the needs of individuals and groups. Recognizing the needs of ethnic minorities was explicitly stated as national policy in the Patients' Charter (DoH 1991). Subsequently, a stronger emphasis on tackling the health inequalities and health needs of black and minority ethnic groups has been stated (DoH 2001).

WHAT ARE ETHNICITY, CULTURE AND RACE?

The search for national, ethnic and cultural identities has become an important quest for both majority and minority communities in the twenty-first century. Yet there is a lot of confusion around these concepts. They are often used interchangeably in an essentialist way, giving the impression that they are fixed, solid and immutable definitions, rather than a product of particular social relationships and conditions.

The example of the census illustrates some of the difficulties in reaching precise and/or workable definitions. In 1971, country of birth was used as a proxy for ethnic origin, thus ignoring the numbers of British-born members of minority ethnic groups. The term 'Asian' belied the great variety of different groups in the Indian subcontinent with different languages, origins and religions. In the 1981 census it was felt that the whole issue of ethnic categorization was so difficult that it should be dropped! Following wide discussion, the 1991 census, adopted nine basic ethnic groups, and people were asked to state to which group they thought they belonged. In the 2001 census, the divisible nature of 'white' ethnicity was recognized by the inclusion of an 'Irish' category for the first time.

As can be seen from Box 10.1, these issues are of more than academic interest. Although there might be difficulties in reaching precise definitions, they relate to very important social questions. Until recently, studies have been divided by a sterile debate between 'multiculturalists' and 'antiracists'. The former were accused of concentrating on 'superficial cultural difference' and of ignoring racist pressures. The latter were criticized for subsuming all minorities under the term 'black' or being 'antiracist' but not 'pro' much else (Gilroy 1998).

BOX 10.1	Definitions (from MacPherson 1999)

- **Ethnicity**: refers to a social group with an identity that is both collective and individual, and a common language, values, religious customs. The members are aware of sharing a common past, possibly a homeland, and might personally be aware of a sense of difference
- **Culture**: often reflects the ethnicity of one, or occasionally several, ethnic groups. Culture is 'what we do' and refers to habits of thought and behaviour, diet, dress, music and art. It is best described as a collective resource for the management of everyday behaviour and challenges and difficulties
- **Race**: is a construct based on a phenotypical biological difference (usually skin colour) although social assumptions (often negative) are attributed to biological difference
- **Racism**: deterministically associates inherent biological characteristics with negatively evaluated behaviours or actions. Racial discrimination is illegal
- **Institutional racism**: 'The collective failure of an organisation to provide an appropriate and professional service to people because of their colour, culture or ethnic origin. It can be seen or detected in processes, attitudes and behaviour which amount to discrimination through unwitting prejudice, thoughtlessness and racist stereotyping which disadvantages ethnic minority people.'

In reality, it is necessary to remember the stressful nature of the experience of racism, and the pressures associated with lacking access to power and material resources, as many ethnic groups will testify. It is also important to recognize cultural resources such as religion, contacts with kin abroad and communitarian ethics, which are also features of minority ethnic groups.

Why did people migrate?

We are over here, because you were over there. (Bangladeshi woman, Forum on Ethnicity and Health 1999)

Migration has been a worldwide phenomenon, involving whole populations since *Homo sapiens* first evolved on earth. The last two millennia are no exception, as far as Europe and Britain are concerned. The earliest black people to arrive in England were North African soldiers in the Roman army, brought to patrol Hadrian's Wall. Over the next two thousand years many migrants, Jews, Portuguese, Roman, French settled in Britain. From the sixteenth century onwards, England's colonial empire expanded. Africans were a common sight in eighteenth century London, where there was a very large community of about 10 000 (Fryer 1985). By the nineteenth century, similar communities existed in Cardiff and Liverpool. To these were added migrants from Ireland, particularly after the potato famine. In the twentieth century, major migration began after the Second World War, with Irish and Caribbean migrants being recruited actively into the expanding British economy. They tended to occupy the least favourable employment, setting a pattern that continues to this day. Migrants for the textile manufacturing industry were actively sought from India and Pakistan. Some groups like Hindus, Gujaratis, Sikhs, Punjabis and Hong Kong Chinese came from relatively well-off commercial backgrounds with experience of running small businesses. East African Asians expelled from Kenya and Uganda in the 1970s were also from professional and business families. People also came – and continue to come – to the UK because of war and displacement in their homeland, or because of rural poverty. These include those from the Sylhet province of Bangladesh, Zaireans, Kosovans, Bosnians, Kurds, Iraquis and Afghanis. Each group brings with it different combinations of economic circumstances, reasons for migration and cultural resources.

The economic expansion receded in Europe in the 1970s; controls on migration became more severe. By the 1990s there were calls for 'a strong perimeter fence around Europe'. The right to claim citizenship has also narrowed – children born in Britain no longer have automatic citizenship rights. There is always a fear that harsher policies towards migrants outside 'Fortress Europe' will impact on those ethnic minority groups inside (Sivanandan 1989).

It should be clear from these observations that all work that concerns ethnic minority groups has a political dimension. For example, it has been argued (Bhopal 1997) that a perception that the health of ethnic minority groups is poor can augment the belief that immigrants and ethnic minority groups are 'a burden'.

WHO ARE THE UK'S ETHNIC GROUPS?

There are now nearly four million people in the UK belonging to the minority ethnic groups listed in Table 10.1. If Irish people are included, the number becomes nearer five million. Until recently, however, government statistics did not provide a separate category of 'Irish', therefore much of the discussion below contrasts a uniform 'white' or 'general' majority (which includes Irish people), with minority ethnic groups from the Caribbean, South Asia and Africa.

TABLE 10.1	Population by ethnic group and percentage born in the UK 1991		
Ethnic group	**% Population**	**Number (000s)**	**% Born in UK**
White	94.5	51 584	95
Black Caribbean	0.9	500	54
Black African	0.4	212	36
Black Other	0.3	178	84
South Asian			
Indian	1.5	840	42
Pakistani	0.9	477	50
Bangladeshi	0.3	163	37
Chinese	0.3	157	28
Other Asians	0.4	198	44
Other	0.5	290	-

Reproduced with permission of Controller of HMSO and the Office of National Statistics from OPCS (1991).

Population structure

The minority population is generally younger than the white population; about one-third are aged below 16 years, compared with about one-fifth of the white population. The proportion of people aged 65 and over in the white group was five times that of the other minority groups. Irish and Black Caribbean groups tend to be older, whereas just under half of the Bangladeshi group were under 16, and three-quarters under 35 (ONS 1991). On average, there is 9 years' difference in the average age of the ethnic minority population compared with the majority.

In the population of the UK as a whole, females outnumber males because, overall, the average life expectancy of females is higher. In the minority groups, there are equal numbers of males and females, but males outnumber females in all three South Asian groups. In the Bangladeshi group there are 10% more males than females. This reflects earlier patterns of migration, where men arrived in the UK first and wives and families came over later (ONS 1991).

Because of its younger age structure, the minority age population is growing faster than the majority. Between 1992 and 1999 this population increased by 15.6%, compared with 1% of the white population. In the same period, the Bangladeshi population grew by 30% (The Times 2001).

Although relatively small, the number of older people – 'ethnic elders' – is also increasing, and stands at about 70 000 (OPCS 1991), around 4% of the most commonly listed ethnic minority groups. The largest number are African–Caribbean and the lowest is the Pakistani/Bangladeshi group. Because many worked in manual jobs, they are likely to have relatively low incomes in old age.

Geographical distribution

There are significant ethnic minority populations clustered in various parts of the UK, mainly in the major cities. Nearly half of the minority ethnic population lives in London (ONS 1996a).

Black Caribbean populations are found mainly in Inner and South London and in Birmingham. For Indians, London, Leicester, Wolverhampton and Slough are the most important; in Leicester, they make up one-fifth of the population. Pakistanis are most likely to live in the West Midlands, West Yorkshire and Lancashire textile towns and North and West London.

Bangladeshis form one-quarter of the population of Tower Hamlets, London, but also live in the West Midlands and towns in the north-west of England.

Family structure

South Asian households tend to be large – on average more than five people. Almost one in ten contains more than one family. One in five black households consists of a lone parent with dependent children, four times higher than white or South Asian households. This reflects different marriage patterns in the Black Caribbean group, where couples tend to live together without being legally married or have children without living together (ONS 1996b). Divorce rates are low and marriage rates high in the South Asian group. The latter also marry earlier, although second-generation women have a later age of marriage than their mothers. Although most marriages take place within the ethnic group, the proportion of young ethnically mixed couples is increasing (ONS 1996c).

Education

Because there is no data on performance prior to GCSE, most of the information relates to higher education. Ethnic groups show a strong commitment to education – over 60% of South Asians and 50% of black teenagers are still in school at 18, compared with 38% of whites. Chinese and white and Indian applicants are most likely to be accepted into higher education (over 70%). Black Caribbean and Pakistani applicants were significantly less likely to be admitted to university. Indians were more than twice as likely as black or other South Asian groups to be studying for a degree. Around half of the black and South Asian groups were studying for a science degree, compared with just under 20% of whites. Social science proved a popular choice, especially in the Indian group. Of all students in higher education, 8% of black, 12% of Indians, 10% of Pakistani/Bangladeshi, 9% of other ethnic groups and 7% of whites were studying medicine (ONS 1996d).

These data suggest a strong and, in some cases, successful involvement among minority ethnic groups for those able to break through the 'GCSE barrier' at age 16. However, type of qualification and likelihood of university admission suggest that social factors like discrimination or lowered expectations on the part of educators are continuing to affect achievement levels for some groups.

Employment and unemployment

Patterns of work vary among ethnic groups. As a whole, they are less likely to be working (especially women) and more likely to be unemployed, than the majority population.

Ethnic minority people tend to work in certain industries. These include hotels and restaurants (34% of Pakistani/Bangladeshi men) (Labour Force Survey (LFS) 1995) and black people are more likely to work in the health or education or public administration. Women from all ethnic groups are more likely to work in the public sector, but Asian women are more likely to occupy senior positions.

A survey of senior civil service positions and positions of seniority in the police and judiciary show slight improvements over 20 years. In 1965 there were no ethnic minority police officers, now these are about 2%. Recruitment to the armed forces and fire services also remains relatively low.

There are marked differences in employment of older men and women between black and other groups, with blacks more likely to continue in employment. In general, ethnic minorities were more likely to be temporarily employed.

Average hourly pay tends to be lower, with Pakistani/Bangladeshi women earning the lowest rates of all.

Self-employment varies a lot; Pakistanis and Bangladeshis are more likely to be self-employed – 22% – and men were more likely to be self-employed than women.

Unemployment rates vary a great deal between groups and are influenced by age, location and the decline in growth of industries. For each age group, unemployment is higher in all of the ethnic minority groups than for whites. There has been a general fall in unemployment; rates are lower for women, and higher for the young – reflecting a more common experience of youth unemployment. The most recent figures show unemployment among young black, Pakistani and Bangladeshi people aged 16–24 is nearly 40%, almost three times the rate for young white people.

In general, the economic position of members of ethnic minority groups has not improved greatly over 30 years. There has been a movement into white-collar jobs, yet most members of ethnic minorities remain concentrated in social classes IV and V. They continue to work in unskilled, low-paid occupations where working conditions are poor or dangerous. There are, however, important differences between ethnic groups, with blacks and Bangladeshis usually in a worse position economically than Indian or Chinese (ONS 1996e,f).

THE HEALTH OF ETHNIC MINORITY GROUPS

The data on the health of ethnic minority groups comes from a number of sources. The data on morbidity (the prevalence of ill health) is more recent and exhaustive than that on mortality (causes of death).

Adult mortality

The data on mortality is based on death certificates, which are classified according to country of birth, not ethnicity. For many years, analysts relied upon the work carried out by Marmot et al (1984) who studied OPCS data from a previous decade, i.e. nearly 30 years ago. A later study by Balarajan & Bulusu (1990) confirmed the finding that people who have migrated to the UK have higher death rates than those born here, but lower death rates than their home country. It is believed that this is because healthier people migrate – the 'healthy migrant factor'. An exception to this is the Irish ethnic minority (only recently examined separately), whose mortality rates are raised relative to home and UK populations. These effects persist into the second generation (Harding & Balarajan 1996, Raftery et al 1990). This suggests that the 'healthy migrant' factor does not fully explain mortality rates for this group. It has been suggested that people bring the risks of mortality associated with their early life and later acquire the risks associated with living in the UK, for example, cardiovascular risk.

Early studies presented a picture in which ethnic minority people were at risk from some of the same causes of mortality as UK-born people – coronary heart disease, stroke and diabetes. There were higher rates of perinatal mortality in some ethnic groups than in the UK-born. Some conditions like the haemoglobinopathics appeared almost exclusively in particular ethnic groups. Recent mortality figures for men and women are given in Tables 10.2 and 10.3.

| TABLE 10.2 | Standardized mortality ratios (SMR) by country of birth, men aged 20–64 years, England and Wales 1991–3 |

Ethnic group	All causes	Ischaemic heart disease	Stroke	Lung cancer	Other cancer	Accidents and injuries	Suicide
Total	100	100	100	100	100	100	100
Caribbean	89	60	169	59	89	121	59
West/South Africa	126	83	315	71	133	75	59
East Africa	123	160	113	37	77	86	75
Indian subcontinent							
India	106	140	140	43	64	97	109
Pakistan	102	163	148	45	62	68	34
Bangladesh	133	184	324	92	74	40	27
Scotland	129	117	111	146	114	177	149
Ireland	135	121	130	157	120	189	135

From Davey-Smith et al (2000).

| TABLE 10.3 | Standardized mortality ratios (SMR) by country of birth, women aged 20–64 years, England and Wales 1991–3 |

Ethnic group	All causes	Ischaemic heart disease	Stroke	Lung cancer	Other cancer	Accidents and injuries	Suicide
Total	100	100	100	100	100	100	100
Caribbean	104	100	178	32	87	103	49
West/South Africa	142	69	215	69	120	–	102
East Africa	127	130	110	29	98	–	129
Indian subcontinent	99	175	132	34	68	93	115
Scotland	127	127	131	164	106	201	153
Ireland	115	129	118	143	98	160	144

From Davey Smith et al (2000).
– no data. 100 = average for the whole population.

Data in these tables confirm that, for all groups except Caribbean men and Indian women, death rates from all causes are higher than for the UK average and, in some cases, are substantially higher. A closer look reveals a more complex picture (Davey Smith et al 2000). Although Caribbean men and women enjoy low rates for most causes of death, this advantage is spoilt by high rates of stroke and, for men, accidents and injuries. Men and women originating in South or West Africa have over three times the average death rate from stroke, as well as above average death rates from cancer. Interestingly, deaths from ischaemic heart disease are lower than average in this group. Men and women from the Indian subcontinent and East Africa have high death rates from heart disease and stroke, with the stroke mortality among Bangladeshi men being the highest among all groups. People from Scotland and Ireland also have very high mortality, particularly from lung cancer, accidents and suicide. A study of second-generation Irish also shows high mortality rates, especially from lung cancer, but other cancers too, and accidental and violent death. Mortality in men of Irish descent in the West of Scotland shows higher rates for heart disease and accidental and violent death. The ancestors of these men had migrated in the nineteenth century. This suggests that patterns of mortality can continue over generations (Abbots et al 1998).

Adult morbidity

The findings above have been strongly supported by morbidity data from several studies; these include the Health Education Authority's (HEA) Black and Ethnic Minority Health Survey (HEA 1992), the Policy Studies Institute Survey 'The Fourth National Survey of Ethnic Minorities' (Nazroo 1997a) and the Health Survey for England's 'Health of Ethnic Minority Groups' (Health Survey for England 1999).

The latest evidence from the Health Survey for England (1999) reveals that there are higher rates of ischaemic heart disease in Indian, Bangladeshi and Irish men and Irish women. Rates of stroke in Black Caribbean men are over two-thirds higher than average. There is a high prevalence of diabetes among South Asians, and high rates of hypertension among Black, Indian and Pakistani women (Box 10.2). Latest evidence shows no clear and consistent evidence between high blood pressure and either social class or household income (Health Survey for England 1999).

General morbidity – as opposed to morbidity from specific conditions – is divided into different categories. These are longstanding and limiting longstanding illness, acute sickness and self-assessed general health. The Health Survey for England (1999) showed that the prevalence of limiting longstanding illness was higher for Pakistani, Bangladeshi and Irish men, and Pakistani and Bangladeshi men reported worse general health than the general population. The ratios for bad/very bad health for men and women were 2.94 and 3.57 (Pakistani) and 3.91 and 3.31 (Bangladeshi). These findings are similar to the earlier study of 1996 (ONS 1996g). In both studies, the prevalence of reported bad health increased with age. Of all groups, the Chinese enjoyed the best health.

Childhood mortality

Data from the 1980s and 1990s showed that deaths were highest in the Pakistani and Caribbean populations. Pakistani babies had a higher risk of congenital malformations;

BOX 10.2	Main Health Issues for Ethnic Minority Groups

- **Coronary heart disease**: higher rates of angina and heart attack among Indian, Bangladeshi and Irish men, and Irish women.
- **Hypertension/stroke**: higher rates of stroke in Black Caribbean, Bangladeshi and Indian men. Women of Black Caribbean and Pakistani origin have higher rates of hypertension.
- **Perinatal mortality**: higher in ethnic minority groups, especially Pakistani, East African and Caribbean babies.
- **Haemoglobinopathies**: sickle-cell disease affects people in the Caribbean and African population.
- **Mental illness**: the diagnosis rates of schizophrenics are high in African–Caribbeans. General psychiatric morbidity rates are highest in Bangladeshis.
- **Diabetes**: South Asians (especially Pakistani and Bangladeshi women) have rates five times higher than the general population. High rates also seen in Black Caribbeans and Indians.

Bangladeshi mothers were more likely to experience a stillbirth. All measures of child mortality have shown declines over the last 20 years. Davey Smith et al's study (2000) shows that, for all measures, mothers born outside the UK have higher rates and Pakistani mothers have the highest rates of perinatal, neonatal and post-neonatal mortality, and Black Caribbean mothers the highest infant mortality (Table 10.4). The link with deprivation is not clear because Bangladeshi mothers are often in the poorest group, but their children enjoy a better mortality experience.

Childhood morbidity

A study from Glasgow compared British Asian 14–15-year-olds with non-Asians and found less limiting illness, accidents, drug-taking, smoking, drinking and fewer accidents in the British Asian group (Williams 1994). These trends were confirmed in the recent Health Survey for England. Indian, Chinese, Pakistani and Bangladeshi boys were less likely than boys and girls in the general population to report long-standing illness or acute sickness. Pakistani and Bangladeshi boys were also less likely to report good health than boys in the general population (Health Survey for England 1999); lower incidences of smoking and drinking were also recorded.

Mental illness

Evidence for the rates of mental illness among the ethnic minority population is derived from hospital admissions and from community studies. Conclusions based on hospital admission rates are of limited value, because not all cases come to hospital and the routes by which people arrive there vary considerably. The highest rates of hospital admissions are found in Irish migrants, whether from Northern Ireland or Eire. The next highest group are people from Caribbean-born populations and, finally, South Asians, whose rates are lower than the population of the UK and, in the case of Pakistan and Bangladesh, considerably lower. There are also large gender differences, with higher rates for women in every category except for the Caribbean-born. The all-admissions rate for the ethnic minority population is 9% higher than the UK population, but admissions for schizophrenia and paranoia are three times greater for men and twice as great for women among the Caribbean-born (Smaje 1995).

TABLE 10.4	Mortality in the first year of life by mother's country of birth			
Country of origin	**PMR**	**NMR**	**PNM**	**Infant mortality**
UK	8.2	3.9	1.9	5.8
East Africa	12.4	4.1	2.0	6.1
Bangladesh	9.5	4.2	2.2	6.3
India	11.2	3.9	1.5	5.4
Caribbean	11.5	4.7	3.6	8.4
Pakistan	15.8	6.5	3.6	10.1

Adapted from Davey Smith et al (2000).
NMR, neonatal mortality rate = deaths in the first 28 days per 1000 live births.
PMR, perinatal mortality rate = deaths in first week of life (including still birth) per 1000 live and stillbirths.
PNM, post-neonatal mortality rate = deaths between 28 days and 1 year per 1000 live births.
Infant mortality rate = deaths in the first year of life per 1000 live births.

Mental hospital admissions among young male African–Caribbeans are more likely to have been a result of police activity and to be related to compulsory detention under the 1983 Mental Health Act. Patients are more likely to be described as violent and detained in locked wards or secure units. They have a greater chance of receiving physical treatments and to be attended by junior staff.

Patterns of admission and treatment have been subject to a great deal of controversy. Some writers have argued that psychiatrists are more likely to diagnose schizophrenia in African–Caribbean patients or to exaggerate the importance of minor symptoms. Research in the USA does suggest that there is evidence of misdiagnosis and that cultural misunderstandings on the part of some psychiatrists might contribute to this. Other writers have argued that the stresses associated with migration, racism and disadvantage are responsible for producing a real schizophrenia epidemic among young African–Caribbeans. Although the definitions of normal and abnormal behaviour differ widely from culture to culture, there are no cultures that do not have some definition of disturbing, threatening or bizarre behaviour, especially when these occur without any obvious cause. Mental illness certainly occurs in ethnic minority groups. Whereas a Western diagnosis might place emphasis on psychological factors and life events or stress, in other cultures alternative explanations such as the breaking of a taboo and punishment or the capture of the soul by a spirit are all seen as explanations of mental illness. These explanations, and the wider social and cultural context, need to be taken into account if treatment is to be successful. In one reported case, religious healing accompanied the conventional psychiatric approaches when dealing with a mentally disturbed child (Hillier & Rahman 1996).

One of the most complete studies of ethnicity and mental health has come from The Policy Studies Institute (Nazroo 1997b). In this study, both psychotic and neurotic illnesses were investigated. The study was one of the first to match the ethnicity of interviewers and interviewees.

Nazroo's study challenged the commonly held view about extremely high rates of African–Caribbean psychosis. Almost all of the difference was attributable to higher rates amongst middle-aged Caribbean women, not young African–Caribbean men, as had been previously supposed. The study also showed a lower prevalence of neurotic illness among South Asian groups, which was statistically significant. Nazroo and his colleagues were suspicious of these findings, suggesting that the instruments used in the study failed to give an accurate assessment of the prevalence of neurotic illness among the South Asians. Strikingly, the prevalence of mental illness among South Asian groups was higher for those who were born in Britain or who had migrated to Britain at an early age than for those who had come to Britain after age 11. Prevalence was also higher for people who were fluent in English. Therefore it would seem that those who were the most 'acculturated' had the highest rates of mental illness. The authors raised the possibility that survey instruments might not accurately record prevalence among the less 'acculturated', rather than displaying a real difference. There was no clear relationship between psychosis and class position for Pakistanis and Bangladeshis, although a slight relationship was found for Indians and Africans; the strongest relationship between class position and mental health remains that for the white population.

The Health Survey for England (1999) considered scores on the general health questionnaire (GHQ12), which is designed to detect psychiatric morbidity in the general population. It is based on 12 questions on levels of happiness, depression, anxiety and sleep disturbance over the previous 4 weeks. Respondents with a score greater than four are identified as having a possible psychiatric disorder. Although it has been validated for the general population, its specific use in minority populations has not been addressed, and issues of translation might have affected the findings. The findings here reversed those of

155

Nazroo, with Bangladeshis and Pakistanis more likely than the general population to have a high GHQ score; Bangladeshis were highest. Black Caribbean and Indian women were also more likely to have a high score, whereas the Chinese were significantly less likely to have high scores than the general population. Nor were differences found to be significantly related to social class, especially when age standardization was applied. A relationship with income was also found. Those in the lowest income group were more likely to have higher GHQ scores.

The picture of ethnic minority mental health, then, is not altogether clear, and some of the problems are likely to be associated with the kinds of schedules that are used to measure mental health. Recently, a new set of research instruments, known collectively as EMIC, has been produced and tested. It seems to provide questions that are more culturally sensitive and therefore may be able to attune us to the subtleties of difference and similarity in the expression of symptoms of mental ill health among minority ethnic groups (Shaw et al 1999).

The data on ethnic variations in suicide rates, however, remain unchallenged. Current figures show that those born in the Caribbean and most of those born in South Asia have low rates of suicide compared to the general population, but that young women born in India and East Africa have much higher rates (Raleigh 1996). One problem is that the data are analysed by country of birth. This gives little knowledge of the impact of more recent cultural factors, particularly for young persons. Much interpretation, including the most recent (Bhugra 2000), draws attention to the presence of cultural conflict between young women and their families as an explanation of these high rates. However, other recent work (Haque & Hillier 2000) questions this assumption, saying that such rates are much less likely to be a result of 'culture' conflict, than of family conflict, which is not very different from that experienced by young white women.

WHY ARE MORTALITY AND MORBIDITY PATTERNS RAISED FOR ETHNIC GROUPS?

Influence of socioeconomic position

It is the case that most members of ethnic groups are to be found among the socioeconomically disadvantaged. Early research did not show a clear-cut relationship between social class and mortality, and for Caribbean men, the normal inverse trend was reversed. More recent analyses have demonstrated differences in stroke and in ischaemic heart disease between manual and non-manual classes, but not for Caribbeans and West/South Africans (Davey Smith et al 2000). Studies of ethnic morbidity (Nazroo 1997b) showed social class differences between manual and non-manual households. Those households without a full-time worker also displayed worse health.

When analyses are made by social class, mortality rates for men show a clear inverse gradient overall with a standardized mortality rate (SMR) of 71 for social classes I and II, compared with 135 for social classes IV and V. The differences are most pronounced for Scotland (82 compared with 186) and Bangladesh (132 compared with 233). Within ethnic groups, however, there are important variations, with the death rates in social class I ranging from 82 (Scotland) and 83 (Caribbean) to 132 (Bangladesh). Measures of current social class do not capture childhood experience, which can show up later as health disadvantage.

A clear relationship with social class comes in childhood deaths, where manual classes have the highest mortality rate (Raleigh & Balarajan 1995). Within ethnic groups, childhood deaths are higher in the socially disadvantaged Pakistani group, yet Bangladeshi mothers, generally of low economic status, have some of the lowest rates.

Pakistani babies have a higher rate of congenital malformations. Marriage between first cousins is common in Pakistani and other Muslim populations. It serves particular social objectives – the preservation of property, more comfortable in-law relationships and the availability of suitable partners – and so it is suggested that the social benefits outweigh the risks (Ahmad 1998).

It should not be thought that because relationships between class, socioeconomic position and ill health are not so clear cut as for the general population, they are unimportant. Clearly, the effects are there and the fact that ethnic minorities experience greater economic disadvantage is likely to add to their health problems.

Social support, social stress and racism

This has affected the way I live my life ... We are not free to go anywhere, especially at night, you would always be afraid of being injured, of having your car damaged or your family hurt. (Gujarati woman)

Experiences of racism and of social stress are sometimes offered as an explanation for the differing rates of ill health among ethnic minority groups. For example, South Asians born in the Indian subcontinent are the only ones to have experienced a rise in mortality from coronary heart disease between 1972 and 1983 (8% for men and 14% for women) when rates for the rest of the world were falling. The risk of greater mortality from heart disease for this group, it is sometimes suggested, lies not in the classical risk factors but in the likely excess of stressful life events (Williams et al 1994). However, it should be remembered that socioeconomic stresses are likely to be as great, if not greater, for the Caribbean population in which the lowest coronary heart disease rates are observed.

The social support data that come from the Health Survey for England, however, show some quite striking data in all minority groups. Except for Indians, men were more likely than women to be classified as experiencing a severe lack of social support. Groups particularly at risk were South Asian and Chinese men and women, who were at least twice as likely as the general population to lack social support. There were class differences, with people in non-manual social classes less likely to suffer from a lack of social support. This applied to all minority ethnic groups except Bangladeshis (Health Survey for England 1999). Lack of support seemed to increase with age for all groups except the Bangladeshis, where the trend was reversed. This applied to men only, not to women.

Racism and discrimination also affect health. The most obvious way is that the experience of racial discrimination and disadvantage make people feel harassed and victimized, resulting in mental distress and poor health. Discrimination can also affect people directly by placing them at a socioeconomic disadvantage (Virdee 1995). Such disadvantage is also quite obvious to individuals and groups and makes them feel unwelcome and unhappy. Research in the USA has confirmed higher rates of hypertension among those who tolerate harassment and discrimination, rather than those who challenge it. The argument here is that anger becomes internalized in those who accept rather than challenge their situation. Evidence from the Fourth National Survey (Nazroo 1997a), however, shows that experiences of racial harassment did not match those of poor health. Bangladeshi groups whose health, on the whole, is worse reported less harassment than African–Caribbeans. However, the admissibility of harassment, as with the African–Americans, is obviously something that requires further investigation.

Bhopal (1997) has written about racism in medicine, showing how current norms in healthcare treatment are based historically on the needs of the 'white' population, leading to an ethnocentric approach. This is why it is important to acknowledge race and ethnicity, but this acknowledgement in itself can form the basis for emphasizing difference and is potentially dangerous. However, the key issue is the equity that lies at the heart of the National Health Service and it is by now well documented that stark inequalities in the health and health-care of minority groups exist. There is discrimination against medical students from ethnic minorities, against overseas doctors and British-trained doctors with foreign names, and harassment of ethnic minority health professionals by managers and patients (Coker 2001).

Biological factors

Many writers are critical of the attempt to identify genetic factors that could link with ethnic differences in health, especially as there is more genetic variation within ethnic groups than between ethnic groups. It still stands that there are differences in some health problems, for example the haemoglobinopathies, which are strongly influenced by genetic factors that alter propensity to disease. However, many writers are agreed that genetics plays only a minor role in the contribution to health differences. In fact, some writers have suggested that the emphasis on genetic factors serves to racialize the problems of health ethnic minorities and draws attention away from the environmental factors (Davey Smith et al 2000).

In some ways, this is another sterile debate, because it is clear that many important determinants of health are physiological but are subject to long-term influence by socioeconomic and other environmental factors. For example, as Barker has shown (Barker 1994) low birth weight, which results from poor material maternal circumstances, is associated with diabetes, coronary heart disease and hypertension and short stature, related to childhood nutrition, carries with it an increased risk of respiratory and cardio-vascular mortality. The association of coronary heart disease with insulin resistance has been suggested by the fact that diabetes, a major risk factor for coronary heart disease, is highly prevalent in expatriate South Asian populations. It is argued that these populations could have experienced childhood nutritional deprivation but that successful migration has altered that. Insulin resistance is particularly associated with certain deposits of bodily fat and the pattern of obesity in South Asian populations shows that they are more likely to have abdominal fat deposition, what is sometimes called an 'apple shape' rather than the 'pear-shaped' body characteristic of Europeans. However, the role of insulin resistance remains unclear, and it is suggested that most South Asian people with coronary heart disease do not have diabetes. Correspondingly, 'pear-shaped' Europeans also suffer from high rates of heart disease.

Cerebrovascular disease (CVD) ranks second after coronary heart disease as a major cause of death amongst white, South Asian and Caribbean populations in Britain. CVD mortality is very much raised for people from the African and Caribbean, with African and Caribbean women having the highest standardized mortality rates.

Hypertension is a risk factor for CVD mortality. Compared with the general population, blood pressure is low for Chinese, Pakistani and Bangladeshi men. On the other hand, Pakistani women and Black Caribbean women were significantly more likely to have high blood pressure than women in the general population.

Behavioural risk factors

Some minority groups smoke considerably more, some less, than the general population. Rates for Pakistanis (25%) and Indians (23%) are about the same as the general population (27%), with only Chinese having a lower rate (17%). The Bangladeshis have the highest risk ratio (44% of men smoke), together with Irish men (33%) and Black Caribbean men (26%).

Irish women are the most likely to be smokers (33%) followed by Black Caribbean women (25%). A very small number of Indian, Pakistani and Bangladeshi women smoke (under 10%), compared with 27% of women in the general population. As well as smoking cigarettes, chewing tobacco is a habit which exists in the Bangladeshi community, among whom 19% of men and 26% of women report chewing tobacco.

With regard to alcohol use, men and women from all ethnic minorities (with the exception of the Irish) have relatively low rates of alcohol consumption compared to the majority population. Minority groups had a far higher proportion of people who were non-drinkers and more of these were women. The amount of alcohol consumed was almost the same between Irish men and the general population, but much lower for men in other groups. Thirty per cent in the general population drank on average more than 21 units a week. The number of women in the general population drinking more than 14 units a week was 16%, but the alcohol consumption of Irish women was higher, with 19% drinking over 14 units a week.

Compared with the general population, South Asian and Chinese men and women are less likely to take exercise. Men from South Asian communities were less likely to be obese, whereas Irish men were more likely. As far as women are concerned, Black Caribbean and Pakistani women were more likely to be obese and Chinese and Bangladeshi women less likely to be. However, when the waist–hip ratio was used as a measure of central obesity, women from all of the minority ethnic groups were more likely than the general population to have a raised waist–hip ratio.

Cultural factors

> Bangladesh is a hot country and the food is different from here. At that time we had dry fish curry and leaf vegetables. The body sweated and we have laboured. We did not have diabetes. (Bangladeshi man)

> Some say sugar is the body's power. I think the fat and the power have led to diabetes. (Bangladeshi man)

Cultural factors are thought to affect health in various ways. Cultural prohibitions on certain kinds of behaviours, such as smoking or drinking, might influence health outcomes, as described above. Similarly, rules about sexual behaviour, family relationships and gender roles can all influence health. Of particular interest are concepts of health and health beliefs, and research is just beginning to investigate different patterns. These can impact on use of health services, preventive activities or attitudes to chronic illness. Some researchers have shown a reluctance to be involved in understanding the cultures in which people live out their experiences of health and illness. This is because of some well-documented misuses of cultural explanations that have, either in a shallow or a racist way, attempted to explain patterns of ill health. In these explanations, culture has almost always been seen in negative terms, and has not usually been based on any in-depth ethnography. Some examples of bias include the assumption that rickets resulted from the Muslim tendency to cover the female body; the belief that those with sickle-cell disease are also 'seeking drugs' the description of 'surgery haunting' isolated Asian women, and the assumption that 'they care for their own', which means that little attention is paid to the needs of ethnic elders. These prevalent stereotypes suggest that cultural differences in terms of values, beliefs and lifestyles need to be paid more thorough attention.

A study by Greenhalgh and colleagues (1998) provides a good contrast. The authors explored the experience of diabetes in British Bangladeshis. They were interested to discover what aspects of patients' underlying attitudes and belief systems could contribute to the effective management of the condition. The authors were able to note some widely held beliefs about the nature of the body, the efficacy of particular types of food and the causes of disease. Large body size was generally viewed as an indicator of more health and thinness with less health. Illness was thought to be caused by events or agents external to the body, rather than to a failure within it. The study population believed that diabetes was caused by too much sugar and also by the Western diet in general. They also laid a lot of emphasis on physical and psychological stress, including poor housing and the fear of crime, as reasons why people develop diabetes, or other forms of ill health.

Diabetes was regarded as serious, chronic and incurable. To deal with it, measures needed be taken to restore the body's internal balance, by finding appropriate food. Food was classified in certain ways: raw foods, and those that had been baked or grilled, were considered indigestible, as were any vegetables that grew under the ground. These were thought to be particularly bad for elderly, sick or young people. Greenhalgh et al (1998) noted that recommendations for diabetic patients to bake or grill foods, rather than fry them, might not accord with cultural perceptions on digestibility. Other researchers (Pearce & Armstrong 1996) have also noted the importance attached to diet among diabetic patients from ethnic minorities. They do not necessarily follow the medically prescribed diet; moderation in consumption and fresh foods were thought to be more important than the one-sided avoidance of particular foods that was often recommended by clinics.

Most patients were knowledgeable about diabetes testing, and understood the need to lose weight and the importance of dietary modification. The authors remark that there is a real danger in assuming that non-compliance with a 'healthy' lifestyle is always attributable to cultural factors. A recent study of admissions for asthma amongst South Asians also pointed out that the main barriers to good asthma care for South Asians were not to be found in cultural attitudes towards asthma. Although notions of 'balance' in health existed, and ideas of prevention were sometimes unclear, poor asthma control was related to the inadequacy of services and poor relationships with those general practitioners who lacked strategies for asthma care (Griffiths et al 2001).

Occasionally, reports surface in the literature about 'fatalism' among ethnic minority patients, particularly Muslim patients. This is sometimes interpreted as a lack of interest or a belief that medical care is of no value. This is a wrong interpretation of Islam, which enjoins people to care for their health. Although there is a clear understanding of God's will operating in all events, individuals are also expected to take responsibility for their health and to understand the need for change.

Access to and use of health services

People from different ethnic groups have different ways of dealing with illness or keeping healthy. One East London study of the Muslim Bangladeshi community stressed the importance of prayer as one way of dealing with behavioural disturbances in children (Hillier & Rahman 1996). The lack of availability of traditional remedies was seen by some African–Caribbean women as contributing to their hypertension. Unani and Ayurvedic practitioners continue in practice, and British and Chinese acupuncturists flourish. Members of ethnic minorities often consult such private practitioners for the same reasons that the majority population do; better control, communication and understanding in the consultation. Going to a traditional practitioner, or one from the same ethnic group, is often explained thus: 'He is the same as us, and understands our situation better.' Creams and oils to keep the skin supple, close attention to diet and a carefully monitored approach to the balance of the body can be found in any or all ethnic minority groups where health, as a value, has considerable salience. However, Griffiths et al (2001) suggest that, in asthma care, although traditional remedies are in widespread use, they are not regarded as substitutes for appropriate medication.

Consultation rates

A number of studies have shown that GP consultation rates are higher in minority ethnic groups, especially South Asian groups. The exception are the Chinese, once again, who have low rates of utilization for all health services. The Health Survey for England looked at the proportion of informants who had used GP, hospital or dental services, or had taken prescribed medicines in the past 2 weeks: 12% of men in the general population had consulted a GP in the past 2 weeks. Among minority ethnic groups the consultation rate was highest for Bangladeshi men (22%) then Indian, Pakistani and Black Caribbean (15–17%). For women, the pattern was similar, with higher consultation rates for Black Caribbean and South Asian women (21–24%) than all women (18%). Rates for men and women increased with increasing age. For Pakistani, Bangladeshi and Chinese men and women, consultation rates were about five times as high at age 55, whereas for men in the general population they were only twice as high, and among women just over once as high. Indian children and young people were more likely to consult a GP than any other ethnic group (Cooper et al 1998). Consultation rates for both men and women tended to be higher in manual than non-manual households. Irish men and women were the exception, with age standardized rates being lower in manual households.

Of course, consultation rates in themselves do not provide an indicator of the quality of services. Work by Nazroo and colleagues (Ahmad 1993) showed that ethnic minorities, especially Pakistanis and Bangladeshis, were more likely to find physical access to the GP difficult. Waiting times in the surgery were long for all ethnic minority groups and the majority of South Asians, whilst they could understand the GP, were less likely to find the time the GP devoted to them adequate and overall less likely to be happy with consultations.

Overall, ethnic group members consulted more for endocrine, nutritional and metabolic disorders, skin and respiratory conditions, circulatory problems and signs and symptoms of ill-defined origin. The numbers of signs and symptoms that remain unexplained suggest that there are areas of health belief or difficulties within the consultation that need to be explored.

Hospital attendance rates

Attendance at outpatient clinics is similar to that of the rest of the population. However, this information conceals some interesting differences. Among young people, levels of attendance were lower in all minority ethnic groups, whereas for those in the older group, aged 35–54, outpatient attendance by Pakistani men and Bangladeshi men and women was seven percentage points higher than the general population. For those aged 55 and over, Indian, Black Caribbean and Irish men showed higher than average rates of attendance. For admission as inpatients, standardizing for age, Chinese men and women were significantly less likely and Pakistani men more likely (1.43), relative to the general population, to have been admitted as inpatients. There were no differences in attendance either at outpatients or at inpatients between social classes, unlike the general population.

Use of prescribed medication

South Asian men, standardized for age, have a significantly higher mean number of drugs per person than the general population, and Bangladeshi men were more likely to be prescribed more drugs per person. The same situation was shown for women and for the elderly group, but at every age South Asians were taking more medicine. For example, more than half the Bangladeshi men aged 55 and over were on four or more drugs.

There were higher ratios for endocrine-related drug usage for Black Caribbean, Indian, Pakistani and Bangladeshi men and more than one-third of all drugs were used in diabetes control, which is consistent with the higher prevalence of diabetes amongst Black Caribbean and South Asian men. The rate of the use of cardiovascular prescriptions among Indian men and Black Caribbean women was significantly higher than that of the general population. Again, both Chinese men and women showed lower drug usage.

Haemoglobinopathy services

> They get suspicious because they can't believe you can be better in 2 days, but if I can look after myself I don't see why I should be there. I feel better. I can stop taking the pain-killers once I didn't have no more pain, but they were giving me tablets which I didn't know were pain-killers. (Sickle cell patient)

Although much of the evidence is anecdotal, work that has been done on patients suffering from the haemoglobinopathies does suggest that institutional racism at the level of care exists. Sickle-cell disease (SCD) is an inherited condition that occurs predominantly in ethnic Caribbean people. The genetic trait for the disease helps to protect the carrier from malaria, and therefore is most likely to be found in populations where malaria is endemic. Researchers (Ahmad 1993, Anionwu 1996) have described the way in which the disease has been marginalized and ignored. Britain is well behind the USA in providing screening services.

SCD is clearly an example of a condition where patients can be 'experts'. Their descriptions of pain, or factors associated with painful crisis can be seen as valuable information to clinicians. A recent study (Maxwell et al 1999) of experiences of hospital care by sickle-cell patients showed that patients were mistrusted and stigmatized, and that there was both under- and overtreatment of their pain. It was clear that experiences of pain and patterns of hospital admission were likely to be influenced by sociocultural and psychological factors, as well as disease severity. The way in which patients are treated in the UK contrasts with the approach in the USA, where most painful episodes are managed at home and patients with SCD do not normally use health services for pain management. The same pattern has been noted in Jamaica.

In Maxwell et al's (1999) study, patients devised various strategies, including assertiveness, self-education resistance and developing relationships with staff, to deal with the difficulties of coping with chronic SCD.

Dental services

Dentists' services are very underused by the minority ethnic groups, but the reasons are not well understood. Black Caribbean men and women were much more likely to have lost all their teeth than the general population, whereas tooth loss among other minority groups was significantly lower for Chinese men and Bangladeshi women. For all minority groups, women were more likely to visit than men, but for all groups, and both sexes, regular dental attendance was significantly lower than for the general population. Informants in minority ethnic groups were more likely to visit a dentist only when having trouble with their teeth. An exception to this was Irish women, but South Asian men and women, and particularly Bangladeshi women, were also two to three times less likely than the general population to visit a dentist.

Maternity and gynaecological care

The pain was unbearable ... they were shouting ... 'Why you never took antenatal class? ... You should have, then there wouldn't be such a problem for you, and us as well'. (Pakistani maternity patient)

Maternity care is another area where problems have been identified. Failure to provide a female doctor might cause an under-reporting of gynaecological conditions, and the necessity of female clinicians, especially in obstetrics and gynaecology, has been repeatedly stressed. However, even if clinicians are female, their behaviour can sometimes be construed as cold and unfeeling. A study by Bowler (1993) showed how midwives viewed South Asian women as attention-seeking, demanding and rude. It would have been valuable to have found out what the patients thought about their carers. People might not complain at the time, but their silence, their 'muted voices' cannot be taken as evidence that all is well (Bowes & Domoko 1996).

Communication

Communication issues are very important in providing appropriate care and there is quite a bit of evidence to suggest that difficulties in communication between ethnic minority patients and carers lower the quality of available care.

Language is an important issue for patients. People of Indian origin are most likely to speak English, whereas people from Bangladesh are least likely. Men are more likely to be able to speak English than women and younger people rather than older people. In the 50–74-year-old age group, Pakistani and Bangladeshi women are very unlikely to speak English because they have been born abroad and, historically, have had little opportunity (Table 10.5).

On the other hand, 20% of Indians, 50% of Pakistanis and 59% of Bangladeshis communicate with their GP in one or other of the Asian languages. A very high proportion of Asians attend a general practice with an Asian doctor and many Asian GPs work in deprived inner-city areas. Yet very few GPs who do not speak an ethnic minority language employ an interpreting service and therefore children or spouses are often brought in as interpreters. The use of children in this context is inappropriate. Hospitals sometimes use health advocates. These are people from the local community who have been trained to empower patients. They help them to get the information from health professionals that

TABLE 10.5	Main language spoken by people aged 16–74 (1992)	
Indian	**Pakistani**	**Bangladeshi**
Gujarati 36%	Punjabi 48%	Bengali 73%
English 32%	Urdu 24%	Silheti 17%
Punjabi 24%	English 22%	English 10%
Urdu 3%	Other 6%	All languages 100
Hindi 2%	All languages 100	
Other 3%		
All languages 100		
From HEA (1992).		

they require to make informed choices and to access the services they need. Their job is to ensure that patients and health professionals understand each other, and that the patient's wishes are known. They are also there to give patients information about health services, make patients aware of their rights and challenge any instances of discrimination. An advocate has an important role in ensuring that professionals understand, respect and acknowledge the patient as an individual and are aware of, and sympathetic to, that patient's culture. Although there is increasing use of health advocates, these services still remain very underfunded and inadequate. Health advocates are only part of the solution, however. It is necessary for all health professionals (many of whom are members of ethnic minorities themselves) to provide culturally competent care to patients.

> I sit there all day watching, but I cannot ask for anything, or express how I feel. I have to wait for my daughter to come so she could tell the nurse or doctor. There were no interpreters; I did not think you could ask for interpreters. I feel terrible that I could not speak to the nurses. So lonely. There were so many people there, but for me it was like being alone in a crowd. (Hindu female patient)

The need for cultural understanding becomes evident in a whole sequence of interactions between clients and practitioners. Culturally competent practitioners are those who have moved from being culturally unaware to being sensitive to cultural issues, understanding how their own values and biases affect different patients and clients. Culturally competent practitioners can value difference; they combine awareness, knowledge and sensitivity in the interpretation of symptoms, understanding of health beliefs, advice to patients, emotional interaction and explaining the purpose of particular health practices or services.

A study of mothers of Bangladeshi children with behavioural problems showed very clear differences in perception of the functions of a child psychiatry service.

> They did not give us any medicine, they talked and asked us if things were getting any better. We did not want them to ask a child to draw and talk. These things are done in school. They should have checked his chest and X-rayed his brain. I went for sickness. He was not eating, he was tearing his clothes, and not at peace. (Bangladeshi mother of patient)

One study showed that when congruence between the expectations of patient and therapist was achieved, satisfaction with treatment was much higher. Two Bangladeshi therapists were appointed to assist the process (Hillier et al 1994).

CONCLUSIONS

In general, the health of people from ethnic minorities tends to be worse than that of the general population, although there are some exceptions. It is quite clear that material circumstances are of great importance in contributing to the development of disease. However, it is equally important to pay attention to the quality of services that are available to members of ethnic minorities. Here, research suggests that all is not well and that further and greater efforts need to be made to design health services that are accessible and appropriate to members of ethnic minorities and which take into account particular cultural needs and requirements. Too often, reference to cultural needs has been done in an atmosphere that blames cultures for many of the problems. This erroneous approach needs to be replaced by one that considers recognition of difference, equality and dignity as important objectives for ethnic minority care in the National Health Service. In practical terms, this means better communication and translation services, better involvement of ethnic minorities in the organization of health services and more careful specialist service delivery for particular disorders that have an ethnic dimension. These, together with ethnic monitoring, will provide a constant input into the changing situation of ethnic minority health and it is hoped that new NHS structures, which allow greater flexibility for localities to respond to the needs of ethnic minorities, will improve their health situation.

References

Abbots J et al 1998 Morbidity and Irish Catholic descent in Britain; an ethnic and religious minority 150 years on. Science and Medicine 45:3–14

Ahmad W 1993 'Race' and health in contemporary Britain. Open University Press, Buckingham

Ahmad W 1998 Ethnicity health and health care in Britain. In: Peterson A, Waddell C (eds) Health matters. Open University Press, Buckingham, p 114–128

Anionwu E 1996 Ethnic origin of sickle and thalassemia counsellors – does it matter? In: Kelleher D, Hillier S (eds) Researching cultural differences in health. Routledge, London, p 160–190

Balarajan R, Bulusu L 1990 Mortality among immigrants in England and Wales1974–83. In: Britton M (ed) Mortality and geography: a review of the mid-1980s. Office of Population Censuses and Surveys (OPCS) Series DS No. 9. HMSO, London, p 103–121

Barker DTP 1994 Mothers, babies and disease in later life. British Medical Association Publishing Group, London

Bhopal R 1997 Is research into ethnicity and health racist, unsound or important science? British Medical Journal 314:1751

Bhugra D 2000 Rates of deliberate self harm in Asians: findings and models. International Review of Psychiatry 12:37–43

Bowes AM, Domokos TM 1996 Pakistani women and maternity care: raising muted voices. Sociology, Health and Illness 18: 45–46

Bowler I 1993 'They're not the same as us' – midwives' stereotypes of South Asian maternity patients. Sociology, Health and Illness 15:157–158

Coker M 2001 Racism in medicine – an agenda for change. The King's Fund, London

Cooper H, Smaje C, Arber S 1998 Use of health services by children and young people according to ethnicity and social class: secondary analysis of a national survey. British Medical Journal 317:1047–1051

Davey Smith G et al 2000 Ethnic inequalities in health – a review of UK epidemiological evidence. Critical Public Health 10(4):375–407

Department of Health (DoH) 1991 The patients' charter. HMSO, London

Department of Health (DoH) 2001 Speech by public health minister, Yvette Cooper. News Archive, 24 January 2001

Fryer P 1985 Staying power. Pluto Press, London

General Assembly Resolution 217 A 111, Article 22. Universal Declaration of Human Rights. United Nations Department of Public Information, New York, 10 December 1948

Gilroy P 1998 The end of race. Ethnic and Racial Studies 21(5):838–847

Greenhalgh T, Helman C, Choudary AM 1998 Health beliefs and folk models of diabetes in British Bangladeshis: a qualitative study. British Medical Journal 316:978–983

Griffiths C et al 2001 Influences on hospital admission for asthma in South Asian and white adults: a qualitative study. British Medical Journal 323: 962–966

Haque R, Hillier S 2000 Evaluation of a schools-based intervention working with Bangladeshi young women. Mimeo. Department of Human Science and Medical Ethics, Queen Mary University of London

Harding S, Balarajan R 1996 Patterns of mortality in second generation Irish living in England and Wales: longitudinal study. British Medical Journal 312:1389–1392

Health Education Authority (HEA) 1992 Black and ethnic minority health and lifestyle survey. HEA, London

Health Survey for England 1999 Health of minority ethnic groups. HMSO/Office for National Statistics, London

Hillier S, Rahman S 1996 Childhood development and behavioural problems as perceived by Bangladeshi patients in East London. In: Kelleher D, Hillier S (eds) Researching cultural differences in health. Routledge, London, p 38–69

Hillier S, Loshak R, Haq A, Marks F 1994 An evaluation of child psychiatric services for Bangladeshi parents. Journal of Mental Health 3:327–337

Labour Force Survey (LFS) 1995 Employment by gender and industry. Office for National Statistics/HMSO, London

MacPherson W 1999 The Stephen Lawrence Inquiry: report. Home Office, London, p 28, paragraph 6.34

Marmot M, Adelstein F, Bulusu L 1984 Immigrant mortality in England and Wales 1970–78. OPCS Studies in medical and population subjects, No. 47. HMSO, London

Mason D 1996 Teaching race and ethnicity in sociology. Ethnic and Racial Studies 19(4):782

Maxwell K, Streetly A, Bevan D 1999 Experience of hospital care and treatment seeking for pain from sickle cell disease: qualitative study. British Medical Journal 318:1585–1590

Nazroo J 1997a The health of Britain's ethnic minorities. Policy Studies Institute, London

Nazroo J 1997b Ethnicity and mental health. Policy Studies Institute, London

Office of Population Census and Surveys (OPCS) 1991 HMSO, London

Office for National Statistics (ONS) 1991 Census. Population by age 1991. In: Social focus on ethnic minorities 1996. HMSO, London, p 10, Table 1.2

Office for National Statistics (ONS) 1996a Social focus on ethnic minorities. HMSO, London, p 16, Table 1.11

Office for National Statistics (ONS) 1996b Social focus on ethnic minorities. HMSO, London, p 21, Table 2.4

Office for National Statistics (ONS) 1996c Social focus on ethnic minorities. HMSO, London, p 21, Table 2.5

Office for National Statistics (ONS) 1996d Social focus on ethnic minorities. HMSO, London, p 37, Table 3.7

Office for National Statistics (ONS) 1996e Social focus on ethnic minorities. HMSO, London, Table 4.14

Office for National Statistics (ONS) 1996f Social focus on ethnic minorities. HMSO, London, Table 4.17

Office for National Statistics (ONS) 1996g Social focus on ethnic minorities. HMSO, London, p 51–62, Section 5, Health

Pearce M, Armstrong D 1996 Afro-Caribbean beliefs about diabetes: an exploratory study. In: Kelleher D, Hillier S (eds) Researching cultural differences in health. Routledge, London, p 91–103

Raftery J, Jones D, Rosato M 1990 The mortality of first and second generation migrants to the UK. Sociology, Science and Medicine 31:577–584

Raleigh VS 1996 Suicide patterns and trends in people of Indian sub-continent and Caribbean origin in England and Wales. Ethnicity and Health 1:55–63

Raleigh VS, Balarajan R 1995 The health of infants among ethnic minorities. The health of our children. Decennial supplement. HMSO, London, p 82–94

Shaw CM et al 1999 Prevalence of anxiety and depressive illness and help seeking behaviour in African Caribbean and White Europeans: two-phase general population survey. British Medical Journal 318:302–306

Sivanandan N 1989 UK commentary: racism 1992. Race and Class 30:3. London Institute of Race Relations

Smaje C 1995 'Race', ethnicity and health: making sense of the evidence. SHARE/The King's Fund, London, p 65

The Times 2001 Boom in British ethnic minority population. The Times, 21 September 2001

Virdee S 1995 Racial violence and harassment. Policy Studies Institute, London, p 45

Williams B 1994 Insulin resistance: the shape of things to come. Lancet 344:521–524

Williams R, Bhopal R, Hunt K 1994 Coronary risk in a British Punjabi population: a comparative profile of non-biochemical factors. International Journal of Epidemiology 23:28–37

166

Older People, Health Care and Society

Paul Higgs

POPULATION CHANGES

The existence of large numbers of older people in countries such as Britain is a relatively recent feature, characteristic only of the last century and a half. This is not to say that there were no old people in the past; many individuals survived until their 70s and 80s, but there were not enough for them to constitute a significant part of the population. Surviving into old age was an achievement – not an expectation – for the majority of the population. By contrast, in modern Britain the vast majority of the population can expect to live beyond the age of retirement; indeed, many will live beyond the age of 80. In 1998, life expectancy at birth in Britain was 74.9 years for men and 79.8 years for women (HMSO 2001) (see Table 9.1, p. 132); in 1841 the figures were 41 years for men and 43 years for women and, according to Victor (1994), it had taken 400 years for these figures to increase by 8 years. This process has been described as squaring the rectangle of survival (Fig. 11.1).

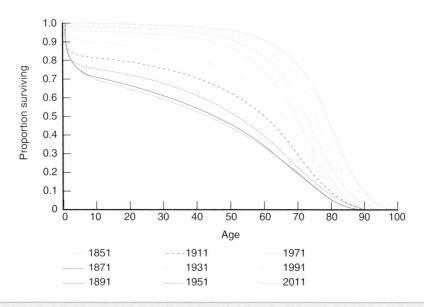

Fig. 11.1 The rectangularization of the life curve in England and Wales.

The increase in life expectancy that accompanied industrialization is not surprising. The advent of public health measures that substantially controlled the impact of infectious diseases had the effect of lowering the infant and maternal mortality rates (see Chapter 1). Consequently, the majority of deaths in England and Wales occur in those aged over 65, with the rate increasing with age.

Not only has life expectancy increased but the nature of the population has also changed. Over 20% of the population is aged 60 or over and this is projected to increase to around 24% in 2051. This increase is caused in part by the relative balance between the birthrates of different generations. As those born during the post-war 'baby boom' grow older they affect the composition of the population, because relatively fewer people were born in the decade that followed. The proportion of those aged over 80 is not set to rise significantly until later in the twenty-first century when, by 2015, this group will have risen from 4% of the population to just over 9%. By contrast, the 16–39 age group, which peaked at 36% of the population in 1986, is projected to fall to 28% by the middle of the twenty-first century.

These changes are not unique to Britain. In 1990, just under 20% of the total population of the European Union was aged 60 or over (Walker & Maltby 1997). In numerical terms, this was about 60 million people. By the year 2020, the corresponding percentage of the population is calculated to be a quarter of all EC citizens. As in Britain, the number of over-80s is also set to increase; by the year 2025 they are projected to rise by up to 115% in Portugal and by nearly an extra million in both Italy and Germany. Life expectancy has also been increasing throughout Europe over the past 30 years, where it has increased by up to 10 years in some countries. In 1989 the average European woman aged 60 could expect to live for another 22 years, and if she was 80 for another 7.5 years.

HEALTH AND ILLNESS

What kind of life can older people expect to lead when they reach retirement age? The answer is: one remarkably similar to that experienced by other people in the population. Although there is a connection between old age and physical disability, the extent of this is not as profound or pervasive as popular image would have it. Acute health problems such as colds or accidental injuries increase with age, but even among the very oldest age groups these only affect 20% of males and 25% of females. On average, people over 75 lost 77 days over a year because of acute sickness. This compares with an average of 21 days for those aged 16–44 (HMSO 2000). Chronic health problems such as arthritis do increase with age. According to the 2000 General Household Survey, 66% of the over-75 age group reporting a long-standing illness in 1998 but this only restricted the activity of 27% of this age group in the 2 weeks before the survey was taken (HMSO 2002).

ACTIVITIES OF DAILY LIVING

Many researchers have looked at the health status of older people from the perspective of their ability to undertake what are called 'activities of daily living' (ADL). There are many different ways of measuring these abilities but most concentrate on a few distinct activities, such as bathing, climbing stairs and cutting toenails (Table 11.1). Again, it should be noted that the majority of older people can undertake these activities. Using data from the 1985 General Household Survey, Johnson & Falkingham (1992) point out that even among those aged over 85, 14% of males and 11% of females are described as having no functional disability. However, nearly half of all women in this age group are deemed to have severe disability.

MULTIPLE PATHOLOGY

One important conclusion acknowledged explicitly by those who construct and use ADL scales is the importance of what is known as 'multiple pathology' among older people. This refers to the fact that an older person is likely to have more than one medical condition, and these will often be of a disabling nature. But, again, although the average number of multiple pathologies increases with age, it should be remembered that nearly two-fifths of older people are not subject to any disabling conditions.

TABLE 11.1	Help needed by elderly people with various tasks: by age (1996–7)					
	65–69	70–74	75–79	80–84	85 and over	All aged 65 and over
Climbing stairs	5	7	11	15	30	10
Bathing/showering	5	6	8	15	24	9
Dressing/undressing	3	2	4	5	8	4
Getting in and out of bed	2	2	1	3	4	2
Getting around the house	1	1	0	1	4	1
Going to the toilet	1	1	1	1	3	1
Eating	0	0	1	1	1	0

From General Household Survey, Office for National Statistics. HMSO (2002)

One common belief about old age is that it is inextricably linked with mental decline, so much so that senile, which is the Latin word for old, has become a pejorative term for mental incapacity. The idea of mental decline as an accompaniment of the ageing process is not supported by the evidence. Senile dementia is probably the most well known organic disorder of the brain to affect old people. Its most common symptoms include memory loss and behavioural disturbances, but the prevalence of dementing conditions is in fact less than 10% for older people living in the community. The incidence of dementia does increase with age but not to a point where more than one-fifth of the oldest age group is severely affected. Affective disorders such as depression do feature highly among the older population, with around one-quarter reporting either a mild or severe clinical affective disorder. Suicide rates seem to increase with age, with people over 65 accounting for 27% of male and 32% of female successful suicides in England and Wales (Victor 1994).

RESIDENTIAL AND INSTITUTIONAL CARE

Another common image of older people is that many of them are residents in some form of institution. This could be an old people's home, a residential or nursing home or a long-stay ward in a geriatric hospital. It is true that nearly 500 000 older people were in some kind of institutional setting by 1990, and that this had grown from 250 000 in 1970 (Henwood 1992). However, such absolute numbers should not be allowed to disguise the fact that these only represent a small fraction of the older population. Even among those aged over 90, nearly three-fifths lived in private households (Bury & Holme 1991). Moreover, the designation of institutional care can be misleading, given that nursing care is not provided by old people's homes (sometimes known as part III homes). Although the numbers of places in institutions nearly doubled between 1970 and 1990, the real growth occurred within the private sector. Places in private residential homes increased from 24 000 in 1970 to 156 000 in 1990, and places in private nursing homes grew from 20 000 in 1970 to 123 000 in 1990. Part of this growth is accounted for by the absolute growth in the numbers of older people, but this can explain only half of the increase. A more plausible explanation is that a massive increase in social security expenditure created major incentives for older people to stay in private residential and nursing homes rather than community-based forms of care (Higgs & Victor 1993). Expenditure on this part of the welfare budget increased from £10 million in 1979 to nearly £1.5 billion by 1993. Curtailing this increase was one of the objectives of the 1993 Community Care Act, which transferred responsibility for funding this group to local councils. Over the latter part of the past decade the financial uncertainty that this has created, alongside an increase in property values, has created problems for the private sector. In certain areas such as London and the south of England, the provision of nursing homes is patchy because many have gone out of business. It has been estimated that there was a fall of 5% in the numbers of places between 1992 and 1999 (HMSO 2001).

USE OF HEALTHCARE SERVICES

Older patients comprise the largest single group of users of hospital services. This is not just confined to those specialisms with an interest in the conditions of old age such as geriatric medicine, but applies throughout most of the major specialities. The admission rate increases with age, with the 1998 General Household Survey (HMSO 2000) showing 21% of men aged over 75 and 15% of women in the same age group reporting an inpatient stay in the previous year. The same survey reported that 17% of those aged over 75 had been inpatients compared with only 12% of those aged 65–74. It is also the case that inpatient length of stay increases with age. Those aged over 75 spend three times as long in hospital than those aged between 16 and 44, with the average length of stay being 12 and 4 days, respectively.

Consulting the general practitioner (GP) also increases with age, as does the average number of consultations made. In 1998, 21% of those aged over 75 had visited a GP in the previous fortnight (HMSO 2000). Women tend to consult the GP more often than men, and they are more likely to receive a home visit. However, Victor (1994) notes that less than 10% of older people in Canada accounted for 35% of all visits to the GP.

Older people are major users of prescribed medicines, having on average more than two-and-a-half times more items than the rest of the population. When non-prescribed drugs are taken into account, only a small proportion of older people are not on medication of any sort. Consequently, one of the notable features of older patients is the existence of what is known as polypharmacy – the taking by one patient of many different medicines. This is a particular problem often associated with the fact that many items are prescribed on repeat prescriptions, leading to a build-up over time. This can lead to problems in acute hospital care, where doctors might not be sure what medication older patients are on when they are admitted.

171

GENERATIONS, AGEING POPULATIONS AND HEALTH POLICY

Ageing might not be synonymous with infirmity and illness but policy makers assume that a population with a high proportion of older people is also one that produces greater demands on its healthcare services. In Britain, the government calculates what is known as a 'dependency ratio' based on the proportion of the population aged under 16 and over 65 to those of working age. It is assumed that the young and the old represent a drain on expenditure that those of working age will have to pay for. As the percentage of older people in the population increases, so does the burden on the working population. This is not just a British phenomenon. A study by the International Labour Organization suggests that, throughout Europe, medical expenditure on health care for the over 65s will increase from 37% of all healthcare spending in 1985 to 58% by the year 2015. Individual countries such as Switzerland could find their expenditure rising to 70% (Walker & Maltby 1997).

Important dimensions of these issues are the similarities or differences that exist between different succeeding generations. Evandrou & Falkingham (2000) have attempted to model the impact on British society of the retirement of different birth cohorts. Most of our experience of old age is derived from cohorts who were born in the 1910s. Their experiences will be very different from those born in the 'baby boom' that occurred between the late 1940s and early 1960s. It is this latter group who will be retiring in the first few decades of the twenty-first century. Evandrou & Falkingham (2000) focus on three areas – living arrangements, health and access to resources. They point out that the proportion living alone is likely to increase because of social factors such as divorce, childlessness and low birth rates. In terms of health, later generations report more long-standing illness than their predecessors at similar ages. However, in mitigation, younger cohorts are less likely to smoke but tend to work more hours. In terms of access to resources, later generations have greater work participation rates for women than earlier ones, and women are much more likely to work full time. This means that both men and women are more likely to have private pensions and to have benefited from the rise in home ownership. Evandrou & Falkingham conclude that the baby boomers are likely to be 'better off in retirement than today's older people' (Evandrou & Falkingham 2000, p 34). Taken together, the evidence suggests a mixed set of implications for social and health policy.

Will expenditure on the coming cohorts of older people continue to rise or will it stabilize as each succeeding generation brings its own experiences into the equation. At a more generalized level, arguments around purely health concerns centre on the prospects for the 'compression of morbidity' in old age (Fries 1983). Is the level of disability and chronic illness among older people stabilizing or increasing as people live longer, or are individuals having a longer active life expectancy? As we have seen above, the evidence is mixed. One argument is that there has been a decrease in morbidity among higher socioeconomic classes in later life. This is seen to relate to the prevention or delayed onset of many non-fatal conditions that increase the age of onset of disability without affecting age of death. This 'squaring of the rectangle of survival' (see Fig. 11.1) reduces the proportions of the population dying before they reach their natural lifespan and results in larger numbers of older people. If this compression of morbidity could be extended to the rest of the population, then the demands created by an ageing population would be different from what they are currently. In this model of 'successful ageing', individual lifestyle and psychological well-being are seen to be crucial. One implication of this view is that an ageing population would not necessarily be the cause of rising costs connected to physical dependency and disability. However, in practice, all European healthcare systems are preparing for a significant rise in demand. This has led Moody (1995) to argue that modern societies face four possible scenarios (Box 11.1). Although each of these scenarios can be assessed separately in terms of their implications, what is probably more likely to happen is that they are all going to happen in tandem. No single approach to the future of ageing is likely to be dominant. Even Moody's preferred solution of the voluntary acceptance of limits assumes that there can be general agreement on the desirability of such an approach. What Moody directs us to is the uncertainty and contradictions facing the future of ageing.

OLDER PEOPLE AND SOCIETY

The only characteristic shared by all older people is chronological age, and even this is not consistent between societies. In Britain, the state retirement age is often used to designate the onset of old age. This has meant that until recently men became old on their 65th birthday whereas women did so on the occasion of their 60th birthday. In countries such as Kenya, employees of the State often retire at 40 and live on their pensions, so that younger

| BOX 11.1 | Moody's (1995) Four Scenarios for the Future of Old Age |

1. **Prolongation of morbidity**: the state whereby an increase in years is not accompanied by an equal increase in quality of life. This prompts demands for the 'right to die' and rationing based on quality-of-life measures
2. **Compression of morbidity**: a situation where the majority of the population experience good health almost up to the end of their lives and are then subject to a 'terminal drop' just before they die. This strategy advocates health promotion and individual responsibility as the way forward in health care
3. **Lifespan extension**: the abilities and successes of modern medicine are such that the natural lifespan can be extended upwards, leading to the delaying or abolition of many of the features of 'normal ageing'. The emphasis is put on basic medical research into the ageing process. Problems of who gets access to discoveries and treatments would emerge
4. **Voluntary acceptance of limits**: recognizes the problems inherent in the other three positions and argues for a shared 'meaning of old age' that maintains the common good by stressing limits beneficial to coming generations. It is accepted that there must be a point where interventions should be appropriate rather than life extending

people can be employed. The arbitrariness of when retirement occurs means that all we can safely say about it is that it marks the end of participation in the formal economy. Even this is being eroded through the increase of people taking early retirement in their 50s, with some not fully leaving the labour market even then. When old age is deemed to begin is therefore increasingly difficult to ascertain.

It is not the case that older people are either richer than the rest of the population or poorer. There are considerable numbers of relatively well off older people, but it is also the case that some of the poorest people in Britain are old. However, it is a situation that it changing over time. In 1979, 47% of pensioners were in the bottom 20% of the distribution of the income distribution for the whole population. By 1999/2000 this figure had fallen to 25%. During the same period, there were increases in the proportion of pensioners falling into the other four-fifths. In 1999/2000, pensioners were most commonly found in the second fifth (Fig. 11.2). One reason for this change is that pensioners' income has grown at a faster rate than other sectors of the population. It has been estimated that pensioners' income has grown by over 60% in real terms between 1979 and 1997 (Department for Work and Pensions (DWP) 2000). By way of comparison, average earnings grew by 36% in the same period.

Obviously, such averages hide considerable differences between different groups of retired people. Household structure has an effect. Pensioner couples receive twice as much gross income as single pensioners. Incomes are 22% higher for younger pensioners under 75 than for those over that age. Sources of income also play a major role. Income from occupational pensions rose by 162% in real terms between 1979 and 1997 whereas that from state benefits rose by 41% (DWP 2000). Among retired households, the poorest seem

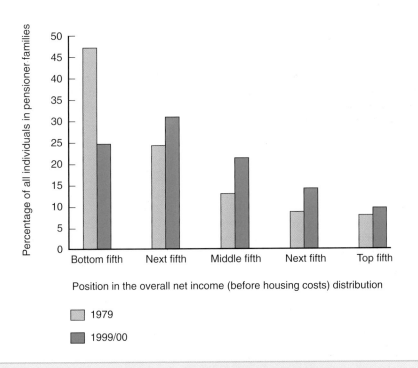

Fig. 11.2   Pensioners' position in the overall net income distribution (1979–99/00).

to be ones comprising older single women. This is sometimes described as the 'feminization of poverty'.

It would be a mistake, therefore, to assume that poverty is a natural state for older people. The poverty of many old people is because many of them rely upon state benefits as their main source of income. Because these entitlements are set very low relative to the standard of living of the rest of the population, it is not surprising that large numbers are poor. It should also be noted that households with children but only one adult are also disproportionately likely to be in poverty. Among recently retired pensioner couples, the proportion of total income received from social security payments amounts to only 37% of their income, as opposed to 53% for pensioner couples over 75. For single pensioners aged over 75 this figure is 68% (DWP 2000).

DOMESTIC CIRCUMSTANCES

The social circumstances of older people also vary greatly. Family structures are dominated by the cultural norm of the nuclear family, where only two generations of a family live under the same roof. This is different from the extended family, where many different generations live together, which is prevalent in some other cultures. Older people who have been married have tended to live in forms of nuclear family when their children have left home. As older people have aged so the chances of them still living with their spouses decreases. This, combined with the relatively high number of women who have never married, means that a substantial number of older people live alone. Social networks therefore become crucial. Although the vast majority of older people do not live with their children, this does not mean that they have little contact. The majority of older people have children and/or a sibling living close to them and contact is frequent. The family does not provide the only source of social contact. Surveys report, unsuprisingly, that friends and neighbours play an important part in maintaining the older person's place in social networks. Age does affect the nature of these contacts, 'younger' old people tend to visit friends whereas 'older' old people tend to be visited. The percentage of reported contact with both family and friends tends to diminish with age, but only a small minority (2%) of older people are actually seen as totally socially isolated. A slightly larger percentage (5%) report that they are lonely.

Most care for physically frail and mentally confused older people is provided by members of such social networks. There are 6 million carers in Britain and 75% are looking after an elderly person. Family relationships are of extreme importance to this process of informal care, with 80% of carers looking after a relative (Henwood 1992). Women, and especially daughters, are the main carers. However, a third of all carers are men, although they often do different things. Sometimes the caring relationship can continue for so many years that the carers themselves become elderly people. The effect of caring on carers can be immense, both in physical and financial terms. The majority receive no help from formal agencies and what help is offered is often designed to stop the informal caring relationship breaking down rather than alleviating stresses. Community care policy depends on informal care 'by the community' to keep costs down.

SOCIOLOGY AND OLDER PEOPLE

The existence of a state of retirement for large numbers of the population is a feature of most industrialized societies. As such, it has prompted the interest of many different sociologists who have constructed a number of different theories to account for the position of older people.

Disengagement theory

One of the first generalized accounts to look seriously at old age was an American approach centred on the theme of 'disengagement' (Cumming & Henry 1961). This was a process whereby older people in industrial societies disengaged themselves from the roles that they occupied in the wider society. This was so younger generations would have opportunities to develop and society could continue. Such disengagement not only occurred in relation to work roles but also in relation to families, when retired generations became much less central to the lives of their children. Seen from this perspective, old age presented the individual with many difficulties. In preindustrial societies, the inheritance of skills and property accorded older people a social function. In industrial societies, the lack of property or skills that could be handed on meant that older people did not have 'scripts' with which to negotiate their new roles. This led many researchers to stress the importance of finding ways to facilitate 'successful ageing' with the priority being psychological adjustment.

A large amount of research was undertaken in the USA during the 1950s and 1960s to provide evidence for this theory. A longitudinal study in Kansas City (Neugarten et al 1964) showed that older people did indeed disengage, although women started this process at widowhood whereas men began on retirement. Again, the processes were seen as involving difficulties in the roles being played by older people and the answers in psychological adaptation. This approach, which for a long time was the dominant paradigm in social gerontology, saw the way in which old age occurred in modern societies as an inevitable and natural process. Questions about whether older people wanted to 'disengage' or were forced to do so by society were not asked. The emphasis on psychological adjustment also avoided looking at the very real social processes that structured old age.

Structured dependency theory

If the disengagement approach centred on the perspective of the individual older person, then the analysis put forward by the predominantly British 'structured dependency' school (Phillipson 1982, Townsend 1981, Walker 1981) stressed the importance of social policy. For the structured dependency writers the most important fact about the ageing process is the existence of the notion of retirement. In most industrial societies the age at which this occurs has been set by the State, and it is from this point that people are entitled to the State retirement pension. Retirement not only marks the withdrawal from the formal labour market but also the shift from making a living to being dependent on the State. In fact, until the 1990s it was a requirement that, to receive a State pension, the recipient was not allowed to undertake paid work, at the risk of having the money deducted from his or her pension. In this way the State pensioner was treated in the same 'punitive' way as the unemployed person on income support.

Consequently, decisions made by the government have a dramatic effect on how older individuals live their lives. A good example is the decision by the post-war government to set different retirement ages for men and women. Women were to retire at 60 because it was estimated that the average age difference between a husband and wife was 5 years. If men retired at 65 it would therefore be intolerable that their wives would still be working and have access to independent income. After all, this might challenge the moral authority of the male head of the household. For similar reasons, many governments allowed married women to opt out of paying a full national insurance contribution on the grounds that they could share their husband's pension rather than having one in their own right.

We know that a significant section of older people experience poverty. For the structured dependency school this is not a coincidence. State retirement pensions are kept at a deliberately low level, even falling in relation to average living standards. One study concluded that they were worth only 20% of average earnings and that their value will drop by half by 2020 (Evandrou & Falkingham 1993). It is suggested, therefore, that the 'disengaged' nature of many old people is the result of low pensions, and not any process brought on by the ageing process. That this can be seen as a continuing feature of modern Britain can be seen by the abolition of the State Earnings Related Pension Scheme (SERPS). This pension scheme had been set up in the 1970s to create a more generous pension for those not covered by private or occupational schemes. It was effectively abolished by the Conservative government in the 1990s after a long period of atrophy. The post-1997 Labour governments have chosen not to reintroduce the scheme, preferring instead to rely on the private sector and 'stakeholder' pensions.

Structured dependency is not just limited to the economic sphere but rather pervades the whole of society as an effect of this inferior status. The association of age with infirmity might not be factually true but it does 'represent' the position of older people, as does the exclusion of older people from various forms of social involvement. Often, lack of resources is the main reason for what are taken to be the characteristics of older people. The cultural emphasis on 'youth' is one that sees ageing in negative terms. This can lead to 'ageism', where it becomes culturally acceptable to discriminate against older people. This can manifest itself in policies seeking to limit medical or healthcare resources to older people, in discriminatory employment practices and in the treatment of physically frail or mentally confused older people.

If, as the structured dependency school argues, the dependency of older people is structured by society then the obvious response to it is to change those policies that most reinforce the inferior position of older people. Increasing the value of State pensions is one obvious answer. This is controversial, given that the general move in policy circles is towards seeing post-retirement income as an individual responsibility. However, structured dependency theorists remain committed to an egalitarian approach to later life and would argue that it is the State's responsibility to provide a good standard of income for all. Otherwise, what is being perpetuated is class inequality, with those whose prosperity in earlier life ensuring prosperity after retirement.

At a wider level, many advocates of the structured dependency thesis argue that there is a need to establish the full citizenship rights of older people. Rather than forcing older people to adopt a position of special pleading, such citizenship rights would establish the rightful basis for high pensions and full access to health care (Bornat et al 1985).

Third ageism

However, the validity of this approach has been challenged by writers such as Laslett (1996), who argues that modern societies create opportunities for a fulfilling 'third age' of relative good health and affluence. He argues that the portion of most people's lives spent in retirement is increasing all of the time. The idea of a fixed retirement is increasingly being challenged by the many individuals who choose early retirement, or who are made redundant. For many, Laslett argues, this provides possibilities for undertaking the self-enriching activities that there was not enough time for when they were preoccupied with the tasks of working or bringing up children. Laslett identifies education as one of the key areas for a successful third age and to this end he has been a proponent of the University of the Third Age.

This theme meshes well with the work of sociologists of culture such as Featherstone & Hepworth (1991), who argue that there has been a blurring of the distinction between 'middle' and 'old' age. This has occurred because of the increasing influence of lifestyle and consumerism on significant numbers of people outside of the younger age groups who have been typically associated with these developments. An important aspect of these processes is that old age becomes seen as a 'mask' detracting from the person beneath. Older people feel that they are just the same as they were when they were younger. The 'mask of ageing' is accentuated in modern societies where the collapse of clear age-appropriate distinctions of clothing has meant that clothing such as jeans can be worn by people of very different ages. This contributes to what has been described as the 'postmodernization of the life course' where the idea of a linear life course, with clearly defined stages, has become more and more problematic. The distinction between adolescence and adulthood has become blurred as teenagers become more adult in their pursuits and adults become used to an extended period of pleasure-seeking non-responsibility, often waiting until their 30s to have children. Similarly, with the popularity of early retirement among the more affluent (and male) members of society, the idea of a simple work and child-rearing trajectory to life suggests an ideal that is no longer the case.

Gilleard & Higgs (2000) have argued that these changes suggest that we need to see later life in the context of what they call the 'cultures of ageing'. It is not just the individualized 'mask' of ageing that needs to be understood but the whole social terrain on which ageing occurs. They argue that the issues of individual ageing are caught up in a number of cultural processes such as not wanting to be identified as 'old' or being seen in terms of a category of 'loss'. This leads to a preponderance in society of the anti-ageing industry's products. These products reach back across all age groups so that the impact of cultures of ageing is felt at earlier and earlier ages. Wrinkles and greying hair are only small examples of the concerns of such 'nutraceuticals'. It is equally important is to establish that there are no activities outside the ambition of older people, whether it is running a marathon or indeed, as the astronaut John Glenn has done (aged 77), going into space. As examples of this it is possible to point to the growing involvement of older people in entertainment and tourist markets, where they are able to enjoy pleasures previously deemed inappropriate for their age group. The importance of consumerism and consumer culture for third-age lifestyles is central to this approach. As the cultural distinctions previously dominated by social class are replaced by individually focused lifestyles, the consequences of ageing become one of the principal arenas where identity is played out. The fragmentation of the ageing process is something everyone becomes involved in, willingly or not.

Obviously, as Gilleard & Higgs (2000) concede, a lot of this depends on older people having the resources to be able to participate in the various cultural activities that are now open to people in later life. This brings in themes associated with the structured dependency approach. The association of age with poverty has been a historical reality for the last two centuries at least. However, is this connection about the nature of poverty rather than of age? The ability to participate is always dependent on having sufficient resources, and is not necessarily a product of reaching retirement age. Industrialization created a class of wage labourers who spent most of their lives in poverty. Only in the late twentieth century did the standard of living of the mass of workers start to approach a degree of affluence. As these cohorts of relatively affluent workers reach retirement they will bring with them some of the benefits they have accrued during their working lives. After all, occupational pensions took off in the 1950s and 1960s and it is now that this delayed expenditure is being utilized.

Gilleard & Higgs (2000) argue that a major difficulty that many studies of later life suffer from is that they assume that old age is a stable phenomenon, rather than being one that is changing constantly. The present generation of retired people, as we have seen, is better off than the ones that preceded it. This might not continue indefinitely as some of the unique factors associated with the 'baby boomer' generation disappear. Each cohort of people entering retirement needs to be studied separately to fully understand the circumstances and experiences that have fashioned them and upon which they will draw.

CONCLUSION

If the twentieth century was the first century to see large numbers of people survive into old age, then it is likely that the twenty-first century will be one where the implications of this transformation will become apparent. Not only will the assumptions of social and health policy be challenged, but so also will the whole of our understanding of the 'stages of life'. How, or whether, these changes will be addressed is unclear, but it is an inescapable fact that they will become a more and more pressing context for all of us.

References

Bornat J, Philipson C, Ward S 1985 A manifesto for old age. Pluto Press, London

Brocklehurst A, Tallis R, Fillet H 1992 Textbook of geriatric medicine and gerontology. Churchill Livingstone, Edinburgh

Bury M, Holme A 1991 Life after ninety. Routledge, London

Cumming E, Henry W 1961 Growing old: the process of disengagement. Basic Books, New York

Department for Work and Pensions (DWP) 2000 The pensioners' income series 1999/2000. National statistics. HMSO, London

Evandrou M, Falkingham J 1993 Social security and the life course: developing sensitive policy alternative. In: Arber S, Evandrou M (eds) Ageing, independence and the life course. Jessica Kingsley, London

Evandrou M, Falkingham J 2000 Looking back to look forward: lessons from four birth cohorts for ageing in the 21st century. Population Trends 99:21–30

Featherstone M, Hepworth M 1991 The mask of ageing and the post-modern lifecourse. In: Featherstone M, Hepworth, Turner B (eds) The body: social process and cultural theory, Sage, London

Fries J 1983 The compression of morbidity. Milbank Quarterly 397–419

Gilleard C, Higgs P 2000 Cultures of ageing: self, citizen and the body. Prentice Hall, Harlow

Henwood M 1992 Through a glass darkly: community care and older people. The King's Fund, London

HMSO 1995 Social trends 1995. HMSO, London

HMSO 2000 Living in Britain 1998. General household survey. HMSO, London

HMSO 2001 Social trends 31. HMSO, London

HMSO 2002 Living in Britain 2000. General household survey. HMSO, London

Higgs P, Victor C 1993 Institutional care and the life course. In: Arber S, Evandrou M (eds) Ageing, independence and the life course. Jessica Kingsley, London

Johnson P, Falkingham J 1992 Ageing and economic welfare. Sage, London

Laslett P 1996 A fresh map of life, 2nd edn. Weidenfeld and Nicholson, London

Moody H 1995 Ageing, meaning and the allocation of resources. Ageing and Society 15:163–245

Neugarten B et al 1964 Personality in middle and late life. Atherton, New York

Phillipson C 1982 Capitalism and the construction of old age. Methuen, London

Townsend P 1981 The structured dependency of the elderly. Ageing and Society 1:5–28

Victor C 1994 Old age in modern society. Chapman and Hall, London

Walker A 1981 Towards a political economy of old age. Ageing and Society 1:73–94

Walker A 1993 European attitudes to ageing and older people. Commission of the European Communities Directorate General V, Brussels

Walker A, Maltby T 1997 Ageing Europe. Open University Press, Buckingham

The Social Process of Defining Disease

CHAPTER 12

The Limits and Boundaries of Medical Knowledge

Paul Higgs

WESTERN MEDICINE

In today's world, the existence of infective agents as a cause of ill health is seen as such as an obvious truth that it hardly needs stating. In a similar fashion, most people are aware that they risk infection if they allow wounds to be exposed to the environment. Two hundred years ago such precautions were not so obvious. The threat to health posed by microorganisms was not part of everyday understanding because such organisms had not yet been identified by science. This did not mean that until the introduction of the theory of sepsis people did not know about the dangers of leaving a wound open to the air. However, an individual's understanding of what was happening was often very different from one centring on the idea of infective agents.

All societies have had ways of dealing with the problems of illness and disease and these ideas made (and in many cases still do make) perfect sense to the people involved. From our vantage point at the beginning of the twenty-first century, the dominant views of earlier centuries or other cultures might seem strange, if not irrational. Modern medicine can seem to be qualitatively different from these other approaches because it is based on the obviously superior rationality of modern science. The evidence to support this view is compelling, given that medical science can diagnose, treat and cure many of the afflictions that have affected human beings for thousands of years. The difficulty with this approach is that it tells only part of the story. Both medicine and science exist in social contexts that can place limits as well as challenges to their activities. This chapter looks at some of the issues involved.

As an example, we can return to germ theory. The discovery of germs is only part of the picture, especially when this particular theory of illness causation can be overextended to account for many other 'social' processes. This can happen because an idea like that of the 'germ' can catch the public imagination and become part of popular mythology (Lupton 1994). It has been used both to label certain individuals or groups as potentially dangerous, and as a metaphor for social persecution where the undesired group are seen as 'germs' infecting the wider society (Bauman 1995).

To understand fully the workings of medicine in the modern world we must look at the circumstances in which medical knowledge comes about. We must also examine how people understand and are influenced by medical knowledge. Our starting point must be the inextricable link between modern medicine and the world of science. Again, this might seem an unnecessary point to make but the history of medicine need not have culminated in the dominance of what has been described as 'western scientific medicine'. Other highly complex systems of medicine have flourished in other cultures, often for thousands of years (Porter 1998).

Conventional accounts of the development of western science stress its emergence out of irrationalism and magic. Applauding prescientific thinkers for their energy in trying to understand and change the natural world, science and the work of scientists starts to come into existence when the metaphysics is replaced by approaches based on observation and experiment. Seeking-out the regularities of phenomena and explaining why they should be so allows science to be both rational and neutral. Such understanding is seen to form the basis for technological innovation.

Normal science and paradigm shifts

However, as some historians and philosophers of science have pointed out, the idea of a simple distinction between irrational prescience and rational science is not always convincing. In his work 'The structure of scientific revolutions', Thomas Kuhn (1970) pointed out that the way in which science operates is often very far from a rigorous objective assessment of evidence. Instead, Kuhn argues, scientific ideas are organized into definable paradigms of ideas that create a state of what he describes as 'normal science'. Such paradigms define the areas of acceptable knowledge and most scientists work within the framework of ideas provided by such approaches. This means that theories that work in accordance with the paradigm are regarded as the common sense of scientific investigation. Where problems concerning evidence occur they are treated as anomalies to the paradigmatic understanding. New phenomena can provide the basis for a new theory only when the conceptual understanding necessary for the new theory has been established. When scientific change does occur it is often the result of a crisis in the existing theory that brings about a radical change in ideas. This change is what Kuhn calls a 'paradigm shift'. This, rather than the empirical 'falsification' of theories, is what happens in the development of science.

The development of hospital medicine

The idea that scientific knowledge can be understood as a series of successive paradigms, each one replacing the last, has been applied to the development of western medicine. As Jewson (1976) has noted, there has been a progressive displacement of the patient from the centre of medical interest. He argues that prescientific medicine can be characterized as 'bedside medicine' because the doctor or physician had to have a very close relationship with the paying patient who provided his income. This ensured a concern with the particular complaints, symptoms and circumstances of individual patients.

The nature of the medical knowledge at the time was based on the notion of imbalances in the four basic humours of the sanguine (blood), the choreric (yellow bile), the melancholic (black bile) and the phlegmatic (phlegm). Diagnosis and treatment were in terms of restoring the appropriate balance between the humours whose disequilibrium had brought about the illness. In this system of medicine, illness was the same thing as the symptoms reported and not the outward sign of something else. Hence, the focus of medical activity had to be individual patients and their concerns.

This system of medicine had its origins in the works of ancient Greeks and Romans and was still the basis of medical knowledge well into the seventeenth century. However, according to the work of the American sociologist Robert Merton (1970), the impact of the Protestant Reformation in sixteenth century Europe provided the impetus for a more experimentally-based theory of how the body worked. Crucially, it allowed the anatomical dissection of corpses, which had been suppressed under conventional Catholicism. This was of tremendous importance because up until this point the knowledge that most physicians had about anatomy was gleaned from Galen's treatise 'On the conduct of anatomy', which was written in the second century AD and was based on the dissection of monkeys rather than humans. Consequently, the publication of works using direct observation to illustrate a human dissection provided one of the bases for an empirical programme of comparative anatomy where the normal could be distinguished from the pathological.

183

Hospital medicine

The ability to look at patients in the context of what was normal allowed medicine to move away from bedside medicine and towards what Jewson described as 'hospital medicine'. The requirement to provide material for scientific investigation resulted in a need for 'cases' to study. Hospitals came to dominate the healthcare scene in the nineteenth century, where the poor would often be allowed access to medical diagnosis if they would offer themselves up for study. Patients' reports of their symptoms became less important than the physical signs their bodies manifested, and both were merely indications of underlying pathological lesions that were the real problem.

Under hospital medicine, the patient's physical body became crucially important in aiding the understanding of illness. The way in which medicine was practised also changed. The physical examination came to be seen by doctors as a more objective method of investigation than the personal accounts provided by the patient. As the nineteenth century progressed, medical science developed a number of methods for investigating the bodies of patients, such as the stethoscope and the X-ray. The invention of the stethoscope by the French physician Rene Laennec in 1816 was particularly important because it allowed the patient to be examined rather than just observed. Pathology could be localized, confirmed by autopsy and compared with the experience of other physicians. In turn, essential bodily activities such as the pulse could be quantified, leading to standardized measures of physical functioning.

Laboratory medicine

To hospital medicine Jewson adds a further development specific to the twentieth century – that of 'laboratory medicine'. Here, the importance of the body and the physical examination is undermined by the molecular processes underlying normal physical functioning. By studying these, and by the patient providing specimens, medicine can diagnose difficulties that might not even give rise to symptoms or expressions of illness, and through pharmacology deal with them.

Surveillance medicine

The development of western biomedicine results in the essential 'dualism' of the body and mind in medical practice (Longino & Murphy 1995), where the individual's body is treated as separate from his or her understanding of it. That such approaches have had a negative effect on the practice of medicine is suggested by the popularity of holistic approaches to medical care. Possibly in response to this, Armstrong (1995) suggests a new development in the emergence of what he describes as 'surveillance medicine'. In this development it is not just the ill patient who is the focus of concern but the whole population. Using the results of health surveys, surveillance medicine starts from the premise that absence of disease is not the same as health. As people go about their everyday lives they exhibit, to varying degrees, many different risk factors, such as diet, weight, behaviour, and so on. Instead of localized pathology occurring at specific moments, all symptoms, signs and diseases become 'factors' of constructed 'risks'. Diets rich in saturated fats allied to obesity (measured by the body–mass index) found among people who smoke are illustrative of factors increasing the risk of coronary heart disease. Unlike the underlying pathology identified by hospital medicine, which would eventually erupt into illness or 'clinical consciousness', all that risk factors identify are propensities to future outcomes, which might in turn be transformed into new risk factors. The time frame for medicine becomes the whole lifespan. This has effects on the form of clinical intervention, which must approach health care through information campaigns and that seeks to encourage the self-monitoring of risk by individuals, as well as behavioural change.

SOCIAL CONSTRUCTIONISM

Michel Foucault and the clinical gaze

The French philosopher Michel Foucault claims that the development of modern medicine has taken the particular route that it has because it simultaneously constructs its own object of inquiry and comes up with ideas to explain and deal with it. To the prescientific physician the evidence for the existence of humours was as compelling as the modern doctor's acceptance of the evidence provided by X-rays. The medieval anatomists using Galen's account of the body could 'see' what he had told them was there because that was what they were supposed to see. Foucault (1976) argued that with the creation of the hospital came what he describes as the 'clinical gaze', which established the idea that disease was a discrete phenomenon of the human anatomy. For Foucault, the gaze is a way of seeing and understanding that becomes identical with the thing itself.

Social constructionism and the sociology of the body

For Foucault, there are no fixed meanings or even the possibility of an appeal to an external reality. For this reason he has often been identified with a theoretical approach known as 'social constructionism'. This approach is marked by an interest in how health and illness are created and understood by society and social processes, rather than seeking to find a biological basis for them. The anthropologist Mary Douglas (1970) has written that in many cultures the body has often been seen as an image of society. As a result, our notions about the body will often relate to prevailing ideas about society.

Consequently, for Foucault, it is not only how medical science sees the body that is affected by discourses of knowledge, but also how people themselves view their own bodies. The shift from traditional agricultural forms of society to modern industrial ones, as Shilling (1993) points out, has also been marked by a transition from a concern with the 'fleshy' body to an interest in the 'mindful body'. What this means is that instead of the body being just an object synonymous with the person, the mind is given a central role in directing what the body does and is made responsible for it. We can see in the emphasis given to health promotion an echo of this approach.

The rise of the 'mindful body' itself also changes the nature of health and illness, as new 'problems' and new 'solutions' become commonplace in medicine. In the nineteenth century, Foucault (1981) argues a concern developed regarding the nature of sexuality and the problem of the 'hysterical woman' and the 'masturbating child'. The worry arose that if these tendencies were not countered then the health of the nation would be harmed. In a different way, current worries regarding fitness and slimming are seen as ways of being desirable and attractive in a consumer society that puts great store on image.

185

The work of Michel Foucault has acted as a challenge to many sociologists to look at how what is taken as normal and benign is in fact the product of our own contemporary imagination. In fields as diverse as dentistry and surgery, Foucaldian analyses have been put forward to account for what is described as the 'fabrication' of discourses and to locate the operation of 'micro-power'. Ultimately, Foucault was interested in how power permeated every aspect of society to such a degree that everybody was involved in the exercise of it. In his studies of madness (Foucault 1973) and penal policy (Foucault 1977) he demonstrated that far from there having been progress to a more humane position, what resulted from psychiatry and penology was more controlling and more invasive. Ironically, one of the dilemmas that resulted from these pieces of research has been the relativization of the subject under study. It can become impossible to see the benefit in any system of knowledge and, as a consequence, impossible to believe there is any point in changing it. This has been particularly true of some feminist researchers who have been influenced by Foucault.

Erving Goffman and bodily idiom

The work of the American sociologist Erving Goffman provides another way in which the body plays a role in constructing our understanding of health and illness. Goffman argues that fundamental to human interaction and communication is the level of non-verbal language in which the body plays a major part. What is called 'body idiom' indicates to all those who share a culture all sorts of important knowledge. What a person says needs to be backed up with the appropriate clothes, gestures, expressions, and so on, if it is to be accepted. Body idiom allows people to classify, label and grade others. It is a continual process that is ever-present in all public interactions. It plays a crucial role in creating individuals' self-identities, as well as their social identities.

Control over the body is therefore important for people in social interactions with strangers. People with physical disabilities are at a disadvantage because if they lack control over parts of their bodies this might interfere with the process of communication. Goffman argues that this can lay the basis for the 'stained' identity that forms the basis of 'stigmatization'. It is not at all surprising, therefore, that many people with disabilities would prefer to 'mask' and 'pass' off their disablement rather than be classified in terms of their disability. However, this strategy also has its drawbacks given the continual need for the individual to be wary of 'leaking' their discredited identity to others. Epilepsy is one condition where this can occur (see Chapter 13).

Goffman's (1968) account of the social construction of disability as stigma is very useful when we look at how the interaction of people in society plays an important role in creating healthcare problems. The existence of stigma leads one part of medicine to become involved in attempting to find ways of countering the visible signs of stigmatizing conditions with techniques such as corrective surgery, whereas another part attempts to find causes and cures. As a result, medicine becomes involved with issues such as erasing face-disfiguring port-wine birthmarks, providing prosthetic limbs and providing growth hormones for children of lower than average height.

MEDICINE, MEDICALIZATION AND SOCIAL CONTROL

The fact that medicine is wrapped inextricably in social processes means that it is continually expected to move into fresh areas and deal with new problems. Part of the reason for this is the very success of medical science and technology. The capacities opened up by drug research, computerization and the new genetics mean that – potentially – most areas of life can be the focus for medical intervention. Although this is widely welcomed as providing more and more sick people with ways of being made better, it also represents problems on a number of fronts. People can feel that many of their own life experiences are being taken over by a detached biomedical elite. The experience of many women giving birth has been precisely this: that pregnancy is treated like an illness and that the procedures involved in giving birth to a child have been constructed with the doctor in mind rather than the mother. A dispute still rages as to whether hi-tech deliveries are less hazardous than ones that perhaps take place in the mother's home and at the mother's pace. However, the very fact that such a debate exists illustrates that there is some unease at the direction taken by modern medicine.

It is not only patients who are wary of the increased expectations placed upon them by both the public and pharmaceutical companies. The British Medical Journal (BMJ) conducted a poll on its website to identify the top ten non-diseases that healthcare workers were supposed to deal with. These included boredom, baldness, bags under eyes and ugliness (Smith 2002). Part of the problem is that biomedicine has become an integral part of what has been termed 'aspirational medicine' (Gilleard & Higgs 2000) where the individual desires of the population are transformed into biomedical priorities. Top of the BMJ list of non-diseases was unsurprisingly, ageing. The research into avoiding the physical signs of ageing crosses over into research on overcoming ageing itself. Expectations on medicine are therefore created and these can lead to disappointment when reality does not match the ideal.

This can become even more of a problem if expectations are combined with a belief that risks to health can be avoided if people are forewarned. Anthony Giddens (1991) has described modern societies as experiencing what he calls 'manufactured uncertainty' in relation to risk. Such uncertainty is the result of too much information about risks and no real way of assessing their true impact. The controversy over the safety of eating beef against its potential for causing the devastating dementia of Creutzfeldt–Jakob disease illustrates this phenomenon. A similar fear arose about the safety of the combined measles, mumps and rubella (MMR) inoculation given to children and its potential to trigger autism. Both examples demonstrate the power of information simultaneously to make individuals aware of an issue but provide no conclusive answers to their concerns.

latrogenesis

Another aspect of the increasing involvement of medicine in many different aspects of social life is what the radical Latin American priest Ivan Illich (1975) calls 'iatrogenesis', or self-caused disease. He claims that there are three distinct types of iatrogenesis: clinical, cultural and social. 'Clinical iatrogenesis' is when medical treatment makes that patient worse or creates new conditions. As the old joke goes, the last place you want to be if you are ill is a hospital because that is where all the other sick people are and you'll catch whatever they have got. Although this might be a gross simplification it is not entirely without foundation. It is also possible that the medical intervention itself could be unnecessary or irrelevant. 'Social iatrogenesis' is the label Illich attaches to the way in which medicine expands into more and more areas, creating an artificial demand for its services. This in turn leads on to 'cultural iatrogenesis', whereby the ability to cope with the issues surrounding life and death is eroded progressively by medical accounts. This leads to a reliance on medicine to solve problems and a corresponding decrease in autonomy. Illich believes that, as a consequence, the scope of modern medicine should be demystified if not curtailed.

Connected to these notions is the fact that medicine can, as we have seen, create its own problems by medicalizing hitherto non-medicalized areas of life. A good example is the case of heroin addiction (Dally 1995). At first sight, this might seem an area of obvious medical action but through most of the nineteenth century it was regarded as a pastime and not a medical concern. This changed when it became a controlled drug in 1906. However, even up to the 1960s a small but significant number of addicts were enabled to maintain their addiction through private prescriptions provided by some GPs in private practice. What this meant was that these addicts were not criminalized and were thus enabled to live lives of relative stability. What problems these individuals had were ones of lifestyle and not necessarily the result of a medical condition. What changed this state of affairs was a number of people abusing the system and the identification of the medical category – 'drug dependency' – as a field of activity for the speciality of psychiatry. Addiction was to be cured rather than controlled. Gradually there was a change in the approach taken towards addicts; now they were to be actively treated to remove their dependency on heroin. Methadone replacement therapy was offered as an alternative. Unfortunately, it did not have a particularly high success rate and many addicts dropped out of the programmes, usually resorting to illegal 'street' heroin. This in turn brought them into conflict with the police and ensured that, to maintain supplies for their addiction, they had to adopt a criminal lifestyle.

In this manner it could be argued that medicine, by being morally pressurized to do something about a social problem, ends up adding to, rather than dealing with, the real issues of drug addiction. Part of this attitude can be seen in the dilemma about the high rates of HIV infection among intravenous drug users. Do you give out syringes and thereby condone illegal drug use, or do you refuse and let infection rates increase?

Mental illness

A way of understanding these issues is to utilize the concept of social control. All societies need to have some form of generally accepted value system if they are to remain relatively stable. This, by definition, creates people who refuse to, or cannot, fit in. These people become seen, and are often treated, as deviants. Various groups at different times can be seen to occupy this category. They could be members of youth subcultures, new-age travellers or criminals but they all play the same role in that they enable the majority to define themselves in terms of who they are not. Medicine can, and has, played a role in defining populations of deviants by finding medical conditions for them. This happened most notoriously in the former Soviet Union, where people opposing the nature of the State were often diagnosed as having severe psychiatric problems necessitating hospitalization.

However, similar things happened in Britain up until the early decades of the twentieth century, where pregnancy outside marriage was regarded as indicative of an absence of morals, which could only have a medical cause.

To this end, a number of 'rebels' within the psychiatric profession, such as Szasz (1966), have argued that psychiatry's main role is to control deviant populations because of the tremendous legal and categorizing powers capable of being invoked. Often, those subject to psychiatric control lose all social and civil rights and are subject to controversial treatments such as electroconvulsive therapy. In addition, those labelled as mentally ill are completely at the mercy of those treating them and can regain their lives only if they agree with these people.

In contrast to the 'anti-psychiatrists', Hirst & Woolley (1982) argue that it would be wrong to assert that there is no real negative context to mental illness. They point out that all cultures have categories to express the idea that a person is not functioning properly. These might be seen as episodic occurrences or more long-term difficulties, but they are identified by most people as problems none the less. Psychiatry does become involved in controlling some members of society, but this is not sufficient reason to claim that this is its only function.

MEDICINE, SOCIAL STRUCTURE AND SOCIAL POLICY

The practice of medicine is not confined to the ideas that determine what is and what is not a medical problem. Modern medicine has come into being at the same time as industrialization and has become an integral feature of it. As countries have become more technologically advanced so has medicine. Since the Second World War, breakthroughs connected to groups of drugs such as antibiotics have meant that many infectious diseases can now be successfully dealt with. Previously deadly diseases such as smallpox have been officially eradicated from the planet. With this success has come a growth in demand for modern health services throughout the world. Because modern medicine is perceived as being capable of achieving great things with people's health, then more and more people want access to it. This has meant that many developing nations are put in impossible situations trying to provide costly hi-tech medicine in environments where there are few resources.

At this point it is useful to remember McKeown's argument that the improvement in the health of the British population during the nineteenth and early twentieth centuries was a result of improvements in diet, sanitation and public health (McKeown 1979). The efforts of doctors did not make much impact until the second part of the twentieth century (see Chapter 1). The impressive strides made by medical knowledge therefore depend crucially on the existence of a wider social infrastructure that can support such advances. In most societies this is formalized into some form of healthcare system. There are many different types of healthcare system (Roemer 1989) (see Chapter 19). Some organize health care on free-market principles with the State playing a minimal role except to provide a safety-net for certain underprivileged groups, whereas others are based on compulsory State insurance, as in France. Britain is quite unusual in the way it organizes its health services because it is funded out of general taxation rather than through individual contributions.

However, the differences between healthcare systems do not just reflect national characteristics but are different solutions to the problems of providing access to medical and health services and being able to pay for it. At its most simple, this accounts for the disparities in healthcare provision in some developing countries. The possession of wealth or being an expatriate of a western nation means that you have access to medical facilities as good as those in the industrialized countries. Correspondingly, if you are poor your access to services is likely to be minimal and might in fact be rudimentary.

Marxist accounts of welfare

The existence of welfare states in the industrialized countries is a relatively recent phenomenon. Britain introduced old age pensions and a limited medical insurance scheme at the beginning of the twentieth century, and the welfare state of which the National Health Service was a cornerstone did not come into being until 1948. Among the reasons put forward for this delay was the belief that State welfare was a victory for the working class because it shifted responsibility for paying for welfare away from the poorest sections of society. Marxist writers such as Vincente Navarro (1994) and Ian Gough (1979) argue that health care is a key battlefield in the conflict between labour and employers in all societies. The working class wants to ameliorate as many of the adverse conditions created by capitalism as it can, whereas the employers want to make as much profit as they can at as little cost. Sometimes, as in post-war Britain, concessions have to be made to allow profitability to continue. At other times, such as during the 1970s, cuts have to be made to this 'social wage' so that money can be diverted to profit. This is not to suggest that health care is only an outcome of political struggle. Marxist theorists have also identified that the role of the welfare state is central to the continuation of a profitable capitalism. The welfare state carries out three roles: to ensure the health and education of the existing workforce; to produce the next generation of workers; and to justify the inequalities of capitalism. Of course, not all of these things can be done successfully all of the time, and this is why the welfare state seems in a constant state of crisis.

It is not only Marxists who have noted the close connection between the economy and the welfare state that has resulted in a crisis for the idea of a welfare state. Mishra (1984) noted that if money is to be spent on welfare the first thing that has to be established is economic prosperity. All welfare states seem to be coming to this conclusion, with governments of all persuasions, from New Zealand to Holland, trying to reduce expenditure. This difficulty is sometimes known as the 'fiscal crisis of the state' and results from the tendency for welfare, and particularly health spending, to increase over time. Many policy analysts believe that a limit to spending is essential if health care is to continue to be publicly funded and organized. Much of the impetus to reform healthcare systems in Britain and throughout the industrialized world has concentrated on finding ways of controlling costs and making the delivery of health care more effective and efficient. The initial solution in Britain was the introduction of what has been known as 'managed competition' or 'quasi-markets'. This has given way under the post-1997 Labour governments to the idea of commissioning health care. The language might have changed but the fundamental issues of limited finances and efficiency remain.

189

The 'third way' and social policy

One important direction in which social policy is going is the development of what has been described as 'third way' politics. Although it is true that this formulation has failed to articulate why it is different to both neo-liberalism and social democracy, the election of 'New Labour' seems to have created a new approach to relations between the State and its citizens. The idea of mass citizenship entitlements, which was fundamental to the creation of the welfare state and of the National Health Service, has become seen as an anachronism not suitable for modern times. The world is no longer made up of people defining themselves in terms of class. Instead, many potential identities can form the basis of our individualized relationship with society. The significance of consumption and consumerism is one major challenge to the traditional view of citizenship.

At its core, the 'third way' approach sees the enabling of individuals as its central role, rather than utilizing the State as a provider of services or security (Giddens 2000). In fields as diverse as pensions, education and unemployment, the onus is on the individual to take responsibility and make choices. This approach accepts that there will be differences of outcome but such differences reflect a complex world where the old ideas of State control can no longer work. The nature of medicine and the provision of health services must also reflect this 'third way' approach. The idea of medical paternalism that has been dominant throughout the whole period of modernity suddenly finds itself challenged. Professional autonomy regarding practice finds itself under public scrutiny. The idea that General Medical Council's (GMC) self-regulation of the medical profession is sufficient has been seriously challenged by the Bristol Royal Infirmary Inquiry into heart surgery on children. The areas of research and the questions that arise from scientific curiosity and progress are no longer only the province of those with professional insight. Developments in assisted conception and cloning have opened areas of public concern as to the acceptable actions of doctors. More significantly, what the public has a right to expect from the providers of health care is now subject to consumer demand and interests. The simple distinction between dealing with disease and enhancing health in its most comprehensive form can be illustrated by the public response to the prescribing of Viagra. These developments are further compounded by government policies that seek to provide information to all involved in making choices about health care, whether this is at a general or individual level. Not only is local consultation seen as necessary in developing services but various performance indicators, such as league tables produced so that individuals can assess institutional activity.

In return for this information and nominal role in decision making, is the constant monitoring and surveillance of both practitioners and patients. The new approach does not appreciate passivity or reluctance to engage. A term coined by Michel Foucault 'governmentality' is useful to describe this process. What it refers to is the guiding of behaviour or organizing the 'conduct of conduct'. The emphasis is on ensuring that individuals choose the 'correct' way to do something. In the arena of health there have always been correct ways to do things such as cleaning your teeth. This has now extended to many other areas such as diet and exercise. The role of the healthcare system becomes increasingly one that is involved in attempting to modify individual behaviours. This role is a double-edged sword because it can easily lead to the conclusion that individual behaviour is the source of many social problems as well as being their solution. An example of this can be found in 'New Labour's' response to the health inequalities debate where recommendations of income redistribution were rejected in favour of promoting health behaviour change.

However, it would be wrong to conclude that the boundaries of health care and medicine are set by the priorities of an increasingly globalized capitalism. Many of the conclusions drawn by politicians and policy makers are not shared by many individuals operating in the fields of health care and medicine. There have been many struggles over the impact of World Bank and International Monetary Fund policies towards the developing world. These policies can particularly affect the provision of health services as Structural Adjustment Programmes, with their priority to privatize, adversely affect investment in the public sector. In a similar fashion, the burden of debt in many countries also puts an impossible set of demands on poor countries. In recent years, developing countries have started to successfully challenge the dominance of some multinational drug companies by demanding that patented drugs to deal with HIV/AIDS be sold more cheaply or produced generically. Antiglobalization movements have also had an effect on the situation faced by many of the world's population. Bringing the demand for 'people before profits' to the attention of the people in the industrialized world has pushed some governments to address the linked issues of poverty and health in the developing world. There might be a considerable distance still to go but the globalization of the world economy can lead to a common awareness of the need for health for all of the world's population.

CONCLUSION

This chapter has attempted to cover some of the boundaries to the practice of medicine that exist in the modern world. It has drawn attention to the social and cultural aspects of the construction of medical knowledge. It has also pointed out that medicine and health care can, and have, been involved in the construction and maintenance of forms of social power through the socially sanctioned authority to define what are medical or health problems. These concerns might seem incidental to the way that modern medicine is practised today with its emphasis on resource allocation and clinical effectiveness. However, to ignore these issues is to neglect in some part the way in which we have reached this point of success. A failure to integrate scientific medicine with its social context, or to face some of the difficult implications of its practice, will in the long term separate medicine from its potential as a humanitarian project.

191

References

Armstrong D 1995 The rise of surveillance medicine. Sociology, Health and Illness 17:393–404

Bauman Z 1995 Life in fragments: essays in postmodern morality. Blackwell, Oxford

Dally A 1995 Anomalies and mysteries in the war on drugs. In: Porter R, Teich M (eds) Drugs and narcotics in history. Cambridge University Press, Cambridge

Douglas M 1970 Natural symbols: explorations in cosmology. Cresset Press, London

Foucault M 1973 Madness and civilisation. Tavistock, London

Foucault M 1976 The birth of the clinic. Tavistock, London

Foucault M 1977 Discipline and punish. Penguin, London

Foucault M 1981 History of sexuality, vol. 1. Penguin, Harmondsworth

Giddens A 1991 The consequences of modernity. Polity Press, Cambridge

Giddens A 2000 The third way and its critics. Polity, Press, Cambridge

Gilleard C, Higgs P 2000 Cultures of ageing: self, citizen and the body. Prentice Hall, Harlow

Goffman E 1968 Stigma. Penguin, Harmondsworth

Gough I 1979 The political economy of the welfare state. Macmillan. London

Hirst P, Woolley P 1982 Social relations and human attributes. Tavistock, London:

Illich I 1975 Medical nemesis. Calder and Boyars, London

Jewson N 1976 The disappearance of the sick man from medical cosmology. Sociology 10:225–244

Kuhn T 1970 The structure of scientific revolutions. University of Chicago Press, Chicago

Longino C, Murphy J 1995 The old age challenge to the biomedical model: paradigm strain and health policy. Baywood, Amityville, NY

Lupton D 1994 Medicine as culture. Sage, London

McKeown T 1979 The role of medicine. Oxford University Press, Oxford

Merton R 1970 Science, technology and society in seventeenth century England. Howard Fertig, New York

Mishra R 1984 The crisis of the welfare state. Harvester Wheatsheaf, Hemel Hempstead

Navarro V 1994 The politics of health policy. Blackwell, London

Porter R 1998 The greatest benefit to mankind: a medical history of humanity. Harper Collins, London

Roemer M 1989 National health services as market interventions. Journal of Public Health Policy 10:62–77

Shilling C 1993 The body and social theory. Sage, London

Smith R 2002 In search of 'non-disease'. British Medical Journal 324:883–885

Szasz T 1966 The myth of mental illness. Harper, New York

CHAPTER 13

Deviance, Sick Role and Stigma

Graham Scambler

Social norms are definite principles or rules that people are expected to observe in a given culture or milieu. Only a tiny minority of norms is likely to be codified as laws. Deviance can be defined as non-conformity to a norm, or set of norms, which is accepted by a significant proportion of local citizens or inhabitants. Deviant behaviour is behaviour that, once it has become public knowledge, is routinely subject to sanctions – to punishment, correction or treatment. Importantly, behaviour that is acceptable in one culture might be deviant in another. For example, smoking marijuana is deviant in British culture whereas consuming alcohol is not; the reverse is the case in some Middle Eastern cultures.

ILLNESS, DEVIANCE AND THE SICK ROLE

Few analysts before the 1950s regarded illness as a form of deviance. The term 'deviance' was reserved for behaviour for which individuals could be held responsible; infractions of the law were seen as paradigmatic. A significant change of outlook dates from the work of Parsons (1951), who defined illness as a form of deviance on the grounds that it disrupts the social system by inhibiting people's performance of their customary or normal social roles. If such disruption is to be minimized then the behaviour associated with illness – which, unlike other forms of deviant behaviour cannot be prevented by the threat of sanctions – must be controlled. Control is exercised through the prescription of social roles for the sick and for physicians (see Chapter 4).

According to Parsons, the sick role consists of two rights and two obligations. The rights are that sick people are exempted: (1) from performing their normal social roles; and (2) from responsibility for their own state. Sick people are at the same time obligated: (1) to want to get well as soon as possible; and (2) to consult and cooperate with medical experts whenever the severity of their condition warrants it. Failure to meet either or both of these obligations could lead to the charge that people are responsible for the continuation of their illness and – ultimately – to sanctions, including the withdrawal of the rights of the sick role. Gerhardt (1987) describes Parsons' sick role as a social 'niche' where 'the incapacitated have a chance to recover from their weakness(es), and overcome their urge to withdraw from rather than actively tackle the vicissitudes of the capitalist labour market'. In fact, it can afford its incumbents a legitimate breathing space from a wide range of social demands, and not only from those associated with the labour market.

The sick role is a temporary role into which all people, regardless of their status or position, can be admitted. It is also 'universalistic', in that physicians are held to draw upon general and objective criteria in determining whether individuals are sick, how sick they are and what kinds of sickness they are suffering from. Its main function is to control illness and to reduce its disruptive effects on the social system by ensuring that sick people are returned to a healthy state as speedily as possible. Physicians serve as 'gatekeepers', policing access to the sick role by authoritatively determining who is sick and who is healthy. They also spur the urge to leave the sick role (Gerhardt 1987). Unlike some other commentators, Parsons is not at all critical of physicians functioning as agents of social control. Indeed, he sees the sick role, and physicians' policing of it, as important contributions to the stability and health of the social system.

Among those who are less sanguine about physicians' social control functions is Freidson (1970), who acknowledges Parsons' pioneering work in linking illness and deviance but insists that the argument must be taken a step further:

> Unlike Parsons, I do not argue merely that medicine has the power to legitimize one's acting sick by conceding that he really is sick ... I argue that by virtue of being the authority on what illness 'really' is, medicine creates the social possibilities for acting sick. In this sense, medicine's monopoly includes the right to create illness as an official social role.

Freidson adds that it is in medicine's interests – because it enhances the demand for its practitioners' skills – to pursue actively 'the proliferation of situations that create "deviant illness roles"'.

It is not necessary to adhere to a thesis of 'medical imperialism' – namely, to claim a conspiracy on the part of physicians to 'medicalize' society – to acknowledge either that a multiplicity of new deviant illness roles were created in the twentieth century (perhaps most conspicuously as a product of the growth of psychiatry) or that this has accorded physicians greater powers and responsibilities as agents of social control. Freidson's contribution is to have pointed out that these powers and responsibilities have social – not merely scientific – origins, and require careful analysis and evaluation. After all, to diagnose disease is to define its bearer as in need of correctional 'treatment' of body or mind (even if in practice this often involves little more than recognizing a disease's self-limiting natural history). Unlike Parsons, Freidson sees physicians' social control functions as extending far beyond the policing of the sick role and as possessing negative as well as positive potential for society.

THE FORCE OF A LABEL

In modern societies, professionally trained physicians are generally responsible not only for (collectively) constructing but also for (individually) selecting and applying diagnostic labels. It is now recognized, however, that the application and communication of some diagnoses can have especially serious and unwelcome consequences for patients. This occurs most conspicuously when the conditions being diagnosed are personally or socially stigmatizing. Stigmatizing conditions can be defined as conditions that set their possessors apart from 'normal' people, which mark them as socially unacceptable or inferior beings. Thus, people experiencing deafness, mental illness, severe burns, diabetes, psoriasis, acquired immunodeficiency syndrome (AIDS) and numerous other diseases or symptoms of disease have been in the past and continue to be avoided, rejected or shunned to varying degrees by others.

Another unhappy consequence of being labelled in this way is that people's stigma can come to dominate the perceptions that others have of them and how they treat them. In the vocabulary of sociology, an individual's deviant status becomes a master status: whatever else he or she might be (mother or father, teacher or school governor) he or she is regarded primarily as a diabetic, cancer victim or whatever. In other words, the individual's deviant status comes to dominate and push into the background his or her other statuses. Even the past might be unsafe and subject to retrospective interpretation. Especially pertinent to this line of reasoning are the concepts of 'cultural stereotyping' and 'secondary deviation'.

Cultural stereotyping

Those afflicted with a stigmatizing condition might be expected to conform to a popular stereotype. An American study, for example, found that blind people are often attributed distinctive personality characteristics that differentiate them from sighted people: 'helplessness', 'dependency', 'melancholy', 'docility', 'gravity of inner thought' and 'aestheticism' (Scott 1969). However far-fetched or misleading such stereotyping might be, the blind person cannot ignore how others expect him or her to behave; to do so might well be to ignore key factors in his or her interaction with them. The author goes on to claim that blind people adapt to cultural stereotyping in five major ways: (1) simply concurring; (2) 'cutting themselves off' to protect their self-conceptions; (3) deliberately adopting a facade of compliance for expediency's sake; (4) making people pay something for a 'performance' (e.g. begging); or (5) actively resisting. It should be mentioned that they might also be obliged to respond to stereotypes of blindness held by physicians and other health professionals.

Secondary deviation

One distinction that has gained currency among those investigating links between crime and deviance is that between 'primary' and 'secondary' deviation (Lemert 1967). Study of the former focuses on how deviant behaviour, for example, stealing, originates. Study of the latter focuses on how people are assigned symbolically to deviant statuses, for example, thief or criminal, and the effective consequences of such assignment for subsequent deviation on their part. The importance of studying secondary deviation has been increasingly acknowledged since the 1960s. It is now accepted, for example, that disapproving cultural and professional reactions to deviant behaviour can often foster rather than inhibit a continuing commitment to deviance.

Similarly, some have claimed that a negative, stereotyped reaction to a stigmatizing illness or handicap can confirm individuals in their deviant status, can constrain them to see themselves as others see them and to behave accordingly. For example, a blind person who is expected to be and is consistently treated as 'helpless' and 'dependent' might actually become so; he or she might find it less exacting to concur with and ultimately adopt the prescribed role than to resist it. Those in institutional or custodial care for long periods are particularly vulnerable in this respect.

Perhaps the area in which 'labelling theory' has had the most controversial impact in relation to medicine has been that of mental illness. In the mid-1960s the American sociologist Scheff claimed that labelling is the single most important cause of mental illness (Scheff 1966). He argued that a residue of odd, eccentric and unusual behaviour exists for which the culture provides no explicit labels: such forms of behaviour constitute 'residual rule-breaking' or 'residual deviance'. Most psychiatric symptoms can be categorized as instances of residual deviance. There is also a cultural stereotype of mental illness. When for some reason or other residual deviance becomes a salient or 'public' issue, the cultural stereotype of insanity becomes the guiding imagery for action. In time, contact with a physician is established, a psychiatric diagnosis made and, perhaps, procedures for hospitalization put into effect. Problems of secondary deviation follow with a degree of predictability.

Scheff's theory has been criticized by others, notably Gove (1970). Gove agreed that there is a cultural stereotype of mental illness, but not that people are treated as mentally ill because they inadvertently behave in a way that 'activates' this stereotype. If anything, he argued, 'the gross exaggeration of the degree and type of disorder in the stereotype fosters the denial of mental illness, since the disturbed person's behaviour does not usually correspond to the stereotype' (Gove 1970). Scheff is also wrong, according to Gove, in suggesting that, once publicly noticed, the person will be routinely processed as mentally ill and admitted for institutional care; public officials, he argued, 'screen out' a large proportion of those who come before them. Finally, Gove claimed that Scheff overstated the degree to which secondary deviation is associated with hospitalization for mental illness. Although the dispute between Scheff and his critics continues, it seems reasonable to conclude that he fell foul of the temptation to explain too much in terms of a single, if important, insight.

LIVING WITH A STIGMATIZING CONDITION

Stigmatizing conditions vary in terms of their visibility and obtrusiveness and of the extent to which they are recognized. Not surprisingly, there is an equivalent degree of variation in their effects on individuals' lives. People who are 'discredited', to use Goffman's (1963) terminology, are those whose stigma is immediately apparent, such as amputees, or widely known, such as someone whose fellow workers know of his suicide attempt. The discredited will often find they have to cope with situations made awkward by their stigma: their problem will be one of managing tension. Davis (1964) found that the physically handicapped typically pass through three stages when meeting with strangers: the first is one of 'fictional acceptance' – they find they are ascribed some sort of stereotypical identity and accepted on that basis; the second stage is one of 'breaking through' this fictional acceptance – they induce others to regard and interact with them normally; and the third stage is one of 'consolidation' – they have to sustain the definition of themselves as normal over time.

One major criticism of Davis' account is that it overestimates people's strength of will and psychological stamina to engage in what he calls 'deviance disavowal'. It was noted earlier that some blind people regard it as less taxing to defer to than to contest cultural stereotypes of blindness. Higgins (1980) found that deaf people sometimes actually 'avow' their deviance, and even extend it by acting mute in order to simplify and smooth their relations with the hearing: written messages can minimize misunderstandings and save time and embarrassment.

People who are 'discreditable' are those whose stigma is only occasionally apparent, such as people with epilepsy who suffer infrequent seizures, or little known, such as someone whose status as human immunodeficiency virus (HIV) positive is known only to his or her doctor. The discreditable will usually find they have to take care to manage information; to 'pass as normal' they will have to censor what others know about them. In Goffman's (1963) words, the main quandary is: 'To display or not to display; to tell or not to tell; to lie or not to lie: and in each case, to whom, how, when and where'. People with epilepsy frequently opt to pass as normal, and hence find themselves having to manage information with extreme caution. The following paragraphs illustrate this, and these and the succeeding sections on rectal cancer and HIV/AIDS afford some indication of the types of factors that affect adjustment to stigma.

Epilepsy

The adults with recurring seizures that Scambler & Hopkins (1986) studied clearly felt that, in an important sense, physicians had 'made them into epileptics' by selecting and communicating the diagnosis of epilepsy. It was a diagnostic label that most found unpleasant and threatening and some openly resented and contested, largely, it seems, because they saw the status of 'epileptic' as highly stigmatizing. Those who had been diagnosed in childhood often seemed to have learned to think of their epilepsy in this way as a result of their parents' behaviour: for example, well-intentioned advice never to use the word 'epilepsy', especially outside the home. Schneider & Conrad (1983), reporting the same finding in the USA, refer graphically to such parents as 'stigma coaches'. They add that careless or overprotective physicians can also function as stigma coaches.

Once applied, diagnostic labels tend to be difficult to shake off. Nevertheless, the stigma of people with epilepsy is dormant between seizures; for much of their time, therefore, they are discreditable rather than discredited. Scambler & Hopkins (1986) found that, fearing discrimination, people tended to conceal their epilepsy whenever possible. Witnessed seizures were often 'explained away' – for example, as faints – and 'stories' constructed to account for the fact that they could not drive – 'because of the law, or drink' – because of their anticonvulsant medication. Two-thirds of those experiencing epileptic seizures at the time of marriage hid the fact from their partners, at least until after the ceremony. Of those with full-time jobs outside the home, 28% had disclosed their epilepsy to their employers, and only 1 in 20 – all of whom were experiencing seizures daily at the time – had done so before taking the job.

The same authors made a distinction between felt stigma and enacted stigma. The former refers to the shame associated with 'being epileptic' and, most significantly perhaps, to the fear of being discriminated against solely on the grounds of an imputed cultural unacceptability or inferiority; and the latter refers to actual discrimination of this kind. Scambler (1989) has utilized this distinction to formulate a 'hidden distress model' in relation to epilepsy. This states that the sense of felt stigma is so strong that people with epilepsy typically do their utmost to maintain secrecy about their symptoms and the diagnostic label: they disclose only when it strikes them as prudent or necessary. Non-disclosure, in turn, reduces the likelihood of encountering enacted stigma. Thus felt stigma leads to a policy of concealment that has the effect of reducing the incidence of enacted stigma. Paradoxically, felt stigma was more disruptive of people's lives and well-being than was enacted stigma, which was in fact rarely experienced. Interestingly, Jacoby (1994) has since shown that felt stigma can remain salient even for people whose seizures are extremely infrequent or who are in remission.

Rectal cancer

If in the nineteenth century tuberculosis stood out as the disease arousing the most dread and repulsion, cancer became its twentieth-century equivalent. Sontag (1977) has argued that it is likely to occupy this role until its aetiology is clarified and its treatments as effective as those of tuberculosis. Rectal cancer accounts for 10% of cancer diagnoses. Two-thirds of those with rectal cancer are left with a permanent colostomy following amputation of the anus and rectum. A colostomy is an incontinent, artificial anus that, with no sphincter to control it, can release faeces and flatus unpredictably, generally into a plastic bag attached to the abdomen. MacDonald (1988) has examined patients' perceptions of what amounts to a family of stigmas: 'the shame, taboos and fears associated with mutilation of the body, with faecal incontinence, with seeing and handling faeces, and with cancer'.

MacDonald found that 49% of her sample reported 'some stigma' and 16% 'severe stigma'; these proportions rose to 54% and 26%, respectively, for those with a colostomy, most of whom said they felt as though they had been assaulted and were unclean. Like those with epilepsy, many opted for concealment as a first-choice strategy, felt stigma once more being the motivating factor. They were ashamed by noise and odours from the stoma and filled with self-disgust at the need to handle bags of faeces and to clean faeces from their bodies. They feared exposure because they thought others would be embarrassed or offended and drift away. Some practised 'withdrawal' rather than confront the potential hazards of passing as normal. Many of those in situations where they were discredited rather than discreditable adopted a strategy of 'covering': they took all possible steps to reduce the salience of their stigma for others, to render it unobtrusive (Goffman 1963). A third had never shown the colostomy to their spouses, and more than four-fifths had never shown it to anyone outside the hospital. MacDonald concludes that, although most people in her study learned to accommodate their stomas fairly well, 'a large fraction' suffered impaired quality of life because of their experiences of the stigma of cancer and colostomy'.

HIV/AIDS

Since its recognition in 1981, the human immunodeficiency virus (HIV) has aroused strong responses. In the USA, where the HIV epidemic emerged among gay men and intravenous drug users, a persistently negative societal reaction has continued to play a vital role in the experiences of individuals with the virus. Alonzo & Reynolds (1995) suggest that individuals' adjustments to HIV/AIDS must be seen against the background of a 'biophysical disease trajectory'. They note that disease progression varies widely among individuals, but suggest that over a period of 12 or more years they will usually experience a number of stages. These are summarized in Box 13.1.

The authors then go on to identify four phases of an 'HIV stigma trajectory', which is linked to, but can vary independently of, the biophysical disease trajectory. These four phases are outlined in Box 13.2. They again stress individual variation, and also add that stigma can on occasions be 'expansive', pervading all corners of an individual's biography and identity, and on other occasions 'containable, limited and controllable in terms of consequences and, more importantly, personal and social identity'.

COURTESY STIGMA

It is apparent that those close to people with conditions like epilepsy, rectal cancer or HIV/AIDS, like partners, family and friends (those Goffman (1963) calls the 'wise') are likely to be deeply affected not only by the impact of the conditions themselves on everyday life but

---

HIV/AIDS Disease Trajectory

1. A transient flu-like syndrome associated with seroconversion, developing within weeks or months of infection
2. An asymptomatic period of more than 4 years average duration
3. Symptomatic HIV infection of more than 5 years average duration
4. AIDS characterized by opportunistic illnesses, HIV wasting syndrome, HIV dementia, lymphomas, and other neoplasms, averaging 9–13 months for treated and untreated individuals combined, and 21 months for those receiving antiviral medical treatments

Reproduced with kind permission from Elsevier Science Ltd from Alonzo & Reynolds (1995).

---

by their stigmatizing connotations. The spread of the stigma associated with the condition from the person directly affected to others close to him or her is known as courtesy stigma (Goffman 1963). A study that illustrates this is MacRae's (1999) investigation of courtesy stigma and Alzheimer's disease, a degenerative organic disorder of the brain for which there is as yet no effective treatment or cure. MacRae interviewed 47 family members of persons diagnosed with probable Alzheimer's disease: 31 of these were primary caregivers (either spouses or children). In response to a direct question, 54% of the spousal caregivers and 53% of the child caregivers said they had on occasions been embarrassed and/or ashamed; rather fewer, 37%, of those family members who were not primary caregivers responded affirmatively to this question. Embarrassment and/or shame tended to be experienced 'where it was apparent that the ill family member's behaviour was clearly in violation of social norms' (for example, rudeness to strangers or lapses of etiquette). MacRae argues that whereas for Goffman courtesy stigma is acquired simply by virtue of the individual's rela-

---

BOX 13.2 Four Phases of the HIV Stigma Trajectory

1. **At risk – pre-stigma and the worried well**: this does not correspond to a stage of the disease trajectory, it denotes a time of uncertainty when an individual thinks behaviours might have put him at risk of HIV. He may cope through denial or disassociation. Much depends on the support available. The phase can end with testing for HIV
2. **Diagnosis – confronting an altered identity**: an individual can be diagnosed early or late in the disease trajectory. A typical stress response involves disbelief, numbness and denial, followed by anger, acute turmoil, disruptive anxiety and depressive symptoms. Identity and self-esteem can be threatened, stigma becomes salient, and decisions on disclosure have to be negotiated
3. **Latent – living between health and illness**: this is when the disease is asymptomatic and perhaps at its least disruptive. Individuals can normalize, conceal and even deny their positivity. They might choose to pass as normal, thereby avoiding enacted stigma, but felt stigma can exact a heavy price
4. **Manifest – passage to social and physical death**: there is often no fixed disease course because of widespread individual variation. However, there are fewer symptom-free periods and opportunistic infections accumulate. Stigma tends to be less salient as matters surrounding social and biological death become paramount. Intense felt stigma may nevertheless be associated with isolation and withdrawal as means of concealing 'abominations of the body'. Courtesy stigma may extend to carers who hesitate to reveal cause of death

Reproduced with kind permission from Elsevier Science Ltd from Alonzo & Reynolds (1995).

tionship to the person who possesses the stigma, her study suggests that this acquisition is in fact far from automatic. She commends further study into why it is that some of Goffman's wise develop strong senses of courtesy stigma whereas others reject or otherwise escape it.

AIDS, STIGMA AND HEALTH POLICY AND PRACTICE

The epidemic of HIV/AIDS raises important issues of health policy and practice. Throughout its brief history, AIDS has been both medicalized as 'disease' and moralized as 'stigma'. Weeks (1989) elaborates on this theme by tracing three distinct phases in social responses to AIDS through the 1980s; these are described below.

The dawning crisis (1981–2)

It was not until the summer of 1981 that the health problems increasingly being experienced in the gay community, and leading to much debate therein, became 'an embryonic public issue' in the USA, with physicians and the press beginning to take note. Exploratory attempts were made to understand the nature of the disease known initially as 'the gay cancer', then GRID (gay-related immune deficiency; the acronym AIDS was finally accepted in 1982). Risk categories outside the gay community were soon identified: heroin users, haemophiliacs and, most controversially, people from the island of Haiti. The Federal Administration, however, remained largely inactive, partly because it was intent on public expenditure cuts at the time and partly because AIDS seemed to be confined to marginal and, with the possible exception of haemophiliacs, 'politically and morally embarrassing' groups.

Moral panic (1982–5)

From about 1982 a moral panic set in, with a rapid escalation of media and public hysteria. This was the period of the New Right and Moral Majority onslaught in the USA, and of stories of the 'gay plague' in the tabloid press. Around the same time, 1983–4, HIV was identified and named, opening up new opportunities for medical engagement. In addition, the communities most affected, notably the gay community, began to organize for self-help, for example through Gay Men's Health Crisis in New York and the Terrence Higgins Trust in London. The identification of the virus and progress in understanding modes of transmission shifted attention from risk categories to risk activities.

Crisis management (1985–9)

The last phase identified by Weeks commenced in 1985, when it was recognized that AIDS as a disease constituted a global threat, and to heterosexual as well as to gay or socially marginal communities. Governments in the USA and Britain, mobilized by the perceived threat to 'the general population', began to commit resources, especially to prevention. It is ironic that in so doing they drew on the experience and expertise of the gay self-help groups. The self-help groups themselves became more professional as public funds became available to them and as demands on their services increased. An uneasy alliance was formed between the self-help groups and the medical profession.

Weeks' brief history of the first decade of AIDS and current debates highlight a number of important issues concerning the role of physicians. First, not only was AIDS – uniquely combining sex, drugs, death and contagion – itself highly stigmatizing, but it was initially discerned in an already markedly stigmatized population, that of gay men. For several years political and popular homophobia meant that both effective research and health interventions were delayed, and that specialist physicians came under some pressure to sanction or facilitate punitive action against 'guilty' HIV/AIDS carriers – like gay and bisexual men and, later, injecting drug users – if not against 'innocent' carriers – like haemophiliacs and babies of infected mothers. Fortunately, such pressure (and the guilty/innocent dichotomy underlying it) was largely resisted by the British medical profession. The evidence of history is that the punitive medical policing of socially marginalized groups, quite apart from infringing civil rights, is counterproductive in that it leads to further marginalization and losses of contact and capacity to influence through health education or 'user-friendly' services.

The profile of those affected by HIV/AIDS has changed since the 1980s. Figures from the Public Health Laboratory Service indicate that 41 000 diagnoses of HIV infection had been reported in the UK by March 2000, among whom 17 000 had developed AIDS and 13 500 had died. The increase in the number of diagnosed cases every year from 1994 is likely to be in part a function of greater awareness and testing. However, it is apparent that the way that those with HIV contracted the infection has changed. In the late 1990s diagnoses of infections acquired through sex between men were surpassed by diagnoses of infections due to sex between men and women. In 1999, 45% of those diagnosed with HIV contracted the virus through heterosexual sex; and three-quarters of these heterosexually acquired infections probably occurred abroad. The number of people becoming infected through injected drugs has more than halved since 1993 (National Statistics 2001).

A second and related issue concerns the reception of patients with HIV/AIDS in healthcare settings, particularly in light of the increasing involvement of general, as opposed to specialist, physicians in their treatment and care. Early studies of primary care revealed a lack of commitment to health education about AIDS and of wide divergences of attitude towards the provision of counselling and treatment and over the issue of confidentiality. In one national study, for example, 70% of GPs reported that they found it difficult to discuss the sexual practices of gay men during consultations (Rhodes et al 1989). More recent research in Scotland, based on the subjective accounts of 61 people with HIV/AIDS, suggests continuing unease (including stigmatization) in healthcare settings, especially around the issue of contagion, although health professionals are becoming more familiar with treating patients with HIV/AIDS (Green & Platt 1997).

STIGMA AND PHYSICIAN–PATIENT ENCOUNTERS

Whether patients have epilepsy, rectal cancer, HIV/AIDS or any other stigmatizing condition, the quality of the care they receive is a major concern. The enhanced salience of medical audit will be important here. But quality of care encompasses more than biomedical thoroughness and numerous studies have documented patient unhappiness at physicians' preoccupation with diagnosis and management and apparent lack of interest in psychological and social aspects of care. Scambler (1989) has noted that the accusation that physicians, especially hospital specialists, lack the time, training or motivation to elicit and address patients' own perspectives on their epilepsy is a common one. He goes on to distinguish analytically between three dimensions to patients perspectives: (1) 'felt stigma' – a sense of shame and apprehension at meeting with discrimination; (2) 'rationalization' – a deep need to make sense of what is happening, to restore cognitive order; and (3) 'action strategy' – a need to develop modes of coping across a diversity of roles and situations. Research suggests that physicians tend to be interested in those aspects of patient rationalization that promise to facilitate diagnosis or management, but not in the process per se. Neither felt stigma nor action strategy tend to be on the medical agenda for consultations, and are typically handled inexpertly and cursorily if raised by patients.

The point has often been made that patients' perspectives need to be respected and explored in their own right. Physicians do not merely need to inform and advise, but also to listen. To do this effectively, particularly in relation to stigmatizing conditions, requires what Schneider & Conrad (1983) have termed 'co-participation in care'. Scambler (1990) has argued that physicians need to provide a competent and up-to-date technical service covering the investigation, diagnosis and management of epilepsy – at optimum cost – and to engage in health education oriented to demythologizing and destigmatizing epilepsy in the community. As far as physician–patient encounters are concerned, he suggests four guiding principles, which are summarized in Box 13.3. The literature suggests that these prescriptions are pertinent to a wide range of chronic and stigmatizing illnesses, and to surgical procedures such as mastectomy and colostomy, which have stigmatizing results.

Finally, it is important to note the emergence of a radical challenge to conventional, biomedical and 'common-sense' thinking in relation chronic illness and disability. This has had an important bearing on appreciations of stigma; in particular, the understanding of chronic illness and/or disability as personal tragedy has been criticized. It has been argued, for example, that the system of knowledge based on such 'natural' dichotomies as normal/abnormal, healthy/pathological, socially acceptable/socially unacceptable, and so on, has arisen through a general cultural commitment to a discourse that dominates thinking and practice in the contemporary developed world. Many advocates of the 'disability politics movement' refuse to accept or respond to conventional notions of what is abnormal, unhealthy and unacceptable (Campbell & Oliver 1996). Moreover, their challenge to orthodox biomedical thinking is in many ways in tune with a changing culture in which identity and 'difference' are becoming key issues. As far as stigma is concerned, it is contended that there is no longer any compulsion or necessity to act out social evaluations that mark some people as imperfect, deviant or disabled, and thus as 'outsiders'. Difference should be a source of celebration rather than a rationale for rejection. What such a perspective suggests is the need for a sociological understanding of the often oppressive ways in which agents of social control, including doctors, sanction and enforce social evaluations which have their historical origins in economic and political interests (Barnes et al 1999; see Chapter 12). It is a perspective that is increasingly likely to require health workers to re-examine and re-appraise the social and moral bases of their 'scientific' programmes of treatment and care.

BOX 13.2 Four Criteria of Good Care

1. Acceptance of the principle of co-participation in care, which involves coming to terms with 'patient autonomy', or the patient as decision-maker
2. Acceptance of an open agenda in physician–patient encounters
3. A holistic rather than exclusively biomedical orientation to care, with the emphasis on informing, advising and helping 'persons in context' rather than merely managing disease
4. The development of counselling skills to complement technical skills, which presupposes both an awareness of the impact of epilepsy on quality of life and learned expertise in advising on coping strategies

Reproduced with permission from the Royal Society of Medicine from Scambler (1990).

References

Alonzo A & Reynolds N 1995 Stigma, HIV and AIDS: an exploration and elaboration of a stigma strategy. Social Science and Medicine 41:303–315

Barnes C, Mercer G, Shakespeare T 1999 Exploring disability: a sociological introduction. Polity Press, Cambridge

Campbell J, Oliver M 1996 Disability politics. Routledge, London

Davis F 1964 Deviance disavowal: the management of strained interaction by the visibly handicapped. In: Becker H (ed) The other side. Free Press, Glencoe, IL

Freidson E 1970 Profession of medicine. Dodds, Mead & Co, New York

Gerhardt U 1987 Parsons, role theory and health interaction. In: Scambler G (ed) Sociological theory and medical sociology. Tavistock, London

Goffman E 1963 Stigma: notes on the management of spoiled identity. Prentice-Hall, New York

Gove W 1970 Societal reaction as an explanation of mental illness: an evaluation. American Sociological Review 35:873–884

Green G, Platt S 1997 Fear and loathing in health care settings reported by people with HIV. Sociology of Health and Illness 19:70–92

Higgins P 1980 Outsiders in a hearing world: a sociology of deafness. Sage, Beverley Hills. CA

Jacoby A 1994 Felt versus enacted stigma: a concept revisited. Social Science & Medicine 38:269–274

Lemert E 1967 Human deviance, social problems and social control. Prentice-Hall, New York

MacDonald L 1988 The experience of stigma: living with rectal cancer. In: Anderson R, Bury M (eds) Living with chronic illness: the experience of patients and their families. Allen & Unwin, London

MacRae H 1999 Managing courtesy stigma: the case of Alzheimer's disease. Sociology of Health & Illness 21:54–70

National Statistics 2001 Social Trends 31. HMSO, London

Parsons T 1951 The social system. Routledge & Kegan Paul, London

Rhodes T et al 1989 Prevention in practice: obstacles and opportunities. AIDS Care 1:257–267

Scambler G 1989 Epilepsy. Tavistock, London

Scambler G 1990 Social factors and quality of life and quality of care in epilepsy. In: Chadwick D (ed) Quality of life and quality of care in epilepsy. Royal Society of Medicine, London

Scambler G, Hopkins A 1986 Being epileptic: coming to terms with stigma. Sociology, Health and Illness 8:26–43

Scheff T 1966 Being mentally ill. Aldine, Chicago

Schneider J, Conrad P 1983 Having epilepsy: the experience and control of illness. Temple University Press, Philadelphia

Scott R 1969 The making of blind men. Russell Sage Foundation, New York

Sontag S 1977 Illness as metaphor. Allen Lane, New York

Weeks J 1989 AIDS: the intellectual agenda. In: Aggleton P, Hart G, Davies P (eds) AIDS: social representations, social practices. Falmer Press, London

Organization of Health Services

CHAPTER

14

Origins and Development of the National Health Service

Nicholas Mays

The organization and financing of health care varies widely in different countries. Each healthcare system is the product of the social, economic, demographic and technological context and the political philosophy of the country. All exhibit their own balance of advantages and limitations when judged on criteria such as equity, efficiency, accessibility, acceptability and relevance to needs (see Chapter 19). The history of health care in the UK in the last 150 years mirrors the trend in all advanced Western countries towards greater government involvement in health care in response to calls for better access to and coordination of services (Thane 1982). However, the National Health Service (NHS) that emerged from the interplay and conflict between the medical profession, government, experts, public opinion, employees and insurers was unique to the UK, providing services that are predominantly free at the point of use, accessible to all and paid for out of general government taxation. It is perhaps the best-known example of a health service solution to the financing and allocation of health care in which the vast majority of health care is publicly financed and provided through a publicly managed system.

The purpose of this chapter is to place recent changes in the NHS in a historical context by briefly surveying the evolution of health care in the UK since the nineteenth century and the development of the NHS since its inception in 1948, including the internal market initiated in 1991, before describing and analysing the Labour government's programme of change, which began in 1997.

HEALTH CARE IN THE UK BEFORE THE NATIONAL HEALTH SERVICE

Health care provision in the UK in the nineteenth century and until the mid-twentieth century comprised a number of disparate elements: GP services, the voluntary hospitals, municipal hospitals and local authority public health measures and related services.

General practitioners

In the nineteenth century, hospitals were used primarily by the poor. They remained dangerous places until the very end of the century when developments in anaesthesia and antiseptic surgery improved the success rate of treatments. For those who could afford it, fee-for-service consultation with a qualified practitioner, either in the surgery or at home, was the main means of obtaining medical care. A variety of insurance schemes, organized by Friendly Societies (non-profit-making, mutual-benefit organizations) and trade unions gradually enabled other groups, mainly skilled workers, to use GPs. Increasing numbers of GPs participated in these schemes, particularly in poorer areas where private fees alone did not provide an adequate income. They were paid an annual sum for each patient enrolled on their lists by the insurer. Providing GPs with a modest but reasonably secure income, and protection against competition from unqualified practitioners, the Friendly Societies and trade unions were able to specify standards of care, such as home visiting, and to limit GPs' clinical freedom in order to control costs on behalf of their working-class subscribers. Ironically, this degree of lay control forced leaders of the medical profession to conclude that State intervention would be preferable to Friendly Society interference, leading eventually to the National Health Service (Honigsbaum 1989).

By the end of the nineteenth century, only about half the working class was covered by these schemes of contributory insurance. The poor physical condition of recruits for the Boer War (1899–1901), one-third of whom were judged unfit to serve, alarmed military planners in the government at a time of international tension. Industrialists were anxious to see a healthier and, therefore, more productive male workforce. The early twentieth century also saw considerable social unrest, with working-class uprisings in Germany and an attempted revolution in Russia in 1905. In Britain, the Labour Party, based on the new mass trade unions and the widening of the franchise in 1885, had gained seats in Parliament. Britain's rulers were seeking ways of halting the spread of Socialist ideas. The German government had already tried to defuse the revolutionary potential of disaffected sections of the working class by social reforms designed to improve living standards and quality of life, including, in 1883, a system of state-run social insurance covering sickness, accidents at work and old age and invalidity pensions. Influenced in part by Germany, Britain introduced old age pensions in 1908 and, in 1911, a National Health Insurance (NHI) scheme that many in the medical profession had opposed because the Friendly Societies remained involved in its administration. Many members of the medical profession were equally suspicious of State schemes, fearing control of their work and lower pay; neither fear was justified in the event.

The NHI scheme, covering manual workers between 16 and 65 years of age whose earnings were below the threshold for payment of income tax, provided funds for sickness, accident and disability benefits in cash, and access to GP services free of charge. Hospital and specialist care were not included. It excluded the self-employed, agricultural workers, many unemployed people and nearly all non-manual workers. It excluded all dependants of the insured person, mainly women and children, who had either to pay directly for care or make their own private insurance arrangements. The employer, the employee and the Treasury made contributions to the NHI fund. Entitlement to benefits and GP services was limited to the level of past contributions, so that in cases of chronic illness and unemployment workers could find themselves without cover. Participating GPs had a list or 'panel' of insured workers and were paid a capitation fee for each. The NHI scheme was administered through the existing Friendly Societies and commercial insurance companies, each of which exercised considerable discretion in deciding the level of and entitlement to benefits.

The NHI improved GP remuneration because it provided additional public funds to subsidize the treatment of many more, poorer patients while still allowing 'panel' doctors to work for other insurers as fee-for-service private practitioners. This strengthened the financial position of the GPs (particularly those in more affluent areas where private practice was more profitable), enabling them to resist the Friendly Societies' previous control over their clinical activities. However, it meant that GPs in poorer areas (usually industrial areas and in the north), although better off than before 1911, were paid less and had far larger patient lists than their counterparts elsewhere.

By 1939, approximately 40% of the working population had some coverage for GP services through the NHI scheme and about two-thirds of GPs were involved in 'panel' work (Carpenter 1984). The economic recession of the 1930s had caused high levels of unemployment, which had, in turn, led the scheme into financial difficulties.

Hospital services

Hospital care was available from two separate sources: the voluntary hospitals and the municipal or local authority hospitals.

The voluntary hospitals

There were 1100 voluntary hospitals with 90 000 beds in Britain before the Second World War. These were charitable foundations and treated 36% of all hospital patients in 1938 (Abel-Smith 1964). They ranged from GP cottage hospitals, financed by local subscription, to the large, prestigious teaching hospitals, which were chartered institutions, established as far back as the Middle Ages in some cases and supported by extensive endowments. The teaching hospitals concentrated on acute medicine and surgery and undertook most of the training of doctors and nurses. Their consultants offered their services at the hospital without payment so that the hospital could provide free care to patients who could not afford private treatment. In return, they were relatively free to choose to treat the complex and 'interesting' cases. Consultants' incomes were derived from private practice undertaken outside the hospital. GPs, and those doctors who worked for Friendly Societies or the municipal hospitals, were largely prevented from admitting and treating their own patients in the voluntary hospitals. In return, consultants agreed only to accept patients when they were referred to them by GPs.

After the First World War, inflation reduced the real value of the income from bequests and donations to the voluntary hospitals. Medical science and technology were becoming increasingly complex and expensive. As a result, the voluntary hospitals found themselves with mounting financial problems. They responded by trading on their reputations to raise money from the public – as well as by means testing and charging the growing numbers of more affluent patients who were now using their services – as the effectiveness of hospital care increased. Hospitals set up their own contributory prepayment schemes for those who had some money but could not afford to pay directly out-of-pocket when they used services. To raise income, voluntary hospitals also undertook work on contract to local authorities, some of which were extending their provision of hospital care in the 1930s. By 1937, at least one-third of the voluntary hospitals were virtually bankrupt (Political and Economic Planning 1937). The government had given them some money in the 1920s to reduce their deficits but had refused to take on responsibility for their finances.

Despite the prepayment schemes, many middle-class people found that acute hospital care between the two World Wars was very expensive because the charges they paid also had to subsidise the care of lower-income patients who still generally received free services. However, poor patients brought no income to the voluntary hospitals and so there was an increasing incentive for the hospitals to neglect them, passing responsibility for their care to the municipal hospitals. Both poor and better off people became dissatisfied with this state of affairs.

Municipal (local authority) hospitals

The nineteenth-century system known as the Poor Law provided public assistance to the very poorest people and the unemployed. The system distinguished between the 'undeserving poor' whose poverty was presumed to be the result of indolence and fecklessness, and the 'deserving poor' made paupers by old age, mental infirmity or sickness. Provision for the first group was the bare minimum available in the workhouse, where conditions were deliberately harsher than those facing the poorest people in work according to the principle of 'less eligibility'. This was to encourage the recipients to find employment and leave. The second group, essentially the sick and elderly poor, were supposed to be treated better in separate infirmaries, which were often attached to the workhouses.

In 1929 the Poor Law hospitals were taken over by the local authority health departments headed by the Medical Officer of Health (MOH). They continued to provide mainly chronic, means-tested care for those unable to obtain treatment in the voluntary hospitals or by private means. By 1939 there were 400 000 beds in public hospitals run by the local authorities: 200 000 in 'asylums' serving the mentally ill and mentally handicapped and 200 000 in a range of tuberculosis sanatoria, isolation hospitals for infectious diseases and former Poor Law infirmaries.

Standards in the local authority hospitals rose appreciably during the 1930s but they tended to be worse equipped than the voluntary hospitals and to have lower status because of their Poor Law origins. Local authorities paid doctors relatively poorly and attempted to control their work, which antagonized the profession. By the early 1940s, the medical profession was almost uniformly hostile to municipal control of health services.

There were big differences in approach by different local authorities to the public hospital system in their areas, with some simply perpetuating Poor Law standards, particularly outside London. Indeed, the economic depression of the 1930s meant that many lacked the money to invest in hospitals. Although the two hospital movements were, in a loose sense, complementary, there was little liaison or coordination between them.

Public health and community health services

The earliest and most significant action to protect the population's health in the nineteenth century was the public health legislation enacted between 1848 and 1875. This had led to major improvements in water supplies and sewerage and, ultimately, the control of infectious diseases, which made a far greater impact on the general standard of health than anything in the field of curative medicine up to that time (see Chapter 1). By the end of the nineteenth century, each local authority was required by law to have a MOH, responsible for environmental health, control of infectious diseases, certification of causes of death and a range of preventive services. By the 1930s, the MOH headed a health department in every local authority, with responsibility primarily for services that were not available under NHI, such as maternity services, child health and welfare (health visiting in modern terminology), the school medical service and services for the support of elderly people in their own homes (e.g. district nursing).

Overview of health care in the UK before the Second World War

Despite a reasonably effective pattern of public health and preventive health services, a series of reports between the two World Wars, both official and unofficial, identified major deficiencies in the other health services:

- financial barriers to the use of health services remained because NHI was not available to more than half the population and it did not cover the dependants of the insured worker
- NHI did not include hospital care
- specialists, GPs and hospital beds were unevenly distributed across the country
- there were wide variations in standards in all services
- there were mounting financial problems, especially in the voluntary hospitals, and shortages of equipment and skilled staff
- the local authority services, the voluntary hospitals and the GP services were uncoordinated.

ESTABLISHING A NATIONAL HEALTH SERVICE

By the late 1930s there was growing support for the idea that everybody should have access to good quality health care, but how this should be accomplished was a matter of hot dispute. Decisions would have to be made about, for example, whether services should be funded from general taxation or local taxes or by extending contributory NHI; whether hospitals should be administered by *ad hoc* bodies or by the existing local authorities; whether doctors should become salaried employees of the state or remain independent contractors; and whether services should be free at the point of use or whether there should be charges and tests of the ability to pay (Webster 1988).

The experience of the Second World War showed how the state could intervene positively in many areas of national life; it also generated demands for a better post-war society. In 1939, a State-run centrally organized Emergency Medical Service (EMS), funded by the Treasury, had been set up to deal with the large numbers of expected civilian war casualties. It was free, organized centrally and took over two-thirds of the hospitals. It established a national blood-transfusion service, coordinated ambulance services and showed that a national health service of some sort was feasible. Working in the EMS, leading members of the medical profession also saw for themselves the weaknesses in the existing services, particularly the poor conditions outside the prestigious teaching hospitals.

As a result, a national, universally available healthcare system administered by the State rather than the insurance industry was a central plank in Beveridge's famous blueprint for a post-war 'welfare state' (Beveridge Report 1942). Box 14.1 sets out the government's ambitious aims for a comprehensive health service (Ministry of Health 1944).

The NHS could not be established without the cooperation of the medical profession. Although the British Medical Association (BMA) had published its own report in 1942 calling for a comprehensive health service, covering all but the 10% of people with the highest incomes, it was at loggerheads with the civil servants in the Ministry of Health over the means of implementation, particularly because officials supported a municipal health service. Between 1942 and 1948 there was continuous negotiation between the government and key interest groups, particularly the representatives of the medical profession, about almost every aspect of the finance, organization and control of a new unified service (Eckstein 1958). The GPs resisted a salaried service to preserve professional autonomy. The hospital specialists refused the proposal for local authority control. Both groups were hostile to anything that hinted at the two nineteenth century systems of lay control – the Friendly Societies and the Poor Law. The system that finally emerged, established by the National Health Service Act, 1946, was the product of skilful compromises by Aneurin Bevan, the Labour Minister of Health after 1945. Although it was never formally agreed to by the BMA, it reflected professional concerns to a considerable degree:

- GPs remained independent contractors but most were made better off by the NHS

- hospital consultants were paid for the hospital work they had previously done for nothing

- consultants were allowed to work part-time in the NHS on good salaries and keep their private practices

- beds for private patients ('pay beds') were permitted in NHS hospitals

---

BOX 14.1	Aims of a Comprehensive Health Service with Free Treatment Paid for from Taxes

'To ensure that everybody in the country – irrespective of means, age, sex and occupation – shall have equal opportunity to benefit from the best and most up-to-date medical and allied services available. To provide, therefore, for all who want it, a comprehensive service covering every branch of medical and allied activity.

'To divorce the case of health from questions of personal means or other factors irrelevant to it; to provide the service free of charge (apart from certain possible charges in respect of appliances) and to encourage a new attitude to health – the easier obtaining of advice early, the promotion of good health rather than only the treatment of bad.'

From Ministry of Health (1944 p 47).

- a system of distinction (merit) awards controlled by the profession was established for hospital consultants but not GPs

- doctors were to play a major role in deciding policy at all levels

- hospitals were not to be controlled by local authorities, but 'nationalized' under the control of local appointed bodies.

From the outset, therefore, despite its apparent radicalism, the NHS represented a compromise between the principles of traditional medical authority and rational public administration (Klein 2000). In terms of overall control, finance and access, however, the system had changed markedly. The NHS was open to the whole population solely on the basis of healthcare need, free at the point of use and funded almost entirely from the general tax revenues of central government. The goal was to secure equality of access throughout the country to a comprehensive range of modern services accessible by referral from a GP except in emergencies.

211

THE NHS, 1948–74

The NHS, which began in 1948, nationalized the existing pattern of services and therefore inherited many of the strengths and weaknesses of the previous arrangements. The historical divisions between general practice, local authority health services, local authority hospitals and teaching hospitals remained, and no significant steps were taken to tackle inequalities in the geographical distribution of hospital beds, staff and equipment. Thus the new NHS fell far short of the ideal of full integration (see Fig. 14.1 and Box 14.2 for the structure of the NHS in England). Similar but separate structures were created in Wales, Scotland and Northern Ireland.

The NHS was immediately very popular with the public and rapidly proved financially attractive to the vast majority of medical practitioners. However, two main sources of discontent marked the first 25 years: (1) the level of expenditure; and (2) the organization of the service.

The original expenditure estimates were relatively modest and assumed that spending would stabilize rapidly, although Aneurin Bevan was in no doubt that the NHS would be expensive because of previous under funding and a backlog of untreated ill health. The planners had reckoned without the popularity of the NHS, rising public expectations, inflation and post-war developments in technology and drugs; all of which drove up the cost of the service. To limit public spending, charges were introduced for spectacles, dentures and, eventually, prescriptions, and have remained ever since. By 1953, expenditure had reached such an unexpectedly high level that the Minister of Health ordered an enquiry into the cost of the NHS (Ministry of Health 1956). The Guillebaud committee could find no evidence of profligacy or inappropriate treatment, and noted that healthcare spending had, in fact, declined as a percentage of the national income. Most of the increase in spending was due to price inflation and necessary pay awards. The committee recommended a further increase in spending to remedy the chronic lack of investment in NHS buildings. In a belated response in 1962, the government announced a Hospital Plan for England and Wales, which aimed to make a modem district general hospital (DGH) available to each population of 250 000 people (Ministry of Health 1962).

The demand for health care continued to rise in the 1960s, fed by professional and public aspirations and supported by economic growth. The period 1960–74 was marked by a steady expansion in spending in real terms and in the volume of services provided through the NHS. Spending rose from 3.8% to 5.7% of gross national product. By the

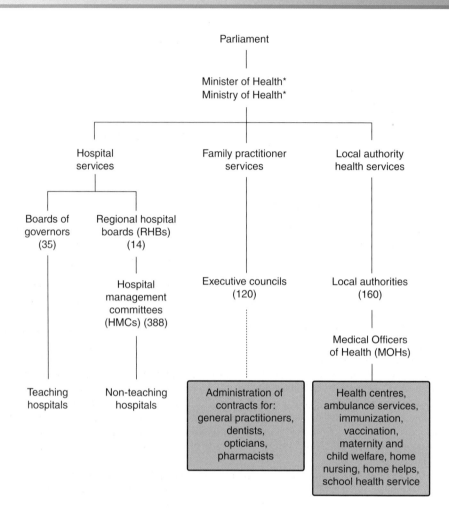

*Secretary of State for Social Services and Department of Health and Social Security (DHSS), respectively, from 1968

—— Direct managerial authority

······ Administrative responsibility

Fig. 14.1 The structure of the NHS in England and Wales, 1948–74.

second half of the1970s, economic growth had slowed down, and with it the growth in NHS resources. The service was having to face up to the dilemmas imposed by the requirement, which faces all health systems, to reconcile seemingly infinite demand for care with inevitably finite resources (see Chapter 19). One possible solution was to get more from the existing level of resources through a more efficient organization. The prevailing view was that the lack of linkage between the different arms of the NHS (see Fig. 14.1) was preventing continuity of care and the most effective use of resources.

BOX 14.2   Tripartite Administration in the English NHS After 1948

1. 14 Regional Hospital Boards (RHBs), appointed by the Minister of Health, were responsible for the Hospital Management Committees (HMCs), which ran the former local authority hospitals. Teaching hospitals outside this system, directly funded by the Ministry of Health
2. Local authorities ran preventive and community health services (e.g. vaccination and immunization, child health services) through departments were led by Medical Officers of Health
3. Executive Councils dealt with the GPs, dentists, opticians and pharmacists who were independent contractors to the NHS

REFORM BY REORGANIZATION, 1974

After lengthy consultation and analysis, the NHS was reorganized in 1974. This produced a new, more integrated structure of 14 Regional Health Authorities (RHAs) whose main function was to allocate finance, plan major capital projects and monitor 90 Area Health Authorities (AHAs), which were responsible for both the hospitals and the community health services formerly managed by the local authorities (Fig. 14.2). The GPs remained independent contractors outside the control of the new authorities. A similar reorganization took place in Wales, Scotland and Northern Ireland.

At RHA and AHA levels, a multidisciplinary team comprising an administrator, an accountant, a senior nurse, a public health physician (now employed by the health authority), a consultant and a GP managed the system. This style of management was devised deliberately to incorporate the main professional groups in the decision-making process, and decisions could be taken only when there was a consensus in favour within the team ('consensus management'). In each area, a Community Health Council (CHC), independent of the health authority, acted as the public's 'watch-dog' and represented the views of patients and the public to the professionals. The CHC had rights of access to information from district managers and to premises, and had to be consulted on major service developments.

The reorganization was designed to facilitate the implementation of an ambitious cyclical process of short- and long-term rational planning and priority setting by region, area and district, which began in 1976. This was accompanied by the introduction of the Resource Allocation Working Party (RAWP) formula to redistribute finance fairly between different parts of the country on the basis of the size and relative needs of the population.

The 1974 reorganization went some way to unifying the NHS and to improving the opportunities for coordination with local authority social services. It failed, however, to reconcile effectively the role of central government in setting policy, overseeing expenditure and monitoring performance, with the requirement for local, delegated authority and freedom to implement policy in the light of specific circumstances. The new structure was criticized for having too many tiers of administration, an overelaborate planning system and too many consultative committees of doctors, nurses and other health workers. Consensus management was said to lead to slow and ineffective decision-making. The effects of redistribution of finance in line with the RAWP formula were particularly painful because it was applied to a now near-static NHS budget.

MANAGERIAL REFORM, 1982–7

From 1979 to 1983 the Conservative government under Margaret Thatcher encouraged those at the local level in the NHS to take decisions in the light of local circumstances.

213

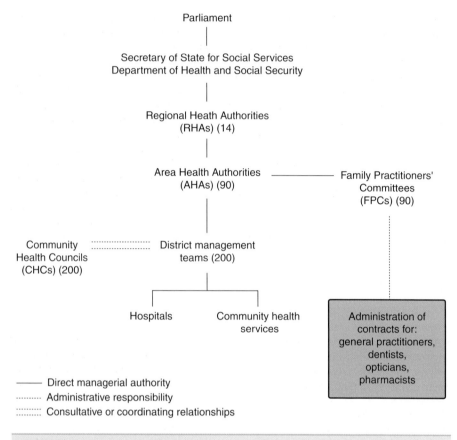

Fig. 14.2   The structure of the NHS in England, 1974–82.

However, this posed the problem of how to ensure that local managers were using resources efficiently and in line with central policy. There was also a pressing need from the government's perspective to find ways of preventing health authorities overspending their budgets.

Whereas previous enquiries had concentrated on the structure of the NHS, a small team of private-sector managers, led by Roy Griffiths of Sainsbury, was asked in 1983 to undertake an inquiry into its management practices. Griffiths found a lack of individual responsibility and accountability for the attainment of objectives among the senior officers in the consensus teams. He concluded that the NHS needed a stronger, clearer management system (Department of Health and Social Security (DHSS) 1983). At every level in the NHS, the consensus teams were replaced by a single general manager with the power to take executive decisions over the resources under his or her control. Two bodies were created within the DHSS: a Health Services Supervisory Board to make strategic decisions about objectives and an NHS Management Board to direct operations in the NHS.

By establishing a hierarchy of general managers on fixed-term contracts and paid according to their performance, the Griffiths reforms enabled the centre to exercise greater control over activity at all levels, increased the powers of managers and reduced the influence of health authority members, particularly those from local authorities. Full-time managers began gradually to introduce more controls over the way traditionally autonomous clinicians used the resources available to them. For example, clinicians became increasingly accountable for delivering an agreed workload efficiently within a set budget through systems of 'resource management' (Packwood et al 1991).

Overall, far greater emphasis was placed on considerations of efficiency and 'value for money' than ever before. The traditional, professional viewpoint that medical services could and should not be susceptible to measurement, external evaluation and control was increasingly challenged (see Chapter 18 for more on this). For example, the NHS Management Board instituted annual RHA reviews of each health authority to ensure that resources had been spent effectively and in line with objectives; set up a system of quantitative performance indicators (PIs) to measure and compare the activity and costs of each district and unit; established a limited list of drugs of proven effectiveness that GPs were allowed to prescribe on the NHS; instituted competitive tendering for support services (e.g. catering, cleaning, portering and security) involving the private sector; implemented new cost–benefit methods for assessing building schemes; and brought in strict cash limits linked to compulsory 'cost improvement programmes' to generate savings for new services.

THE NHS REVIEW, 1988

Why a further review?

Despite the emphasis on greater efficiency in the later 1980s, the NHS still faced the familiar problem of reconciling increasing demand for its services, generated by rising expectations and the availability of new treatments, with the available funds. Total spending was higher than ever in real terms, and more patients were being treated but, by the autumn of 1987, the NHS, and especially its acute hospitals, had entered one of its periodic and severe financial crises. Waiting lists shot into the headlines, along with pressure for more money. At the same time, the medical profession was increasingly reluctant to manage strictly limited resources on behalf of the government. Interest was growing in the potential to make greater use of private health insurance. In January 1988, the Prime Minister, Margaret Thatcher, announced a wide-ranging, confidential review of the NHS by a Cabinet committee. The results were to be published within a year.

The review team was forcibly reminded in the course of its work of the advantages of the existing arrangements, particularly the ability to control the level of expenditure (the lack of such control was a problem in most Western countries) and the cost-effectiveness of the GP system, which allowed many health problems to be dealt with inexpensively without recourse to hospital care. These led to a comparatively low level of overall health spending by international standards (6.5% of the gross domestic product for most of the 1980s). Nevertheless, the whole population was given equitable access to a comprehensive range of high-quality services, regardless of the ability to pay, and with low administrative costs. Although this situation was the envy of many countries: 'the very success of the government in controlling expenditure ... had turned the NHS into a source of political aggravation. Ministers were being constantly (and successfully) pilloried by the medical profession and the political opposition for their failure to fund the NHS adequately' (Klein 1995, p 803).

Evidence was brought forward to show that the NHS was chronically underfunded and that this was reflected in the poor state of repair of its buildings, waiting lists for elective procedures, an inadequate standard of care for people such as those with learning difficulties, and the low pay of its staff.

The most influential economic critique was that the NHS was badly flawed because there were no incentives for healthcare providers to become more efficient (Enthoven 1985). At the same time, studies that demonstrated big variations in patterns of clinical activity (e.g. referral rates to hospital (Andersen & Mooney 1990)) were said to prove that resources were not being used as well as they could be (see Chapter 18). Much of the clinical care in the NHS (and in other systems) appeared to be of unknown effectiveness. It was argued that the near-monopoly position of the NHS in the healthcare market had allowed a paternalistic, professionally dominated and inflexible system to develop with limited patient choice, and managers and clinicians who were insensitive to consumer views (Butler & Pirie 1988).

Options for reform

The review focused on issues relating to the financing and organization of health care rather than the scope or priorities of the NHS.

The main alternative to finance from general taxation was some form of social insurance (see Chapter 19) or, alternatively, an earmarked 'health tax'. The idea behind an explicit 'health tax' was that taxpayers would know where their money was going, and might find it more acceptable than an increase in general taxation. A free-market option was to introduce a basic system of public health care for the poor with private health insurance for the remainder of the population of working age, as in the USA, but there was little support for this type of radical change. The review concluded that general taxation was still the cheapest and fairest way to raise money. General taxation for health services normally redistributes resources away from the healthy and wealthy towards those in poor health and the less well off. It is broadly progressive in that those on higher incomes usually contribute a higher proportion of their income. It also redistributes resources over the lifecycle because children and elderly people are the main users of health services, and most tax revenue comes from people of working age.

The debate about organizational change reflected the influence of American ideas, especially economist Alain Enthoven's proposal in 1985 to create an 'internal market' that would introduce explicit incentives to efficiency into the seemingly monolithic NHS (Enthoven 1985). The basic idea was that it was desirable to separate the role of districts as purchasers of health care from their role as providers (see Box 14.3 for the key features of such an arrangement within a publicly financed service).

BOX 14.3   Key Features of an 'Internal' or Quasi-market in Public Services

- Between the extremes of a fully private, free market and a bureaucratic 'command and control' economy (fully planned hierarchy)
- Some separation of the demand (purchasing) and supply (providing) functions within a service which is still largely publicly financed
- Creation of a network of buyers and sellers linked by more or less binding contracts or service agreements specifying the nature of the service to be provided, to whom, the volume and the timescale
- Purchasers tend not to be individuals (e.g. patients) but agencies acting on behalf of groups (e.g. health authorities) – hence the term 'quasi-market'
- Usually some competition between providers or at least the potential for competition if a provider does not perform well
- Variants were developed in 1980s in UK in state education, public housing, community care and the NHS

'WORKING FOR PATIENTS' (1989) AND THE NATIONAL HEALTH SERVICE AND COMMUNITY CARE ACT (1990)

Although the NHS White Paper of 1989 'Working for patients' (Secretaries of State 1989) was the result of a review by a radical Conservative administration in response to a perceived funding crisis, it was notable, first, for the things that it did not change and, second, because the main changes concerned the means of delivery of health care and not general tax financing or the level of funding (Klein 2000). The only innovation on finance was the introduction of tax relief on private health insurance premiums for the over-60s, which was included at the insistence of Margaret Thatcher.

Despite concerted opposition from the BMA and other NHS trade unions, the main elements in the White Paper became law in the NHS and Community Care Act, 1990, and were implemented rapidly, together with a new GP contract. There were four main areas of change covering: the internal or quasi-market; professional accountability; the management hierarchy; and the development of general practice.

The internal market was introduced in the NHS from April 1991, based on the separation of the roles of purchaser and provider along the lines suggested by Enthoven (1985). The aim was to bring to the NHS the benefits of competition between suppliers, together with business management, without jeopardizing its basic principles. The main elements are set out schematically in Fig. 14.3. District Health Authorities (DHAs) became the main purchasers, financed according to the needs of their populations by a variant of the former RAWP formula, and were free to buy hospital and community health services from any provider, whether in the public, private or voluntary sector. Major acute hospitals and other NHS providers became 'Trusts' free from DHA control. Providers such as hospitals were funded on their ability to win contracts to undertake an agreed amount of work for a DHA. The theoretical incentive for providers, therefore, was to minimize costs and maximize quality in order to stay in business.

At the same time, GP practices with more than 11 000 patients were encouraged to become 'GP fundholders' and to take control of their own budgets for the non-emergency hospital outpatient, diagnostic and pharmaceutical care of the patients on their lists. They were expected to act as informed agents on behalf of their patients and to place contracts, for example for elective surgery, with those providers offering a good standard of service at a reasonable price in line with patients' wishes. It was also believed that fundholders would be more likely to challenge providers to produce better services than staff in health authorities. By 1996, half the population in England was served by GPs involved in fundholding (Audit Commission 1996).

Medical audit (the systematic analysis of the quality of clinical care) was made compulsory in hospitals and general practice. Hospital consultants were to have job descriptions that explicitly set out their clinical time commitments in the NHS. General managers were to be involved in the appointment of new consultants and in the allocation of merit awards.

The Griffiths management reforms were extended with further change towards a private sector management model. Health authorities lost their remaining local authority and professional representatives, were slimmed down to 10 members, and became managerial bodies akin to the boards of directors of private companies. Senior managers became members of the new health authorities in their own right. A Chief Executive was appointed to run the NHS in England, including family practitioner services. Figure 14.4 (p. 219) gives the structure of the Service some years later. Chief Executives were also appointed to run the NHS in Wales, Scotland and Northern Ireland through separate management structures.

217

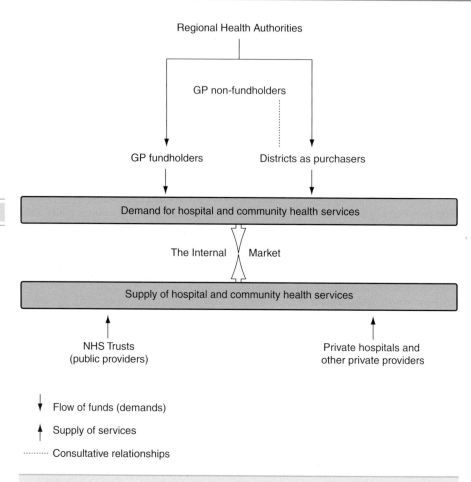

Fig. 14.3 The internal market for NHS services from April 1991.
(*Reproduced with permission from Robinson 1989*).

General practice reforms included a new NHS general practitioner contract introduced in 1990 to: encourage more preventive activities such as screening by GPs; promote a degree of competition between practices for patients; and improve the cost-effectiveness of services delivered in primary care. GPs were required to provide more information about the services they offered and were allowed to advertise their services, and it was made easier for patients to change GP. A higher proportion of GP remuneration was to come from capitation (from 46% to 60% on average) to encourage them to keep their patients healthy. Other elements of GP pay were linked to the attainment of activity targets set by the government (e.g. achieving specified rates of take-up for child immunization and vaccination and cervical cytology). Subsidies enabling GPs to employ additional staff in their practices, such as practice nurses to carry out screening and health promotion work were greatly increased. All GPs were given an official indication of the amount they should

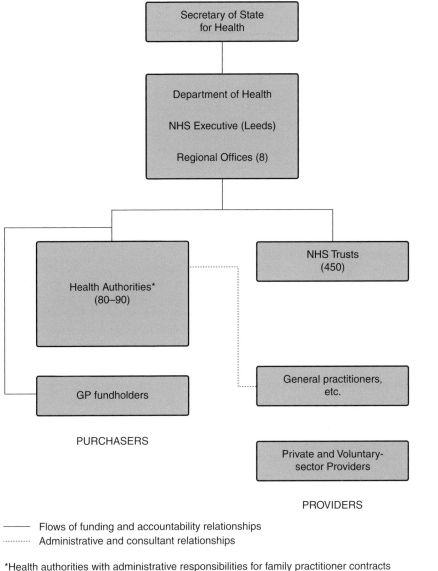

Fig. 14.4 Structure of the NHS in England in April 1996.

be spending on drugs to exert downward pressure on their expenditure. High-prescribing GPs were given advice on how to reduce costs without denying patients the drugs they needed. Family Practitioner Committees (FPCs), which had administered family practitioners' contracts, were renamed Family Health Services Authorities (FHSAs) and given greater powers to audit and monitor the work and spending of family practitioners.

FHSAs were merged with the Health Authorities in April 1996 (see Fig. 14.4 for the structure of the NHS after April 1996).

THE IMPACT OF THE NHS INTERNAL MARKET, 1991–7

Despite the government's radical intentions, the NHS internal market did not produce the degree of measurable change predicted by proponents and feared by opponents (Mays et al 2000). The principal explanation lies in the way the internal market was implemented: the incentives were too weak and the constraints too strong (Le Grand et al 1998, p 130). Central government strictly controlled competition between providers in case the potential efficiency gains from, for example, restructuring hospitals, threatened other goals such as equality of access to services, or caused political embarrassment. As long as the NHS remained publicly financed and the Secretary of State was accountable to Parliament for events within it, it proved impossible to allow competition to take its course. In fact, with the exception of GP fundholders, who were given more freedom to make significant shifts in the pattern of services they purchased (see Table 14.1 for a summary of the impact of the scheme), the NHS was driven at least as much by central directives (e.g. on reducing waiting times) as by the forces of the internal market.

In terms of efficiency, management and administrative costs increased as both purchasers' and providers' roles entailed activities that had not previously existed (e.g. negotiating contracts for services). The numbers of managerial posts increased (from 4610 in 1989 to 12 340 in 1991) but these statistics might overstate the position as the definition of a manager was revised. Even allowing for this increased overhead, the long-term increase in efficiency over the previous 30 years continued, but with relatively little sign of any acceleration after 1991 (Radical Statistics Health Group 1995).

In terms of equity, there was little sign of the discrimination against chronically ill or high-cost patients that had been feared by critics of the internal market. However, there is little doubt (though little good research) that a 'two-tier' system (the preferential treatment of fundholding GPs' patients over patients whose services were purchased by the health authority) did operate in many places. Indeed, it was implicit in the policy that fundholding practices would be able to obtain advantages for their patients through controlling their own budgets for elective treatments.

Although there was little evidence on the quality of care, there were no obvious signs that the market-like system had harmed standards of patient care. GP fundholders used their budgets to provide more accessible services for their patients within their own premises and negotiated shorter hospital waiting times on average than health authorities. However, waits for inpatient treatment (especially long waits over 18 months) for all NHS patients fell during the 1990s. Public dissatisfaction with the NHS is another proxy measure of quality. Dissatisfaction with the NHS rose before the introduction of the internal market, fell during the early 1990s as more money was put into the system and resumed its previous upwards trend in the later 1990s.

On choice and responsiveness to the demands of individual patients – another of the goals of the internal market – the system was designed to empower the purchasers (e.g. fundholding GPs) to act as agents for patients rather than patients themselves as in a more conventional market. Methods of expressing patient 'voice' were little altered by the 1991 system and remained relatively weak.

Whatever else the internal market might have failed to achieve, it did change fundamentally the operating culture of the NHS and the balance of power both between managers and healthcare professionals and between hospital providers and GPs. Providers now have to be far more aware than in the past of the quality and cost of what they provide.

TABLE 14.1	Summary balance sheet of evidence about the benefits and drawbacks of GP fundholding		
Benefits identified (mainly efficiency based)	**Drawbacks (mainly equity based)**	**Areas with little or no hard evidence**	
Shift in balance of power in favour of GPs	Not all fundholders able to make good use of their budgetary power	No direct research on relative efficiency of fundholders and health authorities as purchasers	
Providers more responsive (e.g. shorter waiting times, more information, higher quality standards in contracts) and possibly offered lower prices by hospitals than health authorities	Preferential treatment of fundholders' patients compared with those of other GPs ('two-tier' service), although no evidence that shorter waits for fundholders' patients disadvantaged others	Unknown effect on quality and appropriateness of clinical care purchased (e.g. from hospitals)	
More practice-based services, more accessible to patients	Not clear that all practice-based services are cost-effective (e.g. specialist outpatient clinics)	'Cream-skimming' (i.e. whether fundholders removed potentially costly patients from their lists to protect their budgets) hard to study directly	
Able to make 'savings' from budgets to spend on extra equipment and further patient services. Fundholders more likely to be in surplus than health authorities, but did not deal with emergency services	Not all 'savings' were spent or well spent	Not clear whether funding per capita was fair compared with health authority purchasers	
Rate of increase of prescribing costs lower in fundholding than non-fundholding practices (but difference in rates of change was small and not sustained). Rate of prescribing remained lower in fundholding than non-fundholding practices	Costs of administering fundholding were higher than health authority purchasing because of highly decentralized nature of system		
No difference in referral rates between fundholding and non-fundholding practices despite potential incentive for fundholders to under-refer to protect their budgets	Fundholders had the potential to fragment decisions on local patterns of service and were less publicly accountable than health authorities for their use of funds		
Increased transaction costs in the system due to large number of small purchasers exceeded 'savings' made			

221

Purchasers, after a slow start, came to question traditional ways of providing services and encourage providers to think of new forms of service more relevant to the needs of patients (development in specialist 'outreach' services in the community, early discharge schemes, shared and intermediate forms of care between hospital and general practice, use of skilled nurse practitioners rather than medical staff and so on). Managers in NHS trusts gained greater influence over the pattern of clinical work than before 1991, although this shift in power should not be exaggerated: most managers remained naturally reluctant to confront clinicians head-on over matters of clinical judgement. GP fundholding, however, significantly increased the ability of GPs with budgets for hospital care to influence the way in which hospital specialists provided care to their patients. It also increased the degree of communication between primary and secondary care (Glennerster et al 1994). The experience of fundholding profoundly altered the role of primary care professionals in the system to the extent that the Labour government elected in 1997 chose not only to retain the separation between purchase and provision, but also to organize the NHS in England around Primary Care Groups (PCGs) (see below).

The internal market also exposed long-standing issues, but in new and more noticeable ways (Klein 2000). For example, the purchaser–provider separation and the requirement to contract for specific groups of services drew increasing attention to the fact that purchasers had finite budgets and an ever-lengthening list of demands for services. At the same time, cost-conscious NHS trusts and health authority purchasers came to ask harder questions about where the responsibilities of the NHS for continuing care should end and those of the local authority social services should begin (see Chapter 16). The issue of priority setting (or 'rationing') in health care and the problem of defining the limits of a comprehensive healthcare system have both existed for many years but were largely hidden from view under the previous system.

'NEW LABOUR', NEW NHS?

Eighteen years of Conservative government was brought to an end with the Labour Party's victory in the 1997 General Election. The self-styled 'New Labour' government, determined to find a novel 'third way' between market ideology and old-style Socialism, was critical of many of the changes to the NHS made by its Conservative predecessors under the broad banner of the internal market. In particular, the Labour government argued that the emphasis on markets and incentives to shape the behaviour of providers had undermined the public service ethos of the NHS and had led to an excessive focus on performance measured in terms of the numbers of services delivered rather than the quality or outcomes of care (see Chapter 18 on measuring outcomes). The government resolved to sweep away the internal market and replace it with a system based on 'partnership' and 'collaboration' (Klein 1998a, Secretary of State for Health 1997). The government was also developing proposals for devolution from the national Parliament at Westminster to Assemblies in Wales and Northern Ireland and a Parliament in Scotland, and published separate health White Papers for each country. From 1999, these bodies took responsibility for the NHS in their respective territories although continuing to receive funds from Westminster. The developments in the NHS in England are described in detail in the rest of this chapter.

First, and perhaps surprisingly, the purchaser–provider separation was maintained, although longer-term contracts between purchasers and providers (for 3 years or more) were introduced to help tackle the alleged short-termism of the internal market.

Second, fundholding by individual GP practices was abolished and replaced by a collective form of fundholding for all GPs. Under the new arrangement, all the GPs in an area are members of the local Primary Care Group (PCG) or Primary Care Trust (PCT), which holds the budget for most of the health services used by the patients on their lists and undertakes most of the healthcare purchasing (see Box 14.4). This shift of resources into budgets controlled by primary care professionals continued the process begun under GP fundholding of increasing the influence of GPs on the direction of the NHS. The evolution of PCGs into PCTs ended the separate funding of general medical services (i.e. general practice) and the hospital and community health services, which had existed since the

---

BOX 14.4   Primary Care Groups (PCGs) and Primary Care Trusts (PCTs) in the English NHS

Functions
● Improving the health of the population and addressing health inequalities
● Developing primary and community health services
● Commissioning (purchasing) a range of community health and hospital services for their patients – ultimately responsible for 75% of NHS resources
● PCTs also deliver community health services and fund their constituent GPs/practices from a unified budget

Structure
● Based on groups of general practices with populations of around 100 000 (50 GPs)
● Governed by a board that represents GPs, community nurses, the local community, social services department and the health authority

Levels of PCG (all PCGs to become PCTs by 2004)
● Level 1: PCG is an advisory subcommittee of the local health authority
● Level 2: PCG is a subcommittee that manages a budget devolved to it by the health authority
● Level 3: PCG is a freestanding body accountable to the health authority for commissioning primary, community health and hospital services for its patients
● Level 4: PCG becomes a PCT, a freestanding body accountable to the health authority for commissioning primary, community health and hospital services for its patients and for providing primary and community health services

---

beginning of the NHS. The integration of budgets was intended to improve the coordination of services in and out of hospitals and to improve the overall use of resources (e.g. by encouraging extensions of the scope of primary healthcare services and the development of alternatives to costly hospital care).

The retention of the purchaser–provider separation and primary care-based purchasing suggests that, despite rhetoric to the contrary, the government was prepared to learn from the experience of the internal market (Le Grand 1999). The changes (see Table 14.2 for a summary of what changed and what remained the same) were designed to build on the positive aspects of purchaser–provider separation and fundholding, and to deal with the negative. For example, PCG/PCTs typically have populations of at least 100 000 patients, which are far larger than most of the former fundholding groups and reduces the high management costs of GP fundholding. In addition, GPs and other primary care staff were put in charge of local purchasing and resource management on the grounds that the experience of the previous fundholding scheme had given grounds for believing that they generally understood their patients' needs better than health authority staff (see Table 14.1). The role of health authorities was shifted from purchasing towards work with other, non-health agencies, such as local government, to improve health by influencing the social and economic factors such as unemployment and poor housing that adversely affect population health (see Chapters 2 and 8).

The third main set of changes was designed to ensure greater consistency in the availability and quality of services right across the NHS. A number of widely publicized cases of unacceptably poor quality clinical care, most notably at Bristol Royal Infirmary (Report of the Public Inquiry into Children's Heart Surgery at the Bristol Royal Infirmary 1984–1995, 2001), had demonstrated the need to bolster the systems of professional self-regulation and clinical audit, and to establish accepted external standards against which to measure clinical care:

● The National Institute for Clinical Excellence (NICE) was set up in March 1999 to synthesize the best available evidence on the effectiveness and cost-effectiveness of

TABLE 14.2	Elements of continuity and change in 'The new NHS: modern, dependable' (Secretary of State 1997)
Elements of continuity with the internal market	**Departures from the internal market**
Purchaser–provider split and potential for competition between providers (especially acute hospitals)	Emphasis on collaboration and cooperation rather than choice and competition – NHS as a 'network'
Emphasis on budget capping and integration of separate funding streams	Emphasis on longer-term relationships and service agreements (contracts)
GP-led purchasing of health services on behalf of their patients (volunteer GP fundholding leads to compulsory PCGs/PCTs)	Focus on quality alongside previous focus on efficiency
Central control of overall direction of the NHS with devolved budget management	Increased emphasis on clinical accountability
Consumer focus (e.g. Patient's Charter leads to NHS Plan performance targets and 'star' ratings)	
Rapid institutional change	

treatments, drugs and technologies, particularly new ones, and to produce official guidance on whether they should be funded as part of the NHS.

● In a related initiative, expert groups were commissioned by the Department of Health to develop evidence-based National Service Frameworks for the main diseases and fields of care to identify 'best practice' and optimum service design for use by local purchasers and providers.

● A new and independent inspectorate, the Commission for Health Improvement (CHI), began work in April 2000 to: monitor the quality of services in each NHS Trust; scrutinize local efforts to assure and improve quality; publish the reports of its investigations; and intervene in 'failing' NHS providers if the Secretary of State should decide that serious or persistent problems need to be resolved. The CHI, now called the Commission for Healthcare Audit and Inspection (CHAI), required, in particular, to see how well NHS Trusts, including PCTs, have implemented the concept of 'clinical governance', which is the new shorthand for each NHS organization's responsibility for assuring the quality of its services. Although subject to a number of differing interpretations, 'clinical governance' is probably best defined as 'a system through which NHS organizations are accountable for continuously improving the quality of their services and safeguarding high standards of care by creating an environment in which excellence in clinical care can flourish' (Scally & Donaldson 1998) (see Box 14.5). As an example, the chairperson and chief executive of each NHS trust are now statutorily responsible not only for the financial state of the organization, but also its ability to provide high quality care.

● A National Performance Framework was developed to broaden the basis of quality assessment from activity levels and crude measures of productivity to include indicators of the quality and effectiveness of the services delivered by NHS providers (see Box 14.6 for the areas covered by the performance measures).

These changes to the NHS in England also applied, to varying degrees, to Wales and Northern Ireland, but the new Scottish Parliament has increasingly developed its own

---

BOX 14.5   Clinical governance

What is it?
- The responsibility of all NHS organizations that deliver health services to ensure that their clinical services are of good quality
- It implies that doctors and other clinicians have a duty to ensure that their colleagues are enabled to practise well

Elements at provider level
- A focus on evidence-based practice
- Facilities for continuing professional development
- Clinical audit of care against explicit standards and monitoring of patient outcomes
- The use of quality assurance techniques
- Risk management
- Formal, regular appraisal and re-accreditation of clinicians
- Identification and remedy of poor clinical performance

Elements at national level in England
- National Institute for Clinical Excellence (NICE)
- Commission for Healthcare Audit and Inspection (CHAI)
- National Service Frameworks
- Adverse events monitoring and reporting system
- Modernization Agency
- National Clinical Assessment Authority (NCAA)

---

distinctive policies towards the NHS. For example, the Scottish alternative to PCG/PCTs is known as a Local Health Care Cooperative and has no purchasing responsibility, but is rather a vehicle for improving coordination between local primary care professionals. As a result, whereas GP fundholding lives on in a revised form in England, Wales and Northern Ireland, it has been removed from the system in Scotland.

MAKING THE NHS MORE ACCESSIBLE AND USER-FRIENDLY

One of the Labour government's most frequently articulated desires for the NHS in its first term (1997 to 2001) was to 'modernize' the service. Whereas 'modernization' has tended to be applied loosely to any initiative supported by ministers, it has been linked particularly closely to efforts to make the NHS more responsive to the needs of its users, often regarded as the main weakness of public services delivered by powerful professional groups where competition is limited. The argument runs that with private service industries like banks, supermarkets and travel agencies now accessible 24 hours a day, seven days a week throughout the year on-line, at call-centres or through extended opening hours, the NHS should become more user-friendly in the same way. The main response has been in the field of primary health care with the establishment of NHS Direct (a national, nurse-led telephone help-line) and the emergence of NHS Walk-in Centres designed to supplement the services provided by ordinary NHS general practices by providing quick, initial treatment to patients who cannot visit their family doctor conveniently (e.g. because of work commitments).

The management of waiting lists has also been influenced by rising public expectations and by models from other service industries. For example, targets were set and achieved to increase the proportion of patients given a booked date for admission to hospital for elective surgery rather than being called for treatment at the convenience of the hospital. As a result, the surgical waiting has begun to shift from an uncertain queuing system towards a more predictable system of reservations. Similarly, the wait for patients urgently referred for suspected breast cancer has been reduced to 2 weeks from GP referral to specialist assessment.

> **BOX 14.6** National Performance Assessment Framework and Performance Incentives in the NHS in England
>
> Six areas covered by high level performance indicators ('balanced scorecard')
> - Health improvement – trends in the general health of the population influenced by many factors outside the control of the NHS
> - Fair access – ability of local services to offer fair access in relation to people's needs irrespective of geography, socioeconomic group, ethnicity, age or gender
> - Effective delivery of appropriate health care – effective, appropriate, timely care, in accordance with agreed standards
> - Efficiency – effective care delivered with the minimum of waste and which represents 'value-for-money'
> - Patient and carer experience – assessment of users' experience of services and their views on the quality of care
> - Health outcomes of NHS care – assessment of the direct contribution of NHS services to improvements in overall health
>
> Incentives to improve performance
> - NHS performance ratings given by the Commission for Healthcare Audit and Inspection reward organizations and staff for excellence and improved performance against key targets
> - 'Three star' organizations are rewarded with a high level of autonomy, ability to apply for 'foundation' status and automatic access to resources from the NHS Performance Fund to develop services and reward staff
> - 'Two star' organizations, which are performing well overall but have not reached the same consistently high standards as 'one star' organizations, have a lower level of autonomy and have to agree their plans for spending their share of the NHS Performance Fund with the Modernization Agency
> - 'One star' organizations have still less autonomy than 'two star' organizations and are supported by the Modernization Agency to improve their performance. They have to produce a performance improvement plan and can only spend their share of the Performance Fund with the agreement of the Agency
> - 'Zero star' organizations have the least autonomy, receive intensive support and, where appropriate, intervention from the Modernization Agency, including possibly having their management replaced. Their share of the Performance Fund is used by the Agency to provide external help to improve their performance

There are also increasing numbers of experiments with more explicit algorithms for clinicians to use to place patients in order of priority before they are offered treatment dates (Edwards 1999).

THE NHS PLAN, 2000

Despite the focus on improving service quality and accessibility, the NHS continued to attract adverse publicity in the later 1990s. Further clinical scandals involving unacceptably low standards of care were uncovered. Research was reported that appeared to show that patient survival rates after common cancers were lower in the NHS than in other European countries. This was attributed to both the organization of services and the level of resources in the NHS. It was popularly argued, not for the first time in its history, that the NHS was in 'crisis' due to underinvestment in staffing and infrastructure.

The government, and particularly the Prime Minister, Tony Blair, concluded in 2000 that something must be done to reverse the 'crisis' and to rebuild public confidence in the NHS. In a bold initial move, the Prime Minister promised to bring the level of funding of the NHS as a percentage of national income to the average level enjoyed elsewhere in Europe so as to remedy what he interpreted to be the 'underfunding' of the NHS over many years. At the time, the UK's combined public and private spending on health care was approximately

7% of its gross domestic product, whereas the average for the European Union was 8%. The government committed itself to 6.5% per year growth in real terms (i.e. after allowing for inflation) in NHS spending over a 4-year period (2000–4). This was twice the previous long-term rate of increase. The debate about the level of NHS funding was accompanied by a flurry of discussion about the merits of alternatives or supplements to general taxation as the main source of NHS finance, such as a separate tax to pay for the NHS or more reliance on private insurance. Neither appears to be self-evidently superior to using general taxation to pay directly for health services.

With such an unprecedented large increase in NHS spending in view, it was important to plan how to use the new resources. The 'NHS plan' for England (Department of Health 2000) offered a significant increase in resources in exchange for a tougher regime of rewards and sanctions, backed up by regulation and inspection, to improve the performance of the NHS over a 10-year period. At the core of the Plan were more staff and more hospital beds and a wider range of performance targets relating particularly to outpatient and elective surgery waiting times and focusing effort on priority areas such as cancer and heart disease (see Box 14.7). The first annual report on the implementation of the Plan provided some evidence that progress was being made (e.g. there had been a 25% increase in critical care beds, 10 000 more nurses and the number of people waiting for more than 15 months for inpatient treatment had fallen by more than a third (NHS Modernisation Board 2002)).

There were other innovations, such as the announcement of a Modernization Agency within the NHS to spread 'best practice' in patient care using evaluated pilot schemes. In addition, the CHAI was required to assess the performance of NHS Trusts each year using a system similar to the 'star' ratings awarded to hotels and to publish these as part of an overall report direct to Parliament on the performance of the NHS. Better performers against the performance targets and 'star' ratings (Box 14.7) are rewarded with greater autonomy (e.g. over their use of resources) and allocated part of a discretionary performance-related fund (see Box 14.6). Although the extra money is small compared with Trusts' total incomes, it is designed to reach the frontline staff directly responsible for service improvements. By contrast, poorly performing providers risk having their management taken over by teams from high-performing NHS establishments.

Comparing the performance of entire health care organizations, which produce many different services, is complex. There is the added technical difficulty of having to take into account the fact that Trusts serve different socioeconomic populations. There is also the risk that providers might concentrate on the key indicators at the expense of other important

---

BOX 14.7   Examples of NHS Plan Performance Targets

- No one to wait more than 18 months for any inpatient treatment
- Everyone with suspected cancer able to see a specialist within 2 weeks of their GP deciding that they need to be referred
- Reduction in the number of patients waiting more than 13 weeks for their first outpatient appointment
- Less than 1% of elective operations cancelled on the day
- Cleanliness of facilities
- A satisfactory financial position
- A commitment to improving the working lives of staff
- A low rate of emergency readmissions to hospital
- A low rate of deaths within 30 days of surgery for patients admitted on an unplanned basis

objectives. Nevertheless, performance assessment significantly improves the transparency of the services provided.

Consistent with the government's wider commitment to 'what works' rather than to old Left hostility to the private sector, the NHS Plan included a 'Concordat' with the private sector that encouraged NHS purchasers to use spare private capacity for their patients if this enabled them to meet the government's performance targets (e.g. to reduce waiting times for elective surgery) more cost-effectively than relying on NHS hospitals. The Plan included positive support for public–private partnerships (PPPs) in the NHS, for example, in the case of major hospital building projects. Critics are concerned that such moves are part of a gradual dismantling of the NHS or that they risk leaving the NHS with all the most difficult and costly cases.

Although recognizing the role of the private sector when this could support the achievement of NHS goals, the Plan also made it clear that the government would reduce the influence of the private sector in contrary circumstances. For example, the Plan proposed stronger inducements for hospital specialists to work full-time in the NHS and tighter restrictions on the degree to which specialists could work simultaneously in the public and private sectors in order to minimize any perverse incentives for consultants to favour their private practices over their NHS commitments.

The final strand in the Plan reflected the continuation of the government's desire to strengthen both professional self-regulation and external clinical accountability for national standards of care, particularly in medicine, by introducing new systems to ensure the clinical competence of doctors and other health workers throughout their careers (see Chapter 15 for a discussion of the health professions). The Plan included proposals for the periodic revalidation of doctors' qualifications, and changes to the powers and functioning of the General Medical Council, which deals with the registration (entry into the profession and right to practise) and disciplining of doctors. It also introduced a system for the reporting and monitoring of adverse events and 'near-misses' in clinical practice. This aims to prevent clinical errors in future by identifying current errors comprehensively, learning about what causes them and developing methods of working to avoid them occurring again. Inspired by the safety culture of the aeronautical industry, the focus is on redesigning systems rather than blaming individual practitioners when things go wrong. A National Clinical Assessment Authority (NCAA) was established to help NHS employers assess the small number of 'poorly performing' doctors and make recommendations about whether and under what circumstances they can continue to practice in the NHS.

Whereas the medical profession is subject to increasing external scrutiny, in return, politicians in Britain are increasingly supportive of the idea that, in return, clinicians, should become more directly involved in the design of services at all levels and the Department of Health less so (Milburn 2001). In a number of high-profile clinical areas, such as cancer services, senior clinicians have been appointed with nationwide authority to implement changes to entire systems of service delivery in the hope that this will secure more rapid progress than change led by civil servants and managers.

In addition, power and resources are increasingly being transferred to PCTs, which are planned to control 75% of the NHS budget by 2004 (see Box 14.4). GPs play a major role in PCT decision making. To support this process of devolving responsibility to local clinicians for the way in which resources are used within a framework of standards, the government altered the structure of the NHS in 2002 by reducing the number of health authorities from 90 to 28, reinforcing their recently acquired strategic role to work with non-NHS organizations to improve health and oversee the PCTs. PCTs were given greater operational freedoms to make the local health services' purchasing decisions as they saw fit (see Fig. 14.5). The logic of the new system appears to be that as long as the NHS shows signs of

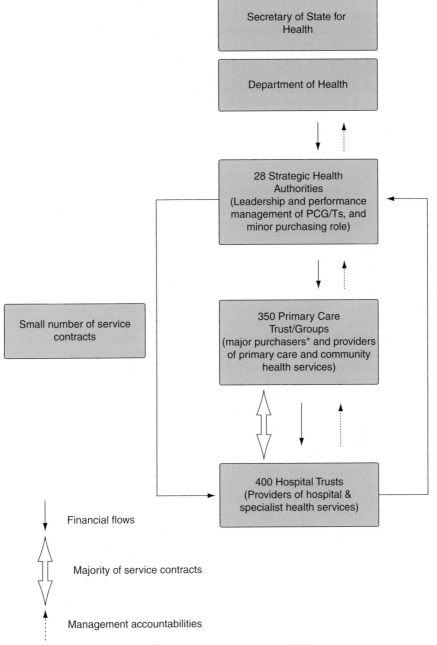

Fig. 14.5   Structure of the NHS in England from April 2002.

meeting the government's key goals, staff at the frontline will be permitted to innovate and be freed from unnecessary central controls (Klein, 2001). Well-performing parts of the NHS will gain autonomy and poorly performing parts will be more strictly controlled.

CONCLUSION: HOW HAS THE NHS CHANGED AND HAS IT A FUTURE?

The history of the NHS can be divided into three phases based on the three basic types of organization said to have prevailed at the time – hierarchies, markets and networks (see Box 14.8 for definitions of these terms):

- the NHS as a hierarchy (1948–79) distinguished by a top-down, command and control planning model led by officials and politicians at national level

- the NHS as a market (1979–97) characterized by the injection of market mechanisms into the NHS, particularly the purchaser–provider split and competitive tendering of support services (e.g. cleaning and catering)

- the NHS as a network (from 1997) marked by an emphasis on collaboration and partnership based on relationships of trust, replacing both market and command-and-control mechanisms (e.g. longer-term contracts).

However, the material in this chapter has shown that the NHS has always been more complex than this neat schema suggests. Most obviously, the NHS market of the 1990s differed substantially from most private markets and was best described as an internal or quasi-market (see Box 14.3). In addition, there is evidence that all three organizational forms have coexisted, to differing degrees, throughout the life of the NHS. For example, one of the paradoxes of the quasi-market period was that hierarchy became more prominent as the government regulated the extent of competition to prevent political embarrassment (see discussion of the impact of the internal market, above). Exworthy et al (1999) argue that although the NHS appeared to be a hierarchy up to the 1980s, the centre had very limited control over the periphery where services were delivered and policy was largely made through professional networks. Similarly, they show how the NHS after 1997 includes strong elements of hierarchical control (e.g. the greater emphasis given to a national framework of performance measurement) as well as allowing residual scope for competition (e.g. the opportunity for private hospitals to bid against NHS hospitals to undertake elective surgery, and for managers from well-performing NHS Trusts to compete to take over the management of Trusts that are performing poorly). They conclude that it is better to think

---

BOX 14.8   Hierarchies, Markets and Networks as Different Forms of Coordination

- Hierarchy: tends to be associated with bureaucracies, typified by a high degree of centralization of policy making and resource allocation; often described as 'command and control'; coordination is by administrative instruction
- Market: form of coordination derived from the exchange between buyers and sellers of a good or service in which quantity and quality determine price, which determines the pattern of consumption. Associated with the notion of the 'invisible hand', which brings supply and demand into balance through rational actors responding to market signals; coordination is by price competition
- Network: form of coordination based on linkages between individuals, often informal and based on a common outlook on life that involves relationships based on trust and reciprocity. Associated with professional groups; coordination is through trust and cooperation

of 'quasi-hierarchies', 'quasi-markets' and 'quasi-networks' in the NHS, as the three basic forms of hierarchy, market and network can coexist.

So much for the past of the NHS, but what of its future? At the beginning of this chapter it was noted that the NHS represents the purest example, worldwide, of a health system in which central government pays for health services for the entire population from general tax revenue, owns most of the facilities and employs most of the staff who deliver care (see Chapter 19). As a result, the NHS is simultaneously criticized endlessly and supported strongly – even cherished – by its patients and the public at large. Table 14.3 attempts to provide a balance-sheet of the current strengths and weaknesses of the NHS, and Box 14.9 gives an indication of some of the trends in the service's performance against common yardsticks of achievement.

Although it is unlikely that the NHS would be set up in the same way as in the 1940s were it to be reinvented today, two leading American commentators have argued strongly that, despite its problems, the fundamental principles of the NHS – universal coverage, general tax financing and the ability to plan nationally – remain correct (Leatherman & Berwick 2000). According to this analysis, the strategy of significant increases in NHS spending begun by New Labour should be sustained and will continue to attract the support of the public.

TABLE 14.3	Strengths and Weaknesses of the NHS in the Twenty-first Century
Strengths	**Weaknesses**
Strong popular support and esteem	Little patient choice, limited responsiveness to patients' views, services still largely professionally-driven
Ability to contain overall spending, including spending on wages, so that other beneficial social programmes are not 'crowded out'	Pressure for increased spending collides with fixed budget determined at national level in competition with other political priorities – budget has tended to increase more slowly than in other European countries
Reasonably efficient system from the point of view of health outcomes in relation to amount spent	Fewer doctors, nurses, etc. than most OECD countries; more restricted access to latest drugs and technology; backlog of investment in facilities; waiting times for non-urgent treatment
Universal access to a wide range of services with few user charges	Variations in quality and availability of specific services with some outcomes poorer than in other European countries
Services largely used in relation to 'need'	Parallel privately financed sector compromises fair access goals of the NHS
Fair finance from general taxation in line with ability to pay	Inability of ministers to avoid 'micromanagement' of the system in response to political pressures
Fair allocation of resources to different parts of the country	
Strong primary medical care, including GP 'gate keeping'	
High quality clinical training and high average competence of staff	
Ability to plan and coordinate services to a degree envied in many other countries	

BOX 14.9   Selected Trends in Health and NHS Performance in England

- Life expectancy at birth increased among males from 71.8 years in 1984 to 75.1 years in 1998 (at age 80 from 5.9 to 6.9 years)
- All-cause death rates among males decreased from 1044.1 per 100 000 (1994) to 1000.7 (1999)
- Cancer death rates in males decreased from 284.7 per 100 000 (1994) to 264.5 (1999)
- Diabetes death rates for males were unchanged at 10.7 per 100 000 in 1994 and 1999
- Cervical and breast cancer screening coverage of women in the target populations was unchanged in the 1990s at approximately 84% and 65%, respectively
- Hospital inpatient activity in 'finished consultant episodes' rose by an average of 3.4% per annum between 1987–8 and 1997–8
- Outpatient waiting times: 75% of patients referred by their GPs waited less than 13 weeks in 1999 and 2000 (and 94% waited less than 26 weeks)
- In-patient waiting time: in December 2000, 74% of patients waiting for elective admission had waited 5 months or less, 21% had waited 6–11 months, and 5% had waited 12 months or more
- Patient care staff in hospitals and community health services increased from 497 300 whole-time equivalents in 1994 to 529 300 in 1999 (and medical and dental staff rose from 52 600 to 60 300 in the same period)
- General medical practitioners (GPs) and practice staff increased from 25 500 whole-time equivalent 'unrestricted principals and equivalents' in 1994 to 25 900 in 1999 and other practice staff from 51 800 whole time equivalents in 1994 to 63 100 in 1999
- Gross expenditure rose from £34 430 million sterling in 1995–6 to £39 883 million sterling in 1998–9, of which Department of Health administration fell from £332 million sterling to £289 million sterling

Source: National Statistics/Department of Health (2001) Health and Personal Social Services Statistics, England. Online. Available: http://www.doh.gov.uk/HPSS

By contrast, Rudolf Klein, a long-time observer of the NHS, is more pessimistic about the ability of a monolithic system such as the NHS to meet the aspirations of an increasingly diverse society and to manage the inevitable conflict between what health professionals believe they should do for their patients and the resources available from taxes to pay for this. Klein argues that the NHS continues to be attractive to governments because it enables the costs of health care to be controlled on behalf of tax payers in ways that other countries struggle to achieve (see Chapter 19), but that this ability comes at an ever-increasing political cost related to 'the NHS's semi-permanent crisis of "under-funding"' (Klein 1998b, p 108). The increased frequency of restructuring and cycles of attempted devolution followed by return to centralization are indicative of the difficulty of managing central financing and accountability against a background of rising expectations and burgeoning technologies. As long as the NHS remains very largely financed from general taxes, it is unlikely that any Secretary of State for Health will ever succeed in becoming distanced from what happens in all parts of the NHS. This is despite repeated calls for the NHS to be run at arm's length from government (King's Fund 2002). As a result, Klein's long-term hunch is that future governments will become more interested than ever before in a system that is more pluralistic and diverse both in its sources of financing and in the distribution of responsibility for the delivery of health care (e.g. making more use of independent suppliers of health services and less of publicly owned providers). Such a system might be more in tune with a society that has less faith in central planning and professional paternalism than was the case in 1946, but it would still need to ensure a reasonably fair pattern of access to services across the population, because the public continues to value fairness in health services. Combining greater pluralism and flexibility with a high degree of fairness in financing and access will not be an easy task.

References

Abel-Smith B 1964 The hospitals 1800–1948. Heinemann, London

Andersen TF, Mooney G (eds) 1990 The challenge of medical practice variations. Macmillan, London

Audit Commission 1996 What the doctor ordered: a study of GP fundholders in England and Wales. Audit Commission, London

Beveridge Report 1942 Interdepartmental Committee on Social Insurance and Allied Services. Cmnd 6404. HMSO, London

Butler E, Pirie M 1988 Health management units. Adam Smith Institute, London

Carpenter G 1984 National health insurance: a case study in the use of private non-profit making organizations in the provision of welfare benefits. Public Administration 62:71–89

Department of Health (DoH) 2000 NHS plan: a plan for investment – a plan for reform. Cmnd 4818. Department of Health, London

Department of Health and Social Security (DHSS) 1983 NHS management inquiry. The Griffiths Report. DHSS, London

Eckstein H 1958 The English health service. Harvard University Press, Cambridge, MA

Edwards RT 1999 Points for pain: waiting list priority scoring systems. British Medical Journal 318:412–414

Enthoven AC 1985 Reflections on the management of the National Health Service. Nuffield Provincial Hospitals Trust, London

Exworthy M, Powell M, Mohan J 1999 The NHS: quasi-market, quasi-hierarchy and quasi-network? Public Money and Management Oct–Dec:15–22

Glennerster H, Matsaganis M, Owens P, with Hancock S 1994 Implementing GP fundholding. Open University Press, Buckingham

Honigsbaum F 1989 Health, happiness and security: the creation of the National Health Service. Routledge, London

King's Fund 2002 The future of the NHS: a framework for debate. Discussion paper. The King's Fund, London

Klein R 1995 Review of Ray Robinson and Julian Le Grand (eds) Evaluating the NHS reforms. Journal of Health Politics Policy and Law 20:802–807

Klein R 1998a Why Britain is reorganizing its National Health Service – yet again. Health Affairs 17:111–125

Klein R 1998b Economic and political costs of the NHS: a changing balance sheet? In: Macpherson G (ed) Our NHS: a celebration of 50 years. BMJ Books, London, p 106–111

Klein R 2000 The new politics of the National Health Service, 4th (revised) edn. Prentice Hall, Harlow

Klein R 2001 Milburn's vision of a new NHS: adopting the missionary position. British Medical Journal 322:1078–1079

Leatherman S, Berwick D 2000 The NHS through American eyes. British Medical Journal 321:1545–1546

Le Grand J 1999 Competition, cooperation, or control? Tales from the British National Health Service. Health Affairs 18:27–39

Le Grand J, Mays N, Dixon J 1998 The reforms: success or failure or neither? In: Le Grand J, Mays N, Mulligan J-A (eds) Learning from the NHS internal market. King's Fund Publishing, London, 117–143

Mays N, Mulligan J-A, Goodwin N 2000 The British quasi-market in health care: a balance sheet of the evidence. Journal of Health Services Research and Policy 5:49–58

Milburn A 2001 Shifting the balance of power in the NHS. Speech delivered on 25 April 2001. Online. Available: http://tap.ccta.gov.uk/doh/intpress.nsf/page/2001-0200

Ministry of Health 1944 A National Health Service. Cmnd 6502. HMSO, London

Ministry of Health 1956 Report of the Committee of Enquiry into the Cost of the National Health Service. Cmnd 9962. HMSO, London

233

Ministry of Health 1962 A hospital plan for England and Wales. Cmnd 1604. HMSO, London

National Statistics/Department of Health (DoH) 2001 Health and personal social services statistics. DoH, London. Online. Available: http:www.doh.gov.uk/HPSS

NHS Modernisation Board 2002 The NHS Plan: a progress report. Department of Health, London

Packwood T, Keen J, Buxton M 1991 Hospitals in transition: the resource management experiment. Open University Press, Milton Keynes

Political and Economic Planning 1937 Report on the British Health Services. PEP, London

Radical Statistics Health Group 1995 NHS 'indicators of success': what do they tell us? British Medical Journal 310:1045–1050

Report of the Public Inquiry into Children's Heart Surgery at the Bristol Royal Infirmary (1984–1995) 2001 Learning from Bristol. Cmnd 5207. HMSO, London

Robinson R 1989 New health care market. British Medical Journal 298:437–439

Scally G, Donaldson LJ 1998 Clinical governance and the drive for quality improvement in the new NHS in England. British Medical Journal 317:61–65

Secretaries of State for Health, Wales, Northern Ireland and Scotland 1989 Working for patients. Cmnd 555. HMSO, London

Secretary of State for Health 1997 The New NHS: modern – dependable. Cmnd 3807. HMSO, London

Thane P 1982 The foundations of the welfare state. Longman, London

Webster C 1988 The health services since the war. Volume 1: problems of health care, the National Health Service before 1957. HMSO, London

CHAPTER 15

Health Professions

Ian Rees Jones

Health care in contemporary Britain is provided by a myriad of professional groups. Ideally, a team working in a hospital will have the patient at its centre and doctors, nurses, radiographers, therapists and laboratory scientific officers all working together and sharing information on the patient. Equally, the primary care team will include general practitioners, midwives, health visitors and community nurses liaising with pharmacists and social workers. Often, however, the reality behind this idealized sense of harmony and cooperation is one of subtle hierarchies, poor communication and misunderstanding. There are tensions and disputes within and between different professional groups. In addition to this, all of these professional groups are facing constant conflict, challenges and change from a variety of different sources including governments, the public and the media. Some have interpreted the situation as one of crisis. Certainly there are deep-seated anxieties about the collapse of trust between the professions and the public. This is particularly the case for the medical profession, whose foundations have been shaken in recent years by a number of high-profile cases of medical negligence and malpractice highlighted by the Bristol Royal Infirmary Inquiry (2001) and the taking of children's organs in Alderhey hospital (Royal Liverpool Children's Inquiry 2001). The Harold

Shipman murders have added to a sense of a profession under siege (DoH 2001a). Indeed, on the 16 January 2001, the president of the General Medical Council (GMC), Sir Donald Irving, stated: 'there are deep-seated flaws in the culture and regulation of the medical profession...' (Irvine 2001, p 1). This statement reflects concerns about the GMC's role in regulating the medical profession, the secrecy involved and the perceived complacency towards poor practice. It also refers to the paternalistic culture of the medical profession, a sense of a lack of engagement with patient rights and growing calls for patient involvement in decision making. It is significant that the National Health Service Reform and Health Care Professions Act 2002 (HMSO 2002) has laid the ground for setting up a Council for the Regulation of Health Care Professions. The function of this body will be to promote the interests of patients and other members of the public in relation to healthcare professional bodies such as the GMC.

How can we understand this sense of crisis among healthcare professions? Drawing in the main on the Anglo-American experience, this chapter will focus on the medical profession. Starting from attempts to define professionalism, the chapter will chart the historical development of the medical profession and its relationships with other healthcare workers before considering theories of professionalism and explanations for changing relations in healthcare work.

PROFESSIONS

Early sociological work on 'the professions' tended to concentrate on definitions of professions and their primary characteristics or traits (Carr-Saunders & Wilson 1933). Sociologists collated a number of features such as the possession of altruistic values, high ethical standards, a service ethos and a body of specialized knowledge attained through lengthy training at universities or medical schools. To these could be added high social status, a monopoly position in the market and high levels of control over conditions of work (see Box 15.1).

Examples of such professions include lawyers, accountants, teachers, priests, doctors, nurses and engineers. The object of this approach was to classify professions on the basis of dimensions of these traits. This would then allow comparisons to be made between professions and with non-professional groups (Goode 1957). These definitional or trait approaches are still useful in that they remind us that professional status is usually accompanied by a privileged position in the labour market, high levels of job interest, job satisfaction, job security and freedom from supervision. In addition, high levels of respect from others accompany high status. However, the trait approach tended to ignore the value judgements underlying many of the ways in which professions were constructed, as well as the underlying conflicts and contradictions within these constructions.

BOX 15.1   Characteristics of a Profession

- Discrete body of knowledge over which members have control
- Monopoly over market for services
- Autonomy over conditions of work and from state and capital
- Code of ethics
- Altruism is a core motive and performance is valued more than financial reward
- Training is lengthy and its quality and content is determined by the profession itself

Professional socialization

Early work on the professions gradually began to be challenged by research that highlighted contradictions within assumed value systems. For example, Becker's work with trainee doctors showed how medical students, who might have started out with a strong sense of altruism, slowly substituted means (passing exams) for ends (helping sick people) and learned to divide patients into good examination material and 'crocks' (Becker et al 1961). This challenged assumptions about a 'trait' of professional altruism because it suggested that the medical profession, in its training, developed a norm of cynicism in conjunction with an abstract ideal of altruism.

Access to medical education involves a highly competitive selection process. This process in itself can be seen as the first step in the path towards professional socialization. Selection processes have been criticized for the incorporation of subjective criteria, particularly a tendency for interview panels to select candidates that mirror the existing image of the profession. Once entry to medical school is secured, medical education involves not only the transfer of knowledge but also the absorption of appropriate attitudes and behaviour towards clients and colleagues. In this sense, the medical profession has, within its training process, a built-in capacity to mould new members in its own image. Studies of medical education have shown how this capacity is maintained through the *formal* educational curriculum, which passes on knowledge and skills and involves periodic formal assessments, and the *informal* curriculum, which transmits attitudes, behaviours and beliefs and where the assessment is based on the approval of performed roles. For example, Simon Sinclair's study of a London medical school shows how the acquisition of formal and informal knowledge, through frontstage and backstage activity, equips medical students with the cultural assets of a professional group (Sinclair 1997). Dingwall (1979), in his study of the development of health visiting, shows how a 'repertoire' of behaviours, norms and mores are instilled in trainees by their tutors. Although this activity often seems trivial and unnecessary to the capacity to practice, it gradually builds up to a style of doing things that is accepted and seen as 'professional'.

The professional project

In response to the limitations of the trait approach, some have argued that 'profession' is a folk concept, constructed in and through social relations. This raises the questions of how and why some occupations are generally viewed to be professions and how these professional groups maintain their status. One way of addressing these questions is to look at processes of professionalization. These occur at different levels but they are connected to the power of the State in that State sponsorship and the sponsorship of power elites is an important condition for professional formation. Developing claims to a privileged social position and the ability to sustain this over time are part of the 'professional project' (Larson 1977). This involves the build-up of assets or capital in three key areas (MacDonald 1995).

In the first place there is the area of economic assets, most clearly apparent in the buildings acquired by professional groups. A visit to the Royal Society of Medicine or the Royal College of Physicians will show how architecture and the aesthetic of buildings reinforce the status of a professional group.

In the second place there is area of organizational assets. Here the relationship with corporate and State health care, as in the USA, or the NHS in the UK, gives professional groups access to and control over large-scale organizational assets.

In the third place there is the field of cultural assets. Here, scientific knowledge, reputation and credentials are promoted and defended by the activities of professional bodies. For example, members of Royal Colleges sit on government advisory panels and contribute to government reports, Royal commissions and independent inquiries. This maintains the standing of a professional group through their role as providers of technical advice and in the process maintains the quality of their technical advice.

A focus on process therefore helps us to understand how so-called 'traits' of professions, such as a specialized knowledge-base and professional ethics, are not fixed but change with society and that these changes can be studied to examine how status and professional boundaries are maintained. The ideology of a successful profession supports its dominance by defining social reality. The specialist scientific and technical expertise of a profession acts as conduit for diffusing its influence. The position and role of the profession is maintained and extended by maintaining standards and influencing the terms of interaction between the profession and the public. The professional project is thus an important contributor to processes of social stratification in that the knowledge and skills-base of the profession are translated into monopolistic practices, restricting of supply and market positioning, which are, in turn, translated into money and power (MacDonald 1995). For these strategies to succeed, the profession needs a stable market that can be fixed in its favour through the maintenance of monopoly. This is achieved through a 'regulative bargain' with the state that restricts access to knowledge, controls the market and supervises the production of producers.

Social closure

The prevailing political culture and the ways in which power networks operate influences the shape of the regulative bargain with the State. The bargain, however, is not achieved easily. The granting of monopoly rights is often the culmination of long-drawn-out battles. In addition, once achieved, the monopoly is not guaranteed. It must be defended and even extended. In other words, the profession must adopt its 'jurisdiction' (Abbott 1988). In this respect, the strategy of professionalism is most clearly understood as a form of 'social closure'. Social closure involves processes of exclusion, usually by means of credentialization supported by state licensing and usurpation, which involve attempts to improve the standing of a subordinate professional group *vis-à-vis* a dominant professional group. Social closure, however, should not be interpreted as a grand conspiracy. Many of these strategies might not be apparent to individuals within a professional grouping who believe and act on principles of altruism and the pursuit of knowledge. Neither should such processes be considered universal or as part of a progressive, continuous development of professional groups. It is important to recognize the social, cultural and historical contingency of professionalism.

HISTORY

The regulatory bargain in Britain

At the beginning of the twentieth century, Britain was a professional society in the sense that the organization of society and its institutions was dominated by the professional classes. This was the culmination of long and often bitter battles between the landed aristocracy and the rising middle classes (Perkin 1989). The rise of medical profession was without doubt central to this process. An understanding of professionalism should therefore be based on macro-historical analysis because the social, cultural and economic contexts within which professions develop influence the form that development takes (Saks 1995). The history of the medical profession in Britain is one of long and sometimes bitter battles to gain monopoly status and to strike a regulatory bargain with the state. This relationship with the State remains the axis on which the development of the medical profession proceeds.

In Britain in the eighteenth century, medicine was practiced by a variety of bonesetters, surgeons, apothecaries, dentists, midwives, herbalists and a host of druggists and so-called 'quacks'. The 'medical profession' was a fragmented rag-tag of interests with as many as 22 licensing bodies. The main divisions were between the apothecaries, honorary physicians and surgeons, and internecine strife was common. Hospitals were mainly voluntary and funded by local subscribers. These subscribers controlled access to hospital services and even had the right to nominate patients to certain hospital beds. In 1815 the Apothecaries Act began a long process of reform. One of the most vocal activists for reform at this time was Thomas Wakeley, surgeon, MP and founder of the Lancet. The reformists were opposed by supporters of *laissez-faire*, who saw any attempt to regulate as an infringement on the workings of 'free individuals to sell their skills in a free market'. Nevertheless, slowly but surely, physicians and surgeons began to wrestle control over admissions to hospital from the subscribers. Control over access to hospital was important because it gave powers of exclusion as well as inclusion.

As the nineteenth century progressed, the categories of patient excluded entry to hospitals were extended to include those with infectious diseases, terminal illness, pregnancy, psychiatric conditions, mental handicap, epilepsy as well as children and elderly people. The medical profession was thus, over time, able to gain sufficient control over hospital access to ensure the patients admitted represented their interests (Abel-Smith 1964). The middle of the century also saw a rapid transformation in the techniques of medicine. A physician at the beginning of the nineteenth century would have practised bedside medicine, treated the patient holistically and relied on crude techniques such as bleeding and purging. By the end of the century, however, the stethoscope, ophthalmoscope and fever thermometer were standard pieces of equipment and hospital medicine had ensured a power base for the profession.

In 1858, after 16 unsuccessful parliamentary Bills and much suspicion from medical practitioners, the Medical Registration Act was passed, thus establishing the General Medical Council and the GMC register. The Act united doctors into a single occupational group and set the foundation for increasing State involvement in health care. Although there was no formal prohibition of practice by the unqualified, the Act conferred an advantage on the emerging medical profession through restricting Poor Law and Friendly Society appointments to GMC registrants. These developments should be placed in the context of a rapidly changing society where the Victorian middle classes were demanding more health care and the mass ranks of the proletarian working class were being exposed to the new health hazards of industrial society.

The British Medical Association (BMA), which represents GPs, had to fight hard to maintain and extend its monopoly powers. For example, in 1896 the BMA secured agreement of medical school deans to discourage students from applying for army posts. This 'boycott' finally won full officer status for doctors in the British Army.

The National Insurance Act of 1911 had support among rank and file doctors because it increased incomes by placing the administration of the previously powerful Friendly Societies in the hands of local health committees that had strong professional representation. However, the Act was not supported by the BMA. Thus changes in the relationship between the profession and the state often exposed tensions within the medical profession.

The development of a nursing profession

In the early voluntary hospitals medical practitioners had domestic servants as their assistants. From the middle of the nineteenth century, the division of labour began to change under influence of reformers like Florence Nightingale, who campaigned for the establishment of nursing schools. Nightingale introduced new forms of discipline and recruited educated women. She emphasized a commitment to care and the role of mediator between the sick and physicians. This ethos, as well as Nightingale's authoritarian methods, produced divisions within nursing that are still evident today. In 1916 the College of Nursing was established, and State registration was instigated in 1918. The professional project for nursing therefore had a trajectory that was heavily reliant on the relationship between nurses and doctors. Today, nurse autonomy is still proscribed and low pay remains endemic. This suggests that the characteristics of professions are not universal, and neither does professionalism develop in predictable or linear ways. Nursing developed in the shadow of medicine (the dominant profession), it lacked a distinctive body of knowledge and the view of nursing as caring and medicine as curing hampered the development of a separate knowledge-base. Nursing also suffered because of weak market status. The presence of nurse auxiliaries, for example, prevented the development of a professional monopoly. It is thus helpful to distinguish between professions that develop within an already established division of labour and dominant professions that are able to influence the form of division of labour itself (Freidson 1970). So, for example, social work and clinical psychology have been able to claim a distinct knowledge-base and work alongside medicine while remaining separate from its division of labour.

The challenge of the welfare state

In 1948 the creation of the NHS, as part of the welfare state, faced considerable resistance by the medical profession. The BMA fought hard to preserve the independent contractor status of general practitioners and consultants fought hard against NHS control of their working conditions. Aneurin Bevan, minister for health in the post-war Labour administration, said of hospital consultants that he got their agreement by 'choking their mouths with gold' (Porter 1997, p 653). The regulative bargain was therefore always an uneasy relationship, and this continues today. In the UK, the profession retained its power within the rigid hierarchical structures of a centralized 'command and control' healthcare system. The role of medical professionals included that of rationing care according to professional definition of clinical need, thus allowing them greater clinical autonomy than their American counterparts.

This status quo came under fire during the 1980s and 1990s as managerial reforms put pressure on the medical profession to change. The introduction of managerialism and internal markets led to calls for more accountability from the medical profession, greater efficiency and greater attention to consumerism.

The dropping of market reforms by the Labour government in the late 1990s did not relieve this pressure. Indeed, the removal of market-based rhetoric might have allowed the State to focus more clearly on increasing central regulation and devolving responsibility. Thus the regulatory bargain shifted during the latter part of the twentieth century as the welfare state evolved into what many have described as a corporatist state.

Comparisons with the USA

The medical profession developed on a different trajectory in the USA. The dominant American ideology of freedom and competition meant that in the first half of the nineteenth century State governments dismantled early attempts to strike a regulatory bargain through licensing. The 'balkanization' of medical practice led to the multiplication of medical schools to meet the growing market for health services and a variety of medical sects were at war with one another throughout the nineteenth century (Starr 1983).

The formation of a strong and more unified medical profession commenced later than in Britain and was heavily dependent on the knowledge-base derived from progress in the techniques of scientific medicine. The Johns Hopkins medical school was founded in 1893 and in 1901 the American Medical Association was reorganized, thus starting the slow exclusion of 'quacks' from the ranks of state licensed medical practice. The Flexner report of 1910 began the process of retrenchment in medical education and led to the closure of large numbers of proprietary medical schools. The American Medical Association, after battling with drugs companies and the federal government, wrested control over dispensation of medicines from pharmacists. Doctors gained control of hospital administration, guided the development of the emerging nursing profession and aggressively usurped the role of midwives. Starr (1983) explains the success of the medical profession in terms of a strategy that involved using doctors in training in the running of hospitals and encouraging professionalism among subservient (mostly women) healthcare workers. This strategy came under threat during the inter-war years as the role of the state and large insurance companies began to expand in the face of economic depression. This trend continued in the post-war years and in 1965 Medicare (health care for social security recipients and the elderly) and Medicaid (healthcare for recipients of public welfare) marked a massive increase in government involvement in healthcare provision. This weakened the profession's hold over the economics of healthcare provision. As corporate medicine began to take hold, physicians moved away from their once prized independent status into group practice, hospital employment and Health Maintenance Organizations (HMOs), thus protecting their incomes and forming bases to protect their collective interests. The capacity of different powerful interest groups to act with and on the medical profession was apparent in the failure of the Clinton healthcare reforms in the 1990s (Skocpol 1997).

The literature on professionalism has been dominated by the Anglo-American experience. The European experience is very different. For example, in France and Germany it is possible to discern the influence of different cultural factors on the ways in which the medical profession developed and practised (Payer 1996). Future comparative studies might change and enhance our understanding and allow us to recognize more clearly that professional development in modern societies is not uniform. This brief historical sketch should, however, give an indication that the relationship between the professions, the state and capital is one that is historically contingent and based on negotiation and conflict.

THEORIES OF PROFESSIONS

In general, therefore, the history of the medical profession has been one of growing power up to the middle of the twentieth century. This power was built around its relationship with the State, social closure and the capacity to dominate other groups. In attempting to explain these developments, sociologists have focused on the concept of professional power.

Professional autonomy and professional dominance

Freidson (1970) drew an important distinction between professional autonomy and professional dominance. He argued that the medical profession's power was based on two interconnected factors: autonomy over one's own work and dominance over the activities of other workers. This approach has been elaborated upon in a model of professional power developed by Elston (1991), which emphasizes the importance of different forms of autonomy in professional formation. These are clinical autonomy, economic autonomy and political autonomy (Box 15.2).

The reach and depth of professional power are dependent on activity in each of these three spheres. In recent years, however, the concern with professional dominance and its effects has been replaced by a focus on the waning of professional power. This sense of decline or a decentring of the medical profession can be related to increasing regulation, a growing concern with quality and accountability and a blurring of boundaries between different professional groups. In other words the intra-professional division of labour is changing. Attempts have been made to try to explain these trends by means of theories of proletarianization and de-professionalization.

Proletarianization

Proletarianization is derived from Marxist interpretations of the professions (Ehrenreich & Ehrenreich 1977, Johnson 1972). From a Marxist viewpoint, professions cannot maintain their autonomy nor be free from wage relationships indefinitely. This is because the logic of capitalism requires that professional classes be reduced to proletarian status. The trend towards incorporating physicians within large corporations in the USA has been cited by some commentators as evidence of proletarianization because this, it is argued, has led to loss of control over work, increasing specialization and rationalization of activity. The development of the physician's assistant is also seen as an example of the way in which the logic of capital strips the medical profession of control over tasks. At its crudest, therefore, the theory of proletarianization sees capital regaining control over the activities of physicians and subordinating them to the needs of capital. Medicine is subsumed under the imperatives of advanced capitalism. Proletarianization of health care can be seen as a tendency for doctors and other healthcare professionals to lose control of a range of work areas. These include the criteria for recruitment to the profession (for example, managerial control over recruitment panels), control over the content of training, control over the terms and content of work, control over the objects of labour (patients), control over the tools of labour (technology and capital equipment) and finally control over the amount and rate of remuneration. The causes of proletarianization have been related to a number of trends in the organization of work under capitalism (Oppenheimer 1973). In particular, the last quarter of the twentieth century witnessed a shift in work relations from those of hierarchical Fordist forms of factory production to post-Fordist flexible working relations and flatter organizational structures.

It is questionable, however, whether such features of proletarianization can be crudely applied to the medical profession. There are a number of clear differences between doctors and proletarianized workers. Doctors still have the power to supervise others. They maintain a range of specialist skills and still have a strong hold over the organization of production. It is simplistic to equate the trend towards wage employment among physicians

---

BOX 15.2   Professional Autonomy

- Clinical autonomy: the capacity of the profession to make independent clinical decisions and monitor its own performance
- Economic autonomy: the capacity to determine enumeration and influence market position
- Political autonomy: the capacity to influence policy

in the USA with proletarianization (Navarro 1988). Two factors need to be kept in mind. In the first place, the capacity of medical elites to manipulate segmentation (the splitting-off of roles and tasks) to their advantage should not be underestimated. In the second place, capitalism is increasingly based around complex networks and information exchange. The logic of information capitalism puts a premium on knowledge and intellectual property and the possession of both maintains class position, privilege, power and status. Thus the credentialized knowledge of the medical profession still maintains power over patients and other healthcare workers. This is so despite the proliferation of free information on the internet. Indeed, it can be argued that rather than threatening professional power, the diffusion of information on risk and health makes additional demands on the profession, members of which are called upon to act as arbitrators of uncertainty who maintain social integration in the face of a new global order (Dingwall 1996).

De-professionalization thesis

The de-professionalization thesis focuses on the medical profession's loss of cultural legitimacy (Haug 1988). Qualities such as professional ethics, monopoly knowledge, authority over clients and autonomy over work are seen to be in decline in the face of public questioning of professional status. The drive towards consumption and client-centred care, better informed clients – what many doctors now refer to as internet-positive patients – are examples of challenges to the cultural legitimacy of medicine captured in the phrase 'the revolt of the client'. The de-professionalization thesis stresses the changes that have occurred in the relationship between doctors and patients. It is argued that the public is increasingly critical of the medical profession and sceptical of medical knowledge. There is also increasing demand for traditional, paternalistic approaches to the lay–professional encounter to be replaced by models of shared decision making, patient involvement and user participation (DoH 1999).

Critics of the de-professionalization thesis argue that it lacks definition and is overdependent on an overstated role for consumerism in health care (Elston 1991). It seems that many things can be referred to as challenges to cultural legitimacy. There is considerable amount of rhetoric around patient empowerment and shared decision making, but increases in rhetoric are not necessarily signs of changes in practice or lay-professional relations.

Contested Domains

Despite the criticisms of proletarianization and de-professionalization, there is broad agreement that medical autonomy and dominance are being challenged. Western healthcare systems are characterized as having increasingly complex organizational structures, increasing rationalization, increasing use of substitution of medical work through employment of other practitioners (nurse/assistants) and increasing hierarchical division within the medical profession. Some have argued that these divisions within medicine strengthen the corporate body of the profession at the expense of some individual doctors or groups of doctors (Freidson 1994). There are divisions, conflicts and tensions both within and between the healthcare professions and these are manifest in inequalities, discrimination and in territorial battles.

Annandale (1998) points out that research on professions has been gender- and race-blind and suggests that increasing stratification within medicine will have disproportionate effects on women and ethnic minority physicians. In the UK, the percentage of medical staff who are women increased from 27% to 34% in the 10 years between 1990 and 2000. In the same period, the proportion of hospital medical consultants who are women grew from 16% to 22%. On the basis of percentages of women doctors in training, it is anticipated that these figures will increase further (DoH 2001b). However, there is still variation in the specialties that employ women at consultant level. For example, the specialty employing the highest percentage of women is paediatrics (38% in 2000) and the lowest is surgery (6% in 2000). These figures do not reveal the continued disparities in pay between men and women doctors. Data for the year 2000 show that the proportion of doctors in all grades who qualified in the UK and reported 'non-white' ethnicity was 17%, whereas the proportion of consultants reporting non-white ethnicity was 9%. There is evidence to suggest that ethnic minority doctors face discrimination at many stages during their careers, from the point of entry to medical schools to applying for senior house officer posts to seeking merit awards (Coker 2001).

The relationship between doctors and nurses has been affected by changes in the old dichotomy of nursing as care and medicine as treatment. The professionalization strategies of nurses have challenged the role boundaries between doctors and nurses as nurses take on prescribing and treatment roles (Weiss & Fitzpatrick 1997). In the UK, the reduction in junior doctors' hours has increased the demand for nurse practitioners to take on some junior doctor roles (Cahill 1996). This has led to calls for the UK to adopt the American physician's assistant model. However, physician's assistants in the USA earn no more than half of what supervisory physicians earn.

The call in the UK for an expanded role for nurses, nurse practitioners, and perhaps even physician's assistants, should be placed in the context of changing labour markets, and in particularly the segmentation of professional work. Healthcare assistants and low-grade staff nurses are arguably shouldering additional responsibility and workloads that went with tasks previously assigned to doctors, without gaining the corresponding autonomy and financial rewards. In the UK, the shift to flexible labour markets and post-Fordist forms of organization has, in the main, affected non-professional groups within health care through processes of contracting-out and competitive tendering. In the USA this has occurred through the exploitation of low benefit, part-time workers. However, in the USA, considerable savings have also been achieved by shifting work form physicians to nurses and physician's assistants (Tilly & Tilly 1998). Segmentation and the development of elites therefore occur between professions and also within professions.

These trends are an illustration of how inter- and intra-professional relations are becoming more complex and that previous analysis of healthcare professions based on boundaries between dominant and other professional groups might be simplistic. As boundaries change and segmentation within professional groups increases, it could lead to the formation of new alliances between elite groups, managerial groups and knowledge-producing groups. These alliances could cut across traditional professional loyalties and allegiances.

These trends highlight another contested domain that has received increasing attention in recent years: the battles for authority between healthcare professions and managers. The enhanced role given to general managers in the NHS from the mid-1980s has been seen by some as a means of reigning in the dominant power of the medical profession (Hunter 1994). It is possible to discern pressures for greater managerial control within the NHS in changes to consultant contracts, GP contracts and devolved budgetary responsibility to Primary Care Trust level. Management of physician activity is more widespread and rigid in the USA through the use of diagnostic related groups (DRG) and clinical review plans. Despite these pressures, physicians can still maintain individual zones of discretion because medicine still has elements of uncertainty and contingency. Patterns of behaviour such as shifting diagnosis, 'DRG creep', and admitting and re-admitting and defensive medicine are common. It is important to remember, therefore, that changes are not wholesale. Doctors still maintain control and discretion in their daily work. However, these developments demand that studies of professions should focus on what work they do, its form and content, its regulation and the relations it reflects with capital and other workers.

Professions, governmentality and the state

In Britain, the medical profession has faced considerable pressure from the State to follow an agenda of quality and efficiency. Examples of this include the setting up of the National Institute for Clinical Excellence (NICE; SIGN in Scotland), the National Clinical Assessment Authority (NCAA) and Commission for Health Improvement (CHI) to monitor service quality and to set national frameworks and guidelines for treatment levels. The GMC's standards of practice GMC (2001) and the emphasis given to revalidation can be seen as an adaptive response to such outside pressures. Doctors still control credentializing and monitor practice standards but they have to fight to maintain this control. In doing so, the rank and file are increasingly subject to surveillance, monitoring and sanctions against unacceptable behaviour, and disciplinary, education and administrative elites maintain and even extend their power.

Regulation of nursing professions in the UK is by the UK Central Council for Nursing Midwifery and Health Visiting (UKCC, the Nursing Midwifery Council (NMC) from April 2002.). The council for Professions Supplementary to Medicine (CPSM) regulates twelve therapy and scientific professions. The UKCC is one of the largest regulatory bodies in the world with more than 634 000 nurses, midwives and health visitors registered. The relationship between the State and these different regulatory bodies is an important feature of the way in which professions maintain their autonomy and status.

Johnson (1996) has drawn on the work of Foucault, to reject the clear distinction between the State on the one hand, and the professions on the other. He argues that modern professions, like medicine, developed in association with the process of what Michel Foucault calls governmentality, in other words, as part of the apparatus of the State. It is through the formal recognition of doctors as experts that they are able to construct and maintain a social reality with universal validity. The point at which this technical autonomy is established is the very same point at which professional practice is indistinguishable from the State. It follows from this analysis that professions become what Johnson terms 'sociotechnical devices' through which the means, and perhaps the ends, of government are expressed. In focusing on the healthcare division of labour, some researchers suggest that the old dichotomy between dominant and non-dominant professions is no longer useful. Rather, professional relationships can be better understood by the concept of 'countervailing powers'. Work relations in health care are characterized as a 'series of moves' between the state, corporations, doctors groups, managers and nurses who engage in phases of harmony, conflict and countervailing actions (Light 1995). This suggests a more complex history of relations between occupational groups, markets and the State. Hanlon (1998) for example, has argued that the redefining of professionalism around commercial issues is a countervailing action in response to loss of trust in social service professionalism. This leads to a cleavage, that cuts across the traditional public sector/private sector divide, perhaps fragmenting what has previously been seen as a homogenous service class. Dingwall (1996) on the other hand emphasizes the State's role in creating market shelters for certain occupational groups. Turning to the problem of trust and uncertainty he argues that successful professions receive state support because they offer ways of managing uncertainty and maintaining social integration in an increasingly uncertain world.

CONCLUSION

It seems that, within health care at least, professionalism is taking on a new hierarchical form with elites exercising authority both in their traditional areas of dominance and over an increasingly emasculated cadre of 'rank and file' (Freidson 1994). In tracking these changes, it is necessary to take account of the nature of the relationship between professions and the State, the status of specialized knowledge, the division of labour and the extent of segmentation within professional groups. In addition, statements concerning changes in professional power and professional roles should be interrogated with respect to four key areas of inquiry. First, the rhetoric of consumerism and lay involvement might not necessarily be accompanied by changes in practice. Second, the linking of changing professional roles to the creation of new institutional forms such as Primary Care Trusts, NICE and new regulatory bodies should not assume either the permanence of these institutional forms or their place in some kind of orderly progression towards better organization of health care. Third, it is important to keep all work relationships (even those of professions) in the context of economic cycles within capitalism. Finally, in the long term we should not underestimate the power of professions to endure, exploit and adapt to new circumstances.

References

Abbott A 1988 The system of professions: an essay on the division of expert labor. University of Chicago Press, Chicago

Abel-Smith B 1964 The hospitals 1800–1948. Heinemann, London

Annandale E 1998 The sociology of health and medicine, a critical introduction. Polity Press, Cambridge

Becker H et al 1961 Boys in white. University of Chicago Press, Chicago

Bristol Royal Infirmary Inquiry 2001 The report of the public inquiry into children's heart surgery at the Bristol Royal Infirmary 1984–1995. Cmnd 5207(1). HMSO, London

Cahill H 1996 Role definition: nurse practitioners or clinician's assistants? British Journal of Nursing 5(22):1382–1386

Carr-Saunders AM, Wilson PA 1933 The professions. Clarendon Press, Oxford

Coker N 2001 Racism in medicine: an agenda for change. King's Fund, London

Department of Health (DoH) 1999 Patient and public involvement in the new NHS. DoH, London

Department of Health (DoH) 2001a Harold Shipman's clinical practice 1974–1998, a clinical audit commissioned by the Chief Medical Officer. DoH, London

Department of Health (DoH) 2001b Hospital, public health medicine and community health services medical and dental staff in England 1990–2000. DoH, London

Dingwall R 1979 The social organization of health visiting. Croom Helm, London

Dingwall R 1996 Professions and social order in a global society. International Sociological Association Working Group 02. Conference, University of Nottingham. Online. Available: http://www.Nottingham.ac.uk/sociology/research/Dingwall.doc

Ehrenreich B, Ehrenreich J 1977 The professional–managerial class. Radical America 2:7–31

Elston MA 1991 The politics of professional power: medicine in a changing health service. In: Gabe J, Kelleher D, Williams G (eds) Challenging medicine. Routledge, London

Freidson E 1970 The profession of medicine, a study of the sociology of applied knowledge. Harper and Row, New York

Freidson E 1994 Professionalism reborn, theory, prophecy and policy. Polity Press, Cambridge

General Medical Council (GMC) 2001 GMC standards of practice. Online. Available: http://www.gmc-uk.org/standards/

Goode WJ 1957 Community within a community. American Sociological Review 22:194–200

Hanlon G 1998 Professionalism as enterprise: service class politics and the redefinition of professionalism. Sociology 32(1):43–63

Haug M 1988 A re-examination of the hypothesis of physician deprofessionalization. Milbank Quarterly 66(2):48–56

HMSO 2002 National Health Service Reform and Health Care Professions Act 2002. HMSO, London

Hunter D 1994 From tribalism to corporatism: the managerial challenge to medical dominance. In: Gabe J, Kelleher D, Williams G (eds) Challenging medicine. Routledge, London

Irvine D 2001 The changing relationship between the public and medical profession. The Lloyd Roberts Lecture, Royal Society of Medicine. Online. Available: http://www.gmc-uk.org/news/lloyd_roberts_lecture.htm

Johnson T 1972 Professions and power. Macmillan, London

Johnson T 1996 Governmentality and the institutionalization of expertise. In: Johnson T, Larkin G, Saks M (eds) Health professions and the state in Europe. Routledge, London

Larson MS 1977 The rise of professionalism: a sociological analysis. University of California Press, Berkeley, CA

Light D 1995 Countervailing powers: a framework for professions in transition. In: Johnson T, Larkin G, Saks M (eds) Health professions and the state in Europe. Routledge, London

MacDonald KM 1995 The sociology of the professions. Sage, London

Navarro V 1988 Professional dominance or proletarianization? Neither. Milbank Quarterly 66(2):57–75

Oppenheimer M 1973 The proletarianization of the professional. Sociological Review Monograph 20:213–227

Payer L 1996 Medicine and culture, varieties of treatment in the United States, England, West Germany, and France. Henry Holt and Company, New York

Perkin H 1989 The rise of professional society, England since 1880. Routledge, London

Porter R 1997 The greatest benefit to mankind, a medical history of humanity from antiquity to the present. Harper Collins, London

Royal Liverpool Children's Inquiry 2001 The report of the Royal Liverpool children's inquiry. HMSO, London

Saks M 1995 Professions and the public interest: medical power, altruism and alternative medicine. Routledge, London

Sinclair S 1997 Making doctors: an institutional apprenticeship. Berg, Oxford

Skocpol T 1997 Boomerang: Clinton's health care reform and the turn against government. WW Norton, New York

Starr P 1983 The social transformation of American medicine. Basic Books, New York

Tilly C, Tilly C 1998 Work under capitalism. West View Press, Oxford

Weiss M, Fitzpatrick R 1997 Challenges to medicine: the case of prescribing. Sociology of Health and Illness 19:297–327

Community Care and Informal Caring

Fiona Stevenson

WHAT IS COMMUNITY CARE?

Community care has been a goal of government policy in the USA, Britain and the rest of Europe since the late 1950s. The overarching aim of a policy of community care is to shift the emphasis of care for dependent groups, such as the elderly, chronically ill, people with learning difficulties and those with disabilities, wherever possible from institutional care to community- or home-based settings.

The term 'community care' is used both in a prescriptive sense to relate to how people should meet the health and social needs of dependent people and also as a description of the set of services that are currently provided.

THE POLITICS OF COMMUNITY CARE

Cowen (1999) suggested that in Britain there was a contrast in the 'spirit of the age' in the period between 1948 and 1978, which he described as the classic welfare state, and the period between 1979 and 1997, which was the period of the new right (or neo-liberal) conservatism. Thus, after the election of the Conservative government in 1979 there was a move from the idea of formal care in the community to an emphasis of care by the community; that is, care by family, relatives, neighbours and friends (informal care) and by voluntary organizations.

On the surface, the ideology of community care appears good and humane, however, when examined at a deeper level the meanings and objectives of community care are associated with confusion and ambiguity. In particular, there is a tension between acting in the interests of vulnerable people in society and the view that successive governments see community care, in particular care by the community with a heavy reliance on the use of informal care, as a way of reducing the financial cost of caring for those who are less able to care for themselves.

249

THE EFFECTS OF COMMUNITY CARE POLICIES

The vast majority of dependant people have always lived outside of institutions, cared for informally at home, usually by family, relatives or friends. In 1986 the Audit Commission investigated the extent to which there had been a change in the balance of care in the previous 15 years, notably the replacement of institutional care by community care. The report concluded that progress had been limited. It suggested that the policies had proved poor value for money in terms of those still in institutions, whereas people in the community might not be getting the support they need (Audit Commission 1986).

Obstacles to the implementation of community care centre on a lack of resources and managerial difficulties. There is also the problem of the coordination between social and health services. The introduction of Primary Care Groups (PCGs) and Primary Care Trusts (PCTs), in April 1999, combining GP and community health services, gives GPs and social services new avenues of cooperation to support carers (Simon 2001). Lewis (1999), however, argued that the continued dominance of general practice in primary care policy might continue to be an obstacle to the integration of community care and primary care. As an initial measure, GPs, members of primary care teams and social services staff were required to have systems in place for identifying carers by April 2000 (DoH 1999). Yet Simon & Kendrick (2001) found that there was a wide variation in the recording of carer status in the notes of carers. They also identified a gap between the expected role envisaged by government and carers' organizations and the actual roles of GPs and district nurses in the support of carers. Simon (2001) provided a list of measures that GPs could take to improve the quality of life of informal carers. This includes measures such as acknowledging the role of carers and providing them with information (Box 16.1).

LEGISLATION

A summary of the key aspects of both legislation and policy documents in relation to carers is presented in Box 16.2.

The NHS and Community Care Act 1990 requires local authority social services and the NHS to work together to prepare, publish and monitor packages of care in concert with other agencies and users. The historical division between health (NHS) and social care (local authorities) has been marked since the inception of the NHS. Collaboration between

---

BOX 16.1   Measures GPs Can Take to Improve The Quality of Life of Informal Carers.

- Acknowledge carers, what they do, and the problems they have
- Flag the notes of informal carers so that in any consultation you are aware of their circumstances
- Treat carers as you would other team members and listen to their opinions
- Include them in discussions about the person they care for
- Give carers a choice about which tasks they are prepared to take upon themselves
- Ask after the health and welfare of the carer as well as the patient
- Provide information about the condition the person the carer is looking after suffers from
- Provide information about being a carer and support available
- Provide information about benefits available
- Provide information about local services available for both the person being cared for and the carer
- Be an advocate for the carer to ensure services and equipment appropriate to the circumstances are provided
- Liaise with other services
- Ensure staff are informed about the needs and problems of informal carers
- Respond quickly and sympathetically to crisis situations

From Simon (2001)

BOX 16.2   Key Aspects of Legislation and Policy Documents in Relation to Carers

NHS and Community Care Act 1990
- Implemented in full in April 1993
- Requires local authority social services and the NHS to work together to prepare, publish and monitor packages of care
- Local authorities also have to involve and consult with users, carers and local organizations
- The active role of the voluntary sector is encouraged

NHS and Community Care Act 1990
- Local authorities have to take the needs of carers into account when undertaking assessments

The Carers (Recognition and Services) Act 1995
- Made the requirement to take the needs of carers into account when undertaking assessments a legal right
- Defines a carer as someone who provided or intends to provide 'a substantial amount of care on a regular basis'
- What is meant by 'substantial' and 'regular' is not defined
- There is no right to services
- Assessments have to be done at the same time as an assessment of the cared for person

Carers and Disabled Children's Act 2000
- Carers have a right to a separate assessment in their own right
- There is a requirement for local authorities to provide services to carers to meet their assessed needs

The report of the Royal Commission on Long Term Care (March 1998)
- Primarily concerned with financing long-term care for elderly people
- Suggested that services to people with a carer should be 'carer blind'
- Recommended the government should consider a national carer support package
- Contained a note of dissent arguing that more emphasis needs to be placed on help for informal carers, in particular the provision of respite care

Caring about Carers: A National Strategy for Carers (1999)
- Carers should receive information, support and care
- A central aspect of the care provision was for short breaks from caring. A special grant of £140 million over 3 years was announced
- Identified the need for flexible working practices from employers
- Identified the need for special help for young carers

health authorities and social services departments is traditionally low as they not only have different organizational structures, but are also based on different ideologies resulting in conflicting perspectives (Cowen 1999). The NHS and Community Care Act also requires local authorities to involve and consult with users, carers and local organizations. Cowen (1999), however, suggested that there has been little advance in real citizenship rights or in the reconfiguring of traditional power relationships in which managers maintain control.

The active role of the voluntary sector, for example the National Association for Mental Health (MIND) and the National Schizophrenic Fellowship (NSF), has been encouraged as a result of the Act and the amount of services they deliver has directly increased. However, Cowen (1999) argued there is a conflict of interests, raising doubts as to the appropriateness of training and the extent to which voluntary agencies should substitute themselves for professional health services.

There has been growing concern expressed for the well-being of carers. The NHS and Community Care Act 1990 requires local authorities to take the needs of carers into account when undertaking assessments. The Carers (Recognition and Services) Act 1995 (Carers Act) made that requirement a legal right. Yet the definition given in the Act of a carer as someone who provided or intended to provide 'a substantial amount of care on a regular basis' is ambiguous. In practice, it is left to the discretion of local authorities to determine what constitutes 'regular' and 'substantial' care (Seddon & Robinson 2001).

Arksey (2002) conducted an analysis tracing the decisions by government, through local authorities and down to individual practitioners to discover how carers' rights under the Carers Act to request an assessment of their ability to care were conceptualized and managed. She showed how carers are filtered out of the assessment process in line with the imperative to remain within budget (Arksey 2002). Moreover, Seddon & Robinson (2001) suggested that separate carer assessments are not an established feature of care management practice and that care managers lack an explicit framework to direct the assessment of carers' needs.

Despite the rhetoric, there were a number of problems with the Carers Act. Under the terms of the Act assessments of carers had to be done at the same time as the cared for person was assessed, if the cared-for person refused an assessment then the carer could not be assessed. Even once assessed there was no right to services under the Carers Act and, crucially, no extra funding was provided to enable assessments to be completed. The right to a separate assessment has since been addressed by the Carers and Disabled Children's Act 2000. This Act contains a requirement for local authorities to provide direct services to carers to meet their assessed needs. However, the Department of Health has indicated that any additional costs are expected to be contained within local authorities' existing allocation (Arksey 2002). Thus it is likely that these potential benefits will not be realized because of pressure on resources.

POLICY DOCUMENTS

In 1999 the government published 'Caring about carers: a national strategy for carers', which contained a package of measures to support carers consisting of three elements: information, support and care. A central aspect of the 'care' provision was for short breaks from caring and a special grant of £140 million over 3 years was announced. The following statement from 'Caring about carers' sums up the approach: 'Helping carers is one of the best ways of helping people to help themselves' (DoH 1999, p 6).

The report of the Royal Commission on Long-term Care, which was established by the government in 1997, published its report in March 1999. The primary concern of the Royal Commission was financing long-term care for elderly people. It suggested that services to people with a carer should be improved and the provision of services should be 'carer blind', thus the existence of a carer should not affect the services provided. It also recommended that the government consider a national carer support package.

The Royal Commission report also contained a note of dissent by two members of the committee. This argued that more emphasis needed to be placed on help for informal carers than was given in the Royal Commission's report, in particular on the provision of respite care. They recommended a budget of £300 million a year to support carers.

The change in terminology from the report published in 1989 entitled 'Caring for people' and the publication of 'Caring about carers' in 1999 demonstrates a shift in government thinking in terms of an increased focus on carers (Pickard 2001). This shift is further illustrated by the inclusion of a question on informal carers for the first time in the 2001 census.

THE IMPLICATIONS OF POLICY DOCUMENTS

Pickard (2001) argued that 'Caring about carers' and the note of dissent draw on two models of carers. On the one hand, they are concerned with the interests of carers *per se*, yet there is also an instrumental concern arising from an interest to ensure that caring continues. The Royal Commission, by contrast, focused on the cared for. Support for the carer is on the grounds of fairness and to relieve carers of the 'burden' of caring by providing support to the person they care for. Thus it is possible, following this model, that informal caring can be at least partially substituted by formal caring. This is a new departure for social policy for carers in the UK and contrasts with the government White Paper 'Growing older', which was published in 1981 and stated that it was the role of public authorities to sustain and where necessary develop, but never to displace, informal care.

Yet, Pickard (2001) pointed out that exclusive focus on the interests of carers might have major drawbacks if this is pursued at the expense of the person being cared for. Thus respite care might prove traumatic for the cared-for person, and therefore also the carer, particularly with regard to mentally alert elderly people who are cared for by their spouse. Thus certain groups might be poorly served by attempts to support carers through increasing access to respite care.

The Royal Commission focused on the interests of the cared-for person on the understanding that such support has advantages for the carer. Aside from concerns about the financial costs of such a policy, it also fails to account for the fact that the cared-for person might want to be cared for by family and friends (McGarry & Arthur 2001). In fact, it raises issues about the proper boundary between family and State care (Pickard 2001).

These two examples – that respite care does not suit everyone and the possible preference for informal care – demonstrate the necessity of considering the effects of proposed schemes on all parties concerned and of recognizing that carers and cared-for people are individuals and therefore their needs and wants are likely to vary.

THE RELATIONSHIP BETWEEN THE FORMAL AND INFORMAL SECTORS

The foundation of community care remains informal care. Services are predominately structured around the dependent rather than the carer and there is confusion over the way the relationship between social care agencies and informal carers should be perceived (Twigg 1989). Twigg (1989) argued that carers occupy an ambiguous position within the social care system. Carers are on the margins of the social care system and not the main focus, therefore concern with carer welfare arguably has something of an instrumental quality to it. Twigg (1989) condensed the relationship between social care agencies and carers into three ideal types: carers as resources, carers as co-workers and carers as co-clients (Box 16.3).

BOX 16.3	Three Models of Carers

1. Carers as resources
   - Represents the 'given', or the taken-for-granted reality against which formal services are structured
   - The informal sector existed prior to and quite separately from formal services
   - Social care agencies, like social services, thus operate, with regard to carers, an essentially residualist model in which the agency responds to the deficiencies of the informal care network
   - The availability of carers remains beyond the influence of agencies.
   - Agencies cannot control or influence carers' decisions about whether or not to take up caregiving.
   - The model places its central focus on the dependant. Although agencies might be concerned to understand caregiving, they are not concerned with the subjective interests of carers
2. Carers as co-workers
   - Agencies work in parallel with the informal sector, aiming at a cooperative and enabling role
   - There are difficulties because of the different normative bases that underpin the formal and informal sectors
   - The model encompasses the carer's interest and the carer's morale within its concerns, but based on what is essentially an instrumental motive
3. Carers as co-clients
   - The general criteria whereby carers do or do not become defined as clients are complex. In practice, the usage tends to be focused on the 'heavy end' of caregiving and on the most heavily stressed individuals
   - Carers' status as clients is never a fully equal one and they remain at best secondary clients rather than fully co-clients
   - The aim is the relief of carer strain

Adapted from Twigg (1989)

Carers can be perceived as resources when social care agencies operate a model in which the agency responds to the deficiencies of the informal care network. Thus the informal sector is perceived as the backdrop to formal provision. In this model, care agencies are not concerned with the welfare of the carers given that they have little control over the supply or activities of informal carers (Twigg 1989).

In the carer as co-worker model, agencies work in parallel with the informal sector, aiming at a cooperative and enabling role. The formal and informal sectors are interdependent (Qureshi & Walker 1986) and complementary (Bulmer 1987). There are, however, crucial differences between the two systems that mean that they do not mesh easily or happily together (Bulmer 1987, Twigg 1989). The co-worker model encompasses the carer's interest and the carer's morale within its concerns but, based on what is essentially an instrumental motive for maintaining high carer morale and involvement, it represents an intermediate outcome on the way to the final outcome of increased welfare for the dependent person.

In the carer as co-client model, the general criteria whereby carers do or do not become defined as clients are complex. In practice, this model tends to be focused on the 'heavy end' of caregiving and on the most heavily stressed individuals. Even here, however, carer status as client is never a fully equal one, and carers remain at best secondary clients rather than fully co-clients. The aim is the relief of carer strain.

Interaction between the formal and the informal sectors therefore varies according to which model is adopted. In the carer as resources model, agencies have no obligation towards the informal sector. In the carer as co-worker model, agencies relate more actively to the informal sector but in an essentially instrumental way. In the model of carers as co-clients, carers become fully integrated into the concerns of the agency (Twigg 1989). In terms of how legislation operates, financial constraints means it is mainly in terms of carers as resources. Policy introduced in the 1990s such as 'Caring about carers' and the note of dissent to the report of the Royal Commission on Long-term Care present a move towards carer as co-worker, while the Royal Commission report itself advocates a model of carer as co-client. However, although there has been an increased focus on carers, change has not been seen in the mainstream services that all the evidence suggests supports carers best (Parker 2002).

THE PROVISION OF CARE

Who cares?

The numbers of people over 16 providing informal care are shown in Box 16.4.

Informal caring rests on personal ties, those of kinship, friendship and neighbourliness (Bulmer 1987). However, all of these have their constraints.

Rhodes & Shaw (1999) underlined the importance of stable communities, strong social networks and local kinship networks, including both immediate and extended kin, for the provision of informal care. Underlying this was the importance of a stable employment base, both in terms of individuals' ability to care and in sustaining the community networks

BOX 16.4	Informal Carers

A series of questions was included in the 1995 General Household Survey to identify people looking after a sick, handicapped or elderly person. The main aim of the questions was to provide national estimates of the number of people who were providing informal care (Rowlands 1998). The data were collected only from people over 16 years of age:

- One in eight (13%) was providing informal care and one in 6 households (17%) contained a carer. Four per cent of adults cared for someone living with them and 8% looked after people living elsewhere. This equates to about 5.7 million carers overall in Great Britain, with about 1.9 million caring for a dependant for someone in the same household. Four percent of adults in Great Britain (about 1.7 million people) devoted at least 20 hours per week to caring and 8% (about 3.7 million people) carried the main responsibility for looking after someone
- Five percent of adults looked after parents and 3% cared for friends and neighbours
- The peak age for caring was 45–64
- Nine out of ten carers looked after someone related to them; four out of ten cared for parents or parents-in-law and two out of ten looked after a spouse
- Among carers with a dependant in their own household, just under 60% helped with personal care. Carers caring for people in other households were far less likely to provide help with personal care
- Of carers devoting at least 20 hours a week to caring; over 60% were women; three-quarters were aged 45 and over and seven out of ten shared their home with their dependant
- Over one-third of all carers reported that no one else helped them look after their dependants. Women were more likely than men to be caring unaided whereas men were more likely to be 'non-main carers'
- Fifty nine percent of all carers had main dependants who did not receive regular visits from health, social or voluntary services. Dependants who lived with their carers were much less likely to receive regular visits from service providers than those who lived in other households

From Rowlands (1998).

and resources on which they can draw. They discussed the implications of the move away from a stable industrial base towards a more flexible and uncertain employment market. This, together with a mobile society and the increasingly transitory and changing nature of local networks and relationships, raises worrying questions about patterns of informal caring in the future (Qureshi & Walker 1986, Rhodes & Shaw 1999,). Yet the vast majority of elderly people care for themselves entirely without help or only minimal support. It is only the 'old' who begin to decline in terms of self care (Qureshi & Walker 1986). Concern has also been voiced about the adverse effect on informal caring of married women's increasing involvement in the labour market, this has been countered by Hirst (2001), who suggested that if having a job increases mobility and other resources then it might enable informal care to be carried out 'at a distance'.

Friends and neighbours can also provide informal caring. Caring can be problematic in friendship because the notion of equivalency tends to be built into the relationship, with a parity of contribution that can be difficult to maintain in a caring relationship (Bulmer 1987). The support offered by neighbours is likely to be general support and social contact rather than more involved care.

Finally, some people have no personal ties and therefore have no access to informal care (Bulmer 1987), thus forcing reliance on formal care from the social services.

Why people care

Proctor et al (2001) conducted a study aimed to provide an in-depth understanding of the process of hospital discharge. They suggested that where the experience of illness is new both the patient and the family members might not have understood the implication of the illness for the carer role. In established illness, family members or the patient might not acknowledge, or be in a position to comply with, the obligations commonly associated with the role of informal carer. Only 11 out of 30 patients in their study at risk of an unsuccessful discharge were willing or able to name an informal carer. Thus carers became defined by the social context of the situation, rather than through personal choice. Having been defined as a carer by either the patient or the professionals, it was then morally difficult for individuals, either professionals or carers, to challenge the obligations associated with the role. When the carers did not conform to professional expectations, they sensed that professionals questioned their moral integrity, thus creating a highly coercive environment within which care was given and received.

People become carers by force of circumstance, a sense of family obligation or as a return for past care and support (Rhodes & Shaw 1999). McGarry & Arthur (2001) reported that some carers saw the support of family members as part of their duty and an expected obligation. Moreover, practical help from the family was preferred to help from formal services, which was perceived as help from 'strangers'.

Finch & Mason (1997) explored people's perceptions of care giving and reported that most people perceive that children should step in and offer assistance, yet there is less broad agreement about what people should actually do. The views expressed as to the type of help that should be offered did not always follow gender stereotypes but there were some normative judgements, for example that sons should provide money and that daughters should care for elderly women (Finch & Mason 1997). Although a poor relationship was not seen as a reason for not offering help, the needs of the younger generation were generally seen to take precedence over those of the older generation. Thus the offer of help was not perceived to be unconditional. The relationship between parents and children is founded on a sense of obligation but one that recognises definite limits. There is no clear consensus as to what it is reasonable to expect, there are, however, well understood principles (Finch & Mason 1997).

Caring can be a source of satisfaction and add a positive and valued dimension to carers' lives (Arber & Ginn 1992). However, care by families can also be problematic because of the generally unequal gender division of caring responsibilities and the past history of the relationship (Qureshi & Walker 1986).

What is a carer?

Arksey (2002) pointed to the reluctance of people to identify themselves as carers, instead seeing themselves as spouses, sons or daughters whose care work reflects marriage vows, family obligations and duty. Rose & Bruce (1995) argued that the term 'care' is rescued from the language of work and reclaimed by spouse carers as 'natural'. Thus, among elderly people caring for spouses the longevity and quality of the relationship prior to the onset of caring means that the boundaries are blurred between caring as part of a close relationship and caring as a more formal role (McGarry & Arthur 2001).

Using data from the 1980 General Household Survey, Arber & Gilbert (1989) described the change in the relationship between couples that were over 65 as moving from reciprocity to dependency. The trend is similar in adult children living with their parents. The transition, they argued, is perceived to be natural. They contrasted the situation with that in which an elderly person moves in with married relations, where there is not the same drift into care.

Caring within a marital relationship can mean that both partners still wish to contribute. Rose & Bruce (1995) provided examples in which the cared-for person performed tasks, such as peeling potatoes or repotting plants, that meant more work for the carer in terms of setting the task up and clearing away afterwards but was important in maintaining at least a show of reciprocity in the relationship. Thus caring and the tasks associated with it have to be seen within the context of the relationship within which they occur. Interestingly, Rose & Bruce (1995) also provided examples to demonstrate how, even when the cared-for person is very dependent, he or she might still have ways of exerting influence.

The idea that elderly people are a care burden not only fails to take account of the fact that most elderly people do not require caring for, it also denies the amount of support that older generations provide for younger, for example in terms of childcare. Thus there is also reciprocity in patterns of intergenerational caring (Martin Matthews & Campbell 1995). Given this reciprocity, it is important not to ignore the experiences of those who receive care; denial of reciprocity in the caring relationship can make caring oppressive (Orme 2001).

Thomas et al (2002) reported how reciprocity and co-dependency between people with cancer and their carers changed in the context of illness. There was greater reciprocity at earlier critical moments in the cancer journey, but greater dependency during periods when patients were undergoing active treatments or were at the palliative care phase.

Caring is not organized along dichotomous lines, for example the carer and the cared for, or women care and men don't (Orme 2001). Thus, in Thomas et al's (2002) study of the care given by informal carers in cancer contexts, 35% of the carers surveyed had a long-standing illness or disability of their own.

Morris & Thomas (2001) suggested that 'carerhood' is a process, rather than a fixed state, and one in which competing needs vie for recognition. Caring cannot necessarily be broken down into a series of identifiable tasks (Martin Matthews & Campbell 1995). Moreover, it can be unpredictable, which makes it hard to manage, particularly for those with other responsibilities such as childcare and employment.

Caring can consist of emotional but not physical support. Thus Thomas et al (2002) divided care into care work and emotion work. Their data suggested that the management of emotions is a crucial aspect of what informal carers do in cancer contexts. They discussed how carers, particularly in spousal relationships, managed the patient's emotions through taking on the illness mantle and symbolically sharing the illness.

Carers put the needs and interests of those they care for above their own and therefore are only likely to take up support services aimed at carers if they feel that these do not divert resources and attention away from those for whom they care (McGarry & Arthur 2001, Morris & Thomas 2001, Thomas et al 2002). Thus, even if services are offered to carers it might be necessary to reassure carers that their needs are legitimate before these services will be taken up.

The needs of carers

Carers are individual people and their responses to caring situations and their needs will vary. Thus, for example, in conditions that affect cognitive function, spouse carers might be mourning the loss of their partner as they have known them as well as coping with physically caring for them, and in such a situation could need psychological support (Addington-Hall et al 1998). Addington-Hall et al's (1998) study concerned the quality of care received in the last years of life by stroke patients, including informal care. They concluded that there was a need for improved support for informal carers, especially for spouses and for those caring for people who are depressed or anxious. They do, however, point out that the data on which the study was based were collected before the implementation of the National Health and Community Care Act (HMSO 1990).

A more recently published study also reported the significant unmet needs of carers. The focus here was a wide range of cancer patients. Needs clustered around aspects of managing daily life, emotions and social identity. Over one in four carers (28%) had three or more significant unmet needs (Soothill et al 2001). Carers with significant unmet needs were more likely to be those where the relationship to the patient was not that of partner or spouse, where the carer had other caring responsibilities, and where the carer did not have friends or relations to call upon for help. They were also likely to be in poor health themselves and caring for a patient who was in the palliative only stage (Soothill et al 2001). Thus those who are already socially disadvantaged are less likely to have all their important needs met. These studies suggest carers have unmet needs despite legislation and government policy focusing on carers.

The general implications of caring

Hubert (1997) examined the lives of carers of young adults with challenging behaviour. She discussed how, by keeping these young adults in the community, families as a whole, but mothers in particular, can become cut-off from the community, leading to social isolation. Thus care in the community can lead to isolation from the community.

Paid employment can have important social and psychological benefits (Glendinning 1992). However, care-giving can have an effect on paid employment. This needs to be taken into account in assessing the overall 'costs' of community care policies (Glendinning 1992). Combining care-giving and paid work is the rule rather than the exception; 49% of carers in Great Britain are working, either full or part time. A further 26% are retired (DoH 1999). Of those carers who are working full time, nearly 20% provide care for more than 20 hours a week and 4% of carers in full-time work also provide care for over 50 hours a week (DoH 1999). Yet among married women – the group most likely to be caring – were those who were economically inactive, followed by those working part-time (Rowlands 1998). It is unclear whether the employment situation is an effect of their situation of providing care, or whether their caring responsibilities are liable, at least in part, for their restricted participation in the labour market.

The mothers of severely disabled young people are half as likely as their counterparts in the general population to be in paid work. Yet mothers with responsibility for a less than severely disabled young person are just as likely to be working as mothers in the general population. Moreover, when mothers do go out to paid work the severity of their son or daughter's condition makes no difference to the kind of job they do and the number of hours they work (Hirst 1992).

There might be economic consequences of constraints on carers' employment at a time when resources are likely to be required for costs such as additional heating. Moreover, caring is likely to have an adverse effect on actual and future employment opportunities and pension provision. These constraints can be substantial and far reaching, although they vary according to factors such as the carer's age, gender, marital status, occupation and amount of time spent caring. The potential long-term effects of a period of restricted labour market participation or withdrawal because of care commitments are of concern because this is likely to occur at a later stage in the lifecycle when there could be greater loss of seniority and less time to 'catch up' before retirement (Glendinning 1992). Glendinning (1992) argued that there is a need for opportunities to work part time or share a job without loss of responsibility, seniority or rate of pay. There is also a need for flexibility; this need for flexibility in the workplace and for offering unpaid leave for family emergencies has been taken up in 'Caring about carers' (DoH 1999).

Both men and women experience workplace and personal costs associated with involvement in the caring role, but gender differences are apparent. Martin Matthews & Campbell (1995) found that when employment and the provision of personal care were combined, both men and women were significantly more likely to experience job effects, career costs and personal costs than their peers without informal caring responsibilities or those only providing instrumental care. Yet women providing personal care experienced more effects than men.

Informal caring varies according to gender, social class, ethnicity and age, all of which affect the likelihood both of caring and of receiving support from the formal sector.

The specific implications of gender for caring

Women figure strongly as both clients and carers (Cowen 1999). Elderly women have more physical impairments and undergo more severe cognitive impairment above the age of 80. Twice as many women over 80 are 'severely' disabled and hence more likely to need both informal and formal caring (Cowen 1999). Both formal (Peace 1986), including work as paid volunteers (Cowen 1999), and informal service provision is dominated by women (Box 16.5).

BOX 16.5   Women as Carers

- Women were more likely to be carers than men, 14% compared to 11%. However as there are more men than women in the total adult population that equates to 3.3 million women compared to 2.4 million men.
- Women were more likely to look after someone outside of the home (10% of women and 7% of men)
- Women were more likely to carry the main responsibility for caring (9% of women and 6% of men)

From Rowlands (1998)

Cowen (1999) argued that community care policies are formulated on the basis that women's caring will automatically support formal caring. Care has traditionally been viewed as coming from the nuclear family, although this has been challenged both by feminists in terms of an assumption of the 'natural' caring role of women and by those who present the reality of who does the caring.

Many of the stresses and strains, or economic costs associated with caring remain unaccounted for. Relatives act as the main carers in a largely unpaid capacity and much of this care is carried out by women in highly stressful situations. These women frequently lack 'know how' and do not have adequate financial support (Cowen 1999). Feminist arguments in particular have focused on the effects on women's physical, and psychological health but also on their long-term employment prospects and future pensions.

Invalid Care Allowance for carers was introduced in 1974 but married women were excluded from receiving the benefit. Campaigning by feminists altered this ruling and married women have been able to claim Invalid Care Allowance since 1986. Yet the focus on getting this allowance might in fact have secured women's place as tied to caring, further entrenching a traditional caring role for women (Annandale 1998). It has been argued that, unlike other issues, there is a general consensus among feminists that community care is resourced through women's unpaid labour, and this consensus is reflected both in empirical studies and theoretical papers (Graham 1997). The arguments have not moved on and continue to present women carers and those they care for as homogeneous. There is a failure to consider the differences and divisions among women, thus masking 'race' and class, sexuality and disability and ignoring the perspective of the cared for (Graham 1997).

Caring by men and women might be perceived differently. Thus what is perceived as admirable in a man might be perceived as the natural duty of a woman (Rose & Bruce 1995). Caring responsibilities might be allocated by default or lack of power or resources, thus men are more able to resist the caring role (Martin Matthews & Campbell 1995). Annandale (1998), however, provides a caution about focusing just on women's experience and the idea that it is *a priori* different to the experience of men, suggesting that this could unintentionally reinforce the idea that caring is women's work. Orme (2001) stressed that a focus on the difference between men and women might have negative consequences for both. Arguably, there should be a focus on the similarities between men and women in terms of caring, rather than on the differences (Fisher 1997).

The focus on women has meant that the role of male carers, particularly as spouse carers, has been ignored. Among older people, traditional gender roles are no longer important, with tasks divided according to ability (McGarry & Arthur 2001, Rose & Bruce 1995). Interestingly, the balance of power within the relationship might remain as before (McGarry & Arthur 2001).

Men participate in caring more than was previously believed (Arber & Gilbert 1989). An analysis of Canadian statistics of informal caring found little gender difference in the amount of informal caring between men and women but that women provided more personal care whereas men provided more instrumental care. Thus the conceptualization of caregiving has a direct influence on the estimate of gender differences in the provision of informal care. The broader the definition the more likely men are to be involved in informal care giving (Martin Matthews & Campbell 1995).

Arber & Gilbert (1989) investigated gender difference in the amount of support carers received. They found that if the level of disability is controlled for then the major source of variation in the amount of support received from formal services was by type of household. People who lived alone received the most from the formal services, people living with a spouse or other elderly person received more formal support than those living with a younger married couple. Those living with a younger married couple received the least support, although they might need support due to pressures such as young children and employment.

Male carers in most households received more help from informal carers than women, although the difference was very small for elderly married couples. Unmarried male carers received slightly more support than unmarried women carers and the least help from informal carers was found when care was provided by a younger married couple (Arber & Gilbert 1989).

Bywaters & Harris (1998) argued that gender inequality in the provision of services might have improved following the fundamental recasting of community care policy culminating in the NHS and Community Care Act 1990. They also argued that social work education has placed significant emphasis on anti-discriminatory practice, which might be expected to have had some impact on the attitudes and behaviour of practitioners carrying out needs assessments. Their study compared the support services that were offered to male clients with female spousal carers and those allocated to female clients with male spousal carers. The assumption that older male clients with female carers would receive less support was supported by their data.

It has been argued that there is an assumption that women will undertake a caring role as part of informal care. However, although more women than men are informal carers and women are more involved in personal care, many factors, such as marital status, the nature of their sibling network and social class, intersected with gender to determine the likelihood of taking on the role of carer (Martin Matthews & Campbell 1995).

The specific implications of social class for caring

The effects of social class are overarching, compounding the difficulties experienced by certain groups in need of community care (Cowen 1999)

Class inequality in informal care reflects the socially structured nature of ill health in British society, because the greatest ill health and disability is suffered by those on the lowest rungs of the class ladder. These families face the greatest burden of providing care, while at the same time possessing fewer material, financial and cultural resources to ease their caring burden (Arber & Ginn 1992).

The need for informal care is not fixed but conditioned by factors that are intimately bound-up with class (Arber & Ginn 1992). The possession of material, financial and cultural resources reduces a physically impaired person's need to rely on informal carers (Arber & Ginn 1992). Moreover, Thomas et al (2002) also found that a carer's material and relational social circumstances had an important bearing on his or her capacity to take on greater quantities of care work.

The poorer health status of the working class results in working-class women being disproportionately disadvantaged by the burdens of informal care provision compared to middle-class women (Arber & Ginn 1992). A higher proportion of lower-working-class than middle-class mothers have to contend with the caring needs of a chronically sick or disabled child. In adulthood, the poorer health of semi-skilled and unskilled men requires correspondingly greater care, generally provided by their wives (Parker 1989 cited in Arber & Ginn 1992). The difference in timing of the need for this care, with middle-class women more likely to be caring in their 60s and working class women caring in their 40s can have profound implications for the development or re-establishment of women's careers (Arber & Ginn 1992).

Informal carers as a whole are drawn equally from all classes, however if co-resident and extra-resident care are examined separately then significant and opposing class differences emerge. Working-class families are more likely than middle-class families to provide care to an impaired or elderly person in the same household. Co-resident care is more time-intensive than extra-resident care and is more likely to constrain the life of a caregiver (Arber & Ginn 1992). Working-class people, however, have fewer financial and material resources (e.g. car ownership) and this increases their likelihood of being a co-resident carer. Moreover, fewer resources also mean less space and less opportunity to manage caring in a way that suits both the carer and the cared-for person (Arber & Ginn 1992).

Arber & Ginn (1992) argued that as the market becomes a more important mechanism in the provision of residential and social care, class could become a key determinant in access to formal private care services, with correspondingly greater burdens of informal care falling on the lower social classes.

Finally class and gender interact, with a stronger class gradient in caring for men than for women. Higher-middle-class men are the least likely to be co-resident carers, whereas semi-skilled and unskilled men are as likely as women in these classes to be co-resident carers (Arber & Ginn 1992).

The specific implications of ethnicity for caring

Gunaratnam (1997) suggested that the literature about caring is ethnocentric, with little information about how ethnicity can shape a caring relationship. Shaky assumptions are adopted about extended family networks supporting elderly and disabled people (Cowen 1999, Gunaratnam 1997). There is variation between the experiences of different ethnic groups as well as within groups. Experiences are affected by class, migration history, gender and the disability of the person needing care (Gunaratnam 1997). Thus there is a need to explore the nature and meaning of care within individual black and ethnic minority communities.

Black and Asian carers figure among the least supported. Diminishing overall family size in Asian communities exacerbates the situation (Cowen 1999). Family care is still strong in British Jewish communities, whereas occupational and social mobility means the Chinese extended family is diminishing in importance (Cowen 1999). The absence of family networks has shaped the domestic lives and health experiences of many black women in Britain (Graham 1997). Family networks govern access to care within the community, yet such resources are not universally available. Poor employment prospects and tightening immigration controls leave many black elders without access to kin (Graham 1997). Although there are voluntary organizations aimed at specific minority communities, not only does family care vary but so does the capacity of such organizations to support family care (Cowen 1999).

Minority ethnic groups experience exclusion from quality public services and community care, regardless of the introduction of anti-racist legislation and the promulgation of anti-racist charters. This might be because of a fear of uncovering demand in an already stretched service (Gunaratnam 1997). Take-up of formal services is low because of a lack of knowledge about services, affected by the inability of some elders to speak English and compounded by illiteracy in their own language (Gunaratnam 1997). There are also insensitivities that alienate minority ethnic elders, for example a lack of dietary awareness, a lack of interpreters and under representation of minority staff within formal services. Crucially, there might also be unfamiliarity among ethnic minority communities with both the word and concept 'carer' (Gunaratnam 1997).

Low social class and poverty are associated with restricted access to informal sources of help, while much formal care is performed by working-class and ethnic-minority groups (Graham 1997). The wider social and economic position of minority communities in terms of class, gender, poverty and racism within employment can interact with ethnic identity to shape the needs of minority carers (Gunaratnam 1997).

The specific implications of age for caring

Thirteen percent of people over the age of 65 provide some form of informal care (Rowlands 1998). Increasing longevity and demographic changes, combined with the continued emphasis on community care, means there will be greater numbers of older people both giving and receiving care (McGarry & Arthur 2001). Far from being a burden on service resources, older people provide a substantial amount of informal care, often alone and with very little formal support (McGarry & Arthur 2001). Of older people in Britain who had help with domestic tasks, 80% relied exclusively on informal help, 10% on both informal and formal sources and 10% exclusively on formal services (Pickard 2001). Hirst's (2001) secondary analysis of the British Household Panel Survey confirmed that spouse care increased more than any other caring relationship during the 1990s, more so for men than for women. As male life expectancy increases, men are now more likely to survive to an age when their spouse or partner needs informal care. By the end of the 1990s, as many men as women were spouse carers.

Many older people meet the demands of being a carer alongside managing their own health difficulties. McGarry & Arthur (2001), in their study of the experiences of informal carers who were aged 75 and over, found that both carers and care recipients were aware of the precarious nature of the relationship. A change in circumstances for either the carer or the care recipient could force the intricate nature of the relationship to collapse.

At the other end of the age continuum, the contributions of children to caregiving have been relatively under-researched (Fox 1998). Fox (1998) reported that children are involved in a range of care activities and often there is a strong emotional component to this caregiving. It has been suggested (DoH 1999) that there are between 20 000 and 50 000 young carers (aged under 18) and that many of these young people receive no support at all from statutory or voluntary services. Fox (1998) suggested that there is a need to acknowledge the practical contribution to informal care that young people are making within the private spaces of family life. The policy document 'Caring about carers' (DoH 1999) contained a chapter on young carers and proposed measures to ensure that these carers receive both recognition and support.

CONCLUSIONS

This chapter has focused on informal care, however, as has been demonstrated, neither care nor informal care are necessarily clear cut and easy to define. There is a blurring of the notion of carer as people 'drift into care', particularly spousal care. The dominance of women in both formal and informal care can also serve to blur the distinction between the two, particularly as formal carers can develop a more personalized relationship with individual clients (Qureshi & Walker 1986). Moreover, the increase in medical technologies that can be administered at home means private space is violated as the home becomes more like the hospital (Kirk & Glendinning 1998, Rhodes & Shaw 1999) also blurring the distinction between formal and informal care.

There is a rhetoric about carers that has yet to be fulfilled. Legislation has provided carers with the right to an independent assessment of their needs. However, the legislation has not been accompanied by additional resources and therefore it is unlikely that assessments for carers will receive priority within a system that is already financially stretched. Resources have been made available for respite care, on the basis that this was effective for carers of people with Alzheimer's and related disorders. Yet caring situations are individual and this might not be the most appropriate way of supporting all carers, particular for people caring for their spouse. It can be argued that the recent policy initiatives are instrumental because they support carers to ensure that they continue to care thus reducing the burden on formal services. Therefore, although the ideology behind policy initiatives appears good and humane they can also be seen as a way of controlling the financial costs of caring for the formal sector, at the expense of informal carers.

References

Addington-Hall J et al 1998 Community care for stroke patients in the last year of life: results of a national retrospective survey of surviving family, friends and officials. Health and Social Care in the Community 6:112–119

Annandale E 1998 The sociology of health and medicine. Polity Press, Cambridge

Arber S, Gilbert N 1989 Men: the forgotten carers. Sociology 23:111–118

Arber S, Ginn J 1992 Research note. Class and caring: a forgotten dimension. Sociology 26:619–634

Arksey H 2002 Rationed care: assessing the service needs of informal carers in English social services authorities. Journal of Social Policy 31:81–101

Audit Commission 1986 Making a reality of community care. HMSO, London

Bulmer M 1987 The social basis of community care. Allen and Unwin, London

Bywaters P, Harris A 1998 Supporting carers: is practice still sexist? Health and Social Care in the Community 6:458–463

Cowen H 1999 Community care, ideology and social policy. Prentice Hall, London

Department of Health (DoH) 1999 Caring about carers: a national strategy for carers. Department of Health, London

Finch J, Mason J 1997 Filial obligations and kin support for elderly people. In: Bornat J et al (eds) Community care: a reader, 2nd edn. Open University, Basingstoke

Fisher M 1997 Older male carers and community care In: Bornat J et al (eds) Community care: a reader, 2nd edn. Open University, Basingstoke

Fox NJ 1998 The contribution of children to informal care: a Delphi study. Health and Social Care in the Community 6:204–208

Glendinning C 1992 Employment and 'community care': policies for the 1990's. Work Employment and Society 6:103–111

Graham H 1997 Feminist perspective on caring. In: Bornat J et al (eds) Community care: a reader, 2nd edn. Open University, Basingstoke

Gunaratnam Y 1997 Breaking the silence: black and ethnic minority carers and service provision. In: Bornat J et al (eds) Community care: a reader, 2nd edn. Open University, Basingstoke

Hirst M 1992 Employment patterns of mothers with a disabled young person. Work Employment and Society 6:87–101

Hirst M 2001 Trends in informal care in Great Britain during the 1990's. Health and Social Care in the Community 9:348–357

HMSO 1990 National Health and Community Care Act. HMSO, London

Hubert J 1997 At home and alone: families and young adults with challenging behaviour. In: Bornat J et al (eds) Community care: a reader, 2nd edn. Open University, Basingstoke

Kirk S, Glendinning C 1998 Trends in community care and patient participation: implications for the roles of informal carers and community nurses in the United Kingdom. Journal of Advanced Nursing 28:370–381

Lewis J 1999 The concepts of community care and primary care in the UK: the 1960's to the 1990's. Health and Social Care in the Community 7:333–341

McGarry J, Arthur A 2001 Informal caring in late life: a qualitative study of the experiences of older carers. Journal of Advanced Nursing 33:182–189

Martin Matthews A, Campbell L 1995 Gender roles, employment and informal care. In: Arber S, Ginn J (eds) Connecting gender and ageing. Open University Press, Buckingham

Morris SM, Thomas C 2001 The carer's place in the cancer situation: where does the carer stand in the medical setting? European Journal of Cancer Care 10:87–95

Orme J 2001 Gender and community care. Palgrave, Basingstoke

263

Parker G 2002 Guest editorial: 10 years of the 'new' community care: good in parts? Health and Social Care in the Community 10:1–5

Peace S 1986 The forgotten female: social policy and older women. In: Phillipson C, Walker A (eds) Ageing and social policy. Gower, Aldershot

Pickard L 2001 Carer break or carer-blind? Policies for informal carers in the UK. Social Policy and Administration 35:441–458

Proctor S et al 2001 Going home from hospital: the carer/patient dyad. Journal of Advanced Nursing 35:206–217

Qureshi H, Walker A 1986 Caring for elderly people: the family and the state. In: Phillipson C, Walker A (eds) Ageing and social policy. Gower, Aldershot

Rhodes P, Shaw S 1999 Informal care and terminal illness. Health and Social Care in the Community 7:39–50

Rose H, Bruce E 1995 Mutual care but differential esteem: caring between older couples. In: Arber S, Ginn J (eds) Connecting gender and ageing. Open University Press, Buckingham

Rowlands O 1998 Informal carers. Results of an independent study carried out on behalf of the Department of Health as part of the 1995 General Household Survey. Office of National Statistics, London

Seddon D, Robinson CA 2001 Carers of older people with dementia: assessment and the Carers Act. Health and Social Care in the Community 9:151–158

Simon C 2001 Informal carers and the primary care team. British Journal of General Practice 51:920–923

Simon C, Kendrick T 2001 Informal carers – the role of general practitioners and district nurses. British Journal of General Practice 51:655–657

Soothill K et al 2001 Informal carers of cancer patients: what are their unmet psychological needs? Health and Social Care in the Community 9:464–475

Thomas C, Morris SM, Harman JC 2002 Companions through cancer: the care given by informal carers in cancer contexts. Social Science and Medicine 54:529–544

Twigg J 1989 Models of carers: how do social care agencies conceptualise their relationship with informal carers? Journal of Social Policy 18:53–66

CHAPTER 7

Health Promotion and the New Public Health

Ian Rees Jones

This chapter describes the evolution of health promotion and the new public health. Different approaches to and models of health promotion will be discussed. The chapter will trace the historical development of health promotion. In doing so, a distinction will be drawn between early attempts at health education and the later development of the new public health and community development based on notions of citizen empowerment. Evidence for preventative interventions will be considered alongside debates on evaluation of health promotion and public policy. Finally, sociological critiques of health promotion and the new public health will be considered.

HEALTH PROMOTION: APPROACHES, PHILOSOPHY AND MODELS

During the early 1970s, western governments experienced what is now referred to as a crisis of welfare. The rising cost of welfare systems, coupled with the devastating fiscal pressures brought about by the oil shock, precipitated calls for controlling government spending. Health care was not immune to these demands. These changes occurred at a time when there was an increasing criticism of the role and effectiveness of medical services: in 1959, Rene Dubos (1959) emphasized the importance of the constraints that modern life and medical science placed on human adaptation. Later, Archie Cochrane (1972) argued that medical care was often ineffective and based on traditional practices rather than on evidence of effectiveness. Ivan Illich (1977) emphasized what he saw as the harmful effects of medicine. This view stressed the role of the medical industrial complex in maintaining a sick society and the colonization of wider world problems with medical viewpoints and medical solutions. A further criticism came from Thomas McKeown (1979), who argued, from an epidemiological standpoint, that improvements in life expectancy could be better related to improvements in standards of living rather than medical science. These criticisms had a profound influence over understandings of health and illness and were part of a growing movement that emphasized the importance of non-medical interventions and prevention.

Definitions of and approaches to health promotion

Health promotion has been defined as:

> Any combination of health education and related organisational, political and economic intervention designed to facilitate behavioural and environmental adaptations which will improve or protect health (Anderson 1983, p 11)

In this sense, health promotion is often presented as an advance on the narrow concerns of health education (Tones 1996). It comprises prevention, health education and public health policy. Prevention is a cornerstone of health promotion because many risk factors associated with disease, such as smoking, are alterable. Thus, it is thought that attempts can be made to reduce or eliminate one or more risk factor to bring about a corresponding reduction in the social and economic burden of illness.

Traditional approaches to prevention are based on interventions at three levels: primary, secondary and tertiary prevention:

- Primary prevention: seeks to prevent the onset of disease, examples include immunization, industrial safety legislation and fluoridation of drinking water.

- Secondary prevention: consists of the early detection and treatment of disease or states likely to lead to disease, examples include screening for diseases such as breast cancer, human immunodeficiency virus (HIV) infection, tuberculosis, or screening for major risk factors such as high blood pressure and cholesterol levels.

- Tertiary prevention: seeks to minimize the disability and handicap from a disease state that cannot be cured or that leaves the individual with some loss of function, examples include the management of diabetes or rehabilitation after stroke.

Screening is an example of the way in which technologies of health promotion increasingly invade people's lives, particularly in primary care, through the introduction of screening clinics, health promotion clinics and health checks at age 75+. Screening programmes have been questioned in terms of their effectiveness in identifying disease. In addition, the psychological costs associated with high rates of false positives and false negatives might not be given sufficient weight in screening decisions.

Contradictions and alternatives

Health promotion aims to prevent illness or maintain health, to reverse or arrest the illness process and to ameliorate the effects of illness. It has grown in strength because to some it emphasizes the importance of government intervention as well as individual responsibility. In this respect, many of the things it promises are appealing to politicians and policy makers. It emphasizes the importance of psychological and social functioning, advocates personal empowerment and questions over-reliance on expensive curative services. However, there are tensions and contradictions between different understandings of health promotion. These derive from it being conceptually dependent on contested understandings of health.

The biomedical model of health had a strong influence over early forms of health education. Indeed, health promotion campaigns still focus on risk factors for disease that are based on epidemiological research. Other notions of health include the 'salutogenic' approach (Antonovsky 1987), which contrasts itself with the 'pathogenic' medical model and its focus on reasons for illness and disease. The salutogenic model sets up an alternative focusing on the reasons for people being healthy. This, it is argued, emphasizes the interaction between people and their environments and seeks ways of creating supportive relationships and conditions that help people cope and remain healthy. Health, it would appear, is a multidimensional concept that has many different definitions that have changed over time. For example, in 1948 the World Health Organization (WHO) defined health as 'a complete state of physical, mental and social well-being' (WHO 1948). By 1978, however, in the Alma Alta declaration, health was defined as more than the absence of disease or infirmity. It was a fundamental human right, that required a concerted effort by 'other social and economic factors in addition to the health sector' (WHO 1978). This reflects the growing influence of the social model of health that sees health being determined by a complex relationship between social, political, cultural, environmental and biological factors. This has been hailed by some as a major advance in thinking about the causes of health and illness and the interventions that should be employed to prevent illness and disease. Others have condemned it as working within the same framework as the medical model merely replacing one set of risk factors (viruses, behaviour) with another set of risk factors (housing, poverty) (Kelly & Charlton 1995).

Public policy versus individual behaviour

Epidemiology has done much to highlight a dilemma at the heart of health promotion. This is often referred to as the prevention paradox (Rose 1992). Rose showed that, with respect to population risk factors for disease, it was more effective to concentrate on shifting the risk levels of the entire population than to concentrate on groups within the population considered to be at high risk of disease. In addition, individual risk factors that appear to explain high levels of variance in a population might be unimportant with respect to determining the population level of any health outcome. This raised questions about the focus of health promotion work or health education that targeted particular groups. It influenced those who called for health promotion approaches that emphasized changes in public policy.

Public policy approaches are concerned with manipulating the social, political and economic environment. They seek changes to advertising codes and the licensing of goods and services (e.g. drugs and alcohol). They also look for changes in government regulation, for example manufacturing regulations and road safety regulations. With wider determinants of health in mind they also look towards changes in the provision of housing education and welfare and fiscal changes such as more progressive tax systems. Such approaches can be contrasted with health promotion work that focuses on behavioural change and is very much grounded in psychological theories, social cognition models and models of health behaviour such as the health belief model (Rosenstock et al 1988). Here, the emphasis is on knowledge, attitudes and changing individual behaviour.

Philosophy

There is considerable disagreement and debate surrounding the philosophical underpinnings of health promotion. Territorial battles abound over the extent of health promotions concerns. Should it exclude negative notions of health and biomedical understandings of disease and illness? Should it be educative or preventive or both? Should it be concerned solely with promoting empowerment and healthy public policy? The flux of the debate is further confused by changing use of terminology over time, reflecting the ebbs and flows of public health activity over the years. For example, early twentieth-century concerns with hygiene were related to health education and prevention in ways that would be considered judgemental and paternalistic today (Armstrong 1995). On the other hand, the concerns of the Health of Towns organization in the nineteenth century have immediate parallels with healthy cities agendas at the end of the twentieth century.

A review of the different models of health promotion reveals an eclecticism that has led to a proliferation of approaches (Katz et al 2000). Ewles & Simnett (1999) developed a five-fold typology of approaches to health promotion ranging from: (1) the medical focus on disease and prevention; through (2) behavioural change, focusing on attitudes and lifestyles; (3) educational, focusing on developing knowledge and decision-making capacity; and (4) client-centred, focusing on empowering individuals; to (5) self-actualization and societal change, focusing on political and social action. This typology is a useful platform for asking why one approach is preferred over another and the extent to which health promotion activity can be a combination of these different approaches.

An alternative analysis is that provided by Tones & Tilford (1994), who describe an interactive model where health promotion has the capacity to raise consciousness and empower individuals, communities and groups to push for social, political and environmental change. At the same time, changes at social, political and environmental levels can equally influence communities, groups and individuals. The variations in models and philosophical underpinnings have been interpreted positively by some as post-modern pluralism, in response to the crude dichotomies of biomedical models of health (Kelly & Charlton 1995). However, although criticisms of the latter still have strong resonance, on their own they do not amount to a reasoned alternative and the contradictions between various health promotion models need to be recognized.

DEVELOPMENTS IN HEALTH PROMOTION

A brief history of public health

The historical development of health promotion is tied to the changing fortunes of public health and public health policy. Public health, as it is understood today, is 'the science and art of preventing disease, prolonging life and promoting health through organised efforts of society' (Acheson 1988). Public health can be traced back to the quarantine and sanitation activities of the ancient Greeks and Romans.

In Britain, four phases of public health have been identified over the last 150 years (Goraya & Scambler 1998). These are the sanitary phase, the preventive phase, the therapeutic phase and the new public health phase. Public health rose to prominence in the nineteenth century with the sanitary idea. In 1842 Edwin Chadwick published his 'Report on the sanitary condition of the labouring population', highlighting how the problems of the industrializing cities – lack of safe water, poor sanitation, overcrowding and poor nutrition – were related to health. However, concern was often focused on ameliorating the 'excesses' of capitalism. The movement was paternalistic, philanthropic and charitable. It worked towards reducing perceived threats to the system and the underlying assumption was that capitalism was still the route out of the problem rather than the problem itself. However, The Public Health Act of 1848 and the activities of the Health of Town's Commission were very much linked to local government. Key elements of this kind of public health work, therefore, were the legitimacy of working locally, an emphasis on resourcefulness and pragmatism, a strong moral tone, populism and the importance of making public health the responsibility of a democratically accountable body. Later in the nineteenth century, John Simon worked to develop a scientific basis for public health.

The Public Health Act 1872 required the appointment of Medical Officers of Health and ensured that public health was based firmly in local government. However, the focus of public health was beginning to change. With advances in medical science and knowledge of disease, preventive measures moved away from an environmental basis to concentrate on the person. This is commonly referred to as the preventative era of public health involving the extension of activities such as mass immunization. In the twentieth century, particularly after the Ministry of Health Act 1919, public health took on more of an administrative role. It was an unfashionable branch of medicine and local Medical Officers of Health were often seen as officious, bullying and bureaucratic. This was the therapeutic era of public health with public health physicians coordinating hospital and non-hospital community services. In 1968, the Todd report led to the establishing of a new specialty of community medicine, defined as a specialty practised by epidemiologists and administrators of medical services. After the 1972 Hunter report, community physicians were integrated into the NHS. The therapeutic era seemed to be increasingly anachronistic in the face of new ideas concerning, health promotion and the new public health. The Public Health Alliance (PHA) was formed in the late 1980s to provide a national focus for discussion of health promotion issues, to set up collaborative networks and to promote research on public health issues. The PHA charter proposed rights for citizens on the basis of an understanding of the wider determinants of health. These included rights to fair incomes, homes, food, transport, public services, education and health promotion and comprehensive health care. In 1988 the first Acheson report set up clearer roles for public health. New posts – Directors of Public Health – were created with responsibilities to survey the health of their local populations, to promote and maintain health and to evaluate existing services. They were also charged with producing 'independent' (often in name only) annual reports on the health of their area. The activism of the new public health movement and government responses to its criticisms of mainstream public health were very much related to changes in ways in which health promotion was viewed.

A brief history of health promotion

A timeline for health promotion is given in Box 17.1. At the beginning of the twentieth century, health education was provided by poorly funded voluntary bodies. The Central Council for Health Education was first established in 1927. Largely paternalistic, it was financed by local authority Medical Officers for Health. It published a magazine called 'Better health' and developed a role of propaganda and instruction around prevailing concerns on sexual health. In 1968 The Health Education Council (HEC) was created. This had a turbulent history. It started by focusing attention on educating women about health (particularly the health of families) but, as it progressed, it began to highlight the role of large corporations such as tobacco companies in affecting population health.

In 1974, Marc Lalonde, the Minister for Health and Welfare in Canada launched the Lalonde Report (Lalonde 1974) with the ambitious claim that 'the goal of the government of Canada will be to not only to add years to life, but life to our years'. The report was a

> ### BOX 17.1   Timeline of Health Promotion
>
> 1927   Creation of the Central Council for Health Education
> 1948   Creation of the World Health Organization
> 1956   Minister of Health refuses to mount a campaign against smoking because he is not convinced that smoking was harmful.
> 1964   Helen Brook sets up the Brook Clinics in London, Bristol and Birmingham to give contraceptive and other advice to unmarried women and young girls
> 1965   Cigarette advertising is banned on TV
> 1968   Creation of the Health Education Council
> 1974   Lalonde Report 'A new perspective on the health of Canadians' is published
> 1976   'Prevention and health: everybody's business' is published in the UK
> 1977   Health for All by the Year 2000
> 1985   World Health Organization publishes 38 targets for health in the European region
> 1986   Ottawa Charter for health promotion
> 1987   Launch of the Healthy Cities project
> 1987   Promoting better health – UK government's programme to improve primary care
> 1992   'The health of the nation' is published
> 1992   Rio Earth Summit – Agenda 21 follows from this
> 1997   Jakarta declaration on health promotion in the twenty-first century
> 1999   'Our healthier nation' is published
> 1998   Health 21 – Health for All policy (21 targets for Europe in twenty-first century)
> 2000   Fifth global conference on health promotion, held in Mexico, emphasizes equity
> 2000   Creation of the Health Development Agency, UK

watershed in that it argued for changes at the level of the environment and lifestyle to improve population health. This was, in many ways, an extension of the medical model rather than a transformation. However, it was a bold challenge to the prevailing orthodoxy and was the launch-pad for the development of health promotion over the next 20 years. The World Health Organization (WHO) launched its health promotion programme in 1981. In 1986, Ireland set up its Health Education Bureau and in 1987 Hungary promised a broad strategy that was never fully implemented because of political and economic changes. The UK tended to lag behind. In 1976 the government published 'Prevention and health: everybody's business' (DHSS 1976). This shifted the emphasis from treatment to prevention, but it focused largely on preventive services such as screening, and most significantly on individual behaviour and personal responsibility for health.

By contrast, 'Health for all by the year 2000' was launched in 1977 at the World Health Assembly. A year later, the Alma Ata declaration (WHO 1978) emphasized the role that diverse sectors such as agriculture, education, industry had in improving health. In the 1980s the health promotion movement increasingly emphasized intersectoral collaboration and the importance of inequalities in health. By 1984 the WHO Regional Office for Europe had set out key principles for health promotion. These were to address the population as a whole, to act on causes of health, to encourage diverse approaches, to foster public participation and to develop the role of health professionals as enablers (WHO 1984). WHO also set out five means of making this happen: (1) improving access to health; (2) the development of an environment conducive to health; (3) the strengthening of social networks and social supports; (4) promoting positive health behaviour and appropriate coping strategies; and (5) increasing knowledge and disseminating information. This work informed the Ottawa Charter (WHO 1986), which emphasized the need to empower local communities and create supportive environments. In 1985 the WHO launched its 38 targets for 'Health for all in Europe'. The WHO targets made reduction of inequalities in health the primary target without which the other targets could not be achieved. Responses to the WHO targets were mixed. Some countries such as Germany and Sweden established national targets early on. The UK had a more limited response. This official lethargy concealed more energetic responses at local levels. For example the city of Liverpool was a vigorous supporter of the WHO Healthy Cities project. This was an attempt to implement the principles outlined in the Ottawa Charter in a number of European cities. In the main, however, such activities were marginal and underfunded (Dooris 1999).

Strategies for health

Slowly some of the ideas of the health promotion movement began to be taken up by governments, although usually in a limited way. The UK produced national strategies in the 1990s: 'health promotion Wales' (1990) and 'the health of the nation' (DoH 1992) for England. 'The health of the nation' had specific measurable targets and emphasized the government's role in prevention alongside individual responsibility for risk. It was criticized for being a prescribed view of the WHO targets, with easily achievable outcomes that possibly contradicted local needs and downplayed the role of inequality and poverty. Wider environmental and public health policy was not addressed. Meanwhile, the health promotion movement at an international level was evolving and taking on ecological and environmental ideas. The notion of sustainability was increasingly adopted, as were the notions of human rights, social justice, empowerment and feminist goals. Emphasis was also on process and not just outcomes and the notion of 'social capital' began to be introduced. For example, Agenda 21 came out of the 1992 Rio Earth Summit and set a framework for sustainable development at a local level. Sustainable development has one eye on the future in demanding interventions that address present day needs without compromising the needs of future populations. The Jakarta declaration in 1997 replaced the regional targets of 'Health for all' with 21 targets for Europe (WHO 1997). These initiatives marked a shift away from disease reduction to targeting and reducing inequalities between countries and regions and between social groups. Thus the social model of health came increasingly to the fore. WHO also began to advocate health promotion in settings such as healthy schools, healthy workplaces and healthy hospitals (WHO-EC-CE 1997). The developments in health promotion at European and global scales throughout the 1990s suggest a greater awareness of the wider determinants of health and the need for intersectoral activities to improve health. However, it is still argued that the commitment, at national level, in terms of resources and institutional change has been marginal (Ziglo et al 2000).

Our healthier nation

In the UK, the Labour government that came to power in 1997 acknowledged the link between poverty, inequality social exclusion and health. It prioritized greater integration of health and social services and produced a raft of key government initiatives. These started with the Acheson report on inequalities (Acheson 1998), a White Paper on tobacco (Smoking kills; HMSO 1998) and the publication of 'Saving lives: our healthier nation' (DoH 1999), which set out targets in key areas (Table 17.1). Based on its 'third way' rhetoric, government documents seemed to move beyond victim blaming but, at the same time, emphasized the language of rights and responsibilities. The focus was on targeting areas through initiatives such as health action zones (HAZ). Meanwhile, mainstream health promotion had experienced restructuring during the 1990s with the introduction of greater competition and competitive tendering. In April 2000 the Health Education Authority was replaced by the Health Development Agency (HDA), which took on a more strategic role. It defined health development as 'the process of engaging everyone in the

TABLE 17.1	Targets for 2010 under 'Saving lives: our healthier nation' (DoH 1999)
Problem	**Target**
Cancer	Reduce the death rate from cancer in people under 75 by at least one-fifth – saving 100 000 lives
Coronary heart disease and stroke	Reduce the death rate from coronary heart disease and stroke and related diseases in people under 75 by at least two-fifths – saving 200 000 lives
Accidents	Reduce the death rate from accidents by at least one-fifth and reduce the rate of serious injury from accidents by at least one-tenth – saving 12 000 lives
Mental health	Reduce the death rate from suicide and undetermined injury by at least one-fifth – saving 4000 lives

promotion of health and well-being'. It focuses its activities on assessing and disseminating information about the evidence on interventions to improve public health (HDA 2001). The Labour government has set in train a host of activities from the funding of healthy living centres, to regeneration, health improvement programmes, health skills programmes and new deals for communities. The 'idea' of health and health promotion has now become a core part of government policies.

HEALTH PROMOTION, EVIDENCE AND POLICY

Evidence-based medicine has become increasingly dominant in recent years. Indeed the British government has made a commitment to apply health impact assessments to its relevant key policies (DoH 1999). This applies as much to health promotion interventions as to any other form of policy intervention and the future of health promotion work depends on being able to demonstrate the effectiveness of interventions both in terms of their efficacy and efficiency. The importance of basing public policy interventions on evidence becomes clear if interventions that produce adverse effects on health are considered. For example, government advice to parents in the past was to place infants in the prone position to sleep. This advice was changed in light of evidence that it led to increased risk of cot death (McKee et al 1996). Some have bemoaned the lack of empirical evidence on the effectiveness of interventions. Indeed, existing evidence tends to be clearer with respect to 'downstream' interventions that are focused on individual behaviour, and there is a paucity of studies evaluating the effectiveness of 'upstream' community- or population-based interventions (MacIntyre et al 2001).

Demonstrating the value of health promotion interventions is often difficult and contentious. Some have argued that the movement towards evaluation imposes managerial and economic rationality on health promotion work (McQueen 2000). Others have argued that effective practice needs to be based on a more complex understanding of social life than orthodox evaluative approaches allow (Connelly 2001). This raises important questions about the appropriateness of evidence for public policy decision making. For example, a study of an intervention that improves the presentation skills of job applicants might show a significant effect in terms of improvements in selection chances but the intervention would have no real effect on the wider social economic forces that periodically lead to large increases in unemployment rates. By confining evidence-based assessment to individualized interventions, health promotion and public health policy might downplay the importance and appropriateness of interventions that address root causes (Smith et al 2001).

SOCIOLOGICAL CRITIQUES OF HEALTH PROMOTION

Sociological critiques of health promotion have questioned its ideological foundations. In so doing some fractures and contradictions have been exposed. Primarily, it is argued that the glossing over of the problem of structure and agency has led to the re-introduction of individualistic and 'victim blaming' tendencies, albeit in new discriminatory forms. Health promotion workers might be the unwitting vehicles for new forms of social control and regulation within advanced liberalism. These problems have been documented by Bunton et al (1995), who categorize sociological critiques as sociostructural, surveillance and consumption based. A fourth that could be added is system-based critiques. Table 17.2 summarizes the main elements of the different critiques of health promotion.

Sociostructural critiques

Sociostructural critiques highlight the neglect within health promotion of the importance of social, political and physical environments on peoples lives. By emphasizing the individual, health promotion ultimately supports the hold of powerful groups on socioeconomic and political structures. Bunton et al (1995) cite examples of such criticisms applied to individualistic approaches to prevention and smoking (Graham 1984) and naïve and one-sided attempts to promote community empowerment (Farrant 1991).

Surveillance critiques

Health promotion programmes have come under the scrutiny of surveillance critiques where they relate to the monitoring, regulation and surveillance of populations. Health promotion and public health workers are involved in population surveillance and this is seen to mark an expansion of the medical gaze from individuals and bodies to communities (Armstrong 1995). These criticisms raise questions about the empowering nature of health promotion work in that, by encouraging self-surveillance of health behaviour, it simultaneously encourages the development of new identities based around the 'technologies of the self'. These critiques draw on Foucault's concept of governmentality (Foucault 1991) and mark a shift in the role of the state in late modernity away from welfare provision towards the conduct of conduct; that is, the promotion of self-regulation, self-surveillance and individual responsibility.

Consumption critiques

Consumption critiques draw on the work of Pierre Bourdieu (1984), who identified forms of social distinction and differentiations constructed around lifestyles and the patterns of

TABLE 17.2	Sociological critiques of health promotion
Critique	**Main elements**
Sociostructural	Health promotion tends to neglect the importance of social, political and physical environments
Surveillance	Health promotion unwittingly expands population surveillance and the 'medical gaze'
Consumption	Health promotion privileges certain lifestyles and is consumerist in its approach
System	Health promotion is contradictory and has little effect on existing structures

consumption of particular collections of goods, leisure and cultural activities. These patterns heavily shape, and are shaped by, consumer cultures. Some researchers have noted that 'healthism' is a central part of consumer society witnessed by the proliferation of goods and services that are marketed on the basis of their healthy qualities. This collapses previous distinctions between the roles of health promoters working in the public sector and promoters of private sector consumption (advertisers, marketing companies, etc.). From this perspective, health promotion workers begin to resemble Bourdieu's 'new cultural intermediaries' promoting, privileging and giving cultural kudos to certain lifestyles.

System critiques

A fourth critique of health promotion looks at the extent to which health promotion and public health work is oriented towards system needs. This criticism has been developed by Scambler & Scambler (1995), who argue that health promotion work is mainly limited to securing change at the level of operational work, leaving factors at political and structural levels unaddressed. Moreover, the efforts of frontline workers might contradict or be contradicted by activities at political and structural levels. To illustrate this, they considered health promotion work with sex workers. They found examples of operational change (defined as formal health promotion work run by professionals and experts). These included health education and outreach work on the streets. They defined political change as something that was beyond the remit of individual health workers, was dependent on governmental action and posed a possible threat to core institutions. They listed a number of factors under different legislation relating to sexual offences and street offences and found these antithetical to the operational health promotion work they observed at the time. For example, the possession of condoms and safe sex literature was seen to be dangerous because of the possibility of it being used in court as evidence of sex work. They highlighted widespread support among sex workers for decriminalization of sex work. They defined structural change as something that required mass public support and possibly extra parliamentary action, and highlighted the dependence of the sex industry on the continuation of poverty and the structural inequalities arising from patriarchy and capitalism. The tensions and contradictions between these different levels place health promotion and public health workers in what Goraya & Scambler (1998) call a 'location paradox'. That is, their mainstream activities work towards system-oriented operational change whereas their rhetoric and sometimes non-mainstream activities aspire towards political and structural change. This is particularly problematic if the latter forms of activity are mainly rhetorical, because this allows the language of radical change to support and legitimize what are exercises in damage limitation.

CONCLUSION

Health promotion has come a long way since its early twentieth century concerns with sexual health. It has been central to the development of socioecological models of health and these ideas remain influential in terms of local, national and international public policies. However, the tensions within health promotion remain. Individualized notions of health behaviour are still powerful and there are a number of barriers to community development and intersectoral work, not least of which is lack of investment. Criticisms of health promotion reflect concerns about its role in social control and maintaining system needs. These are a continual reminder of the need to be aware of the context in which health promotion activity takes place.

References

Acheson D 1988 Public health in England: the report of the committee of inquiry into the future development of the public health function. Department of Health, London

Anderson R 1983 Health promotion: an overview. WHO Regional Office for Europe, Copenhagen

Antonovsky A 1987 Unravelling the mystery of health: how people manage others and stay well. Wiley, New York

Armstrong D 1995 The rise of surveillance medicine. Sociology of Health and Illness 17(3):393–404

Bourdieu P 1984 Distinction: a social critique of the judgement of taste. Routledge, London

Bunton R, Nettleton S, Burrows R 1995 The sociology of health promotion. Routledge, London

Cochrane A 1972 Effectiveness and efficiency. Nuffield Provincial Hospital Trust, London

Connelly J 2001 Critical realism and health promotion: effective practice need an effective theory. Health Education Research 16:115–120

Department of Health (DoH) 1992 The health of the nation. HMSO, London

Department of Health (DoH) 1999 Saving lives: our healthier nation. HMSO, London

Department of Health and Social Security (DHSS) 1976 Prevention and health, everybody's business. HMSO, London

Dooris M 1999 Healthy cities and local agenda 21: the UK experience – challenges for the new millennium. Health Promotion International 14(4):365–375

Dubos R 1959 Mirage of health. Harper, New York

Ewles L, Simnett I 1999 Promoting health, 4th edn. Balliere Tindall, Edinburgh

Farrant W 1991 Addressing the contradiction: health promotion and community health action in the United Kingdom. International Journal of Health Services 21(3):423–449

Foucault M 1991 Governmentality. In: Burchell R (ed) The Foucault effect. Harvester Wheatsheaf, Hemel Hempstead

Goraya A, Scambler G 1998 From old to new public health: role tensions and contradictions. Critical Public Health 8(2):141–151

Graham H 1984 Women, health and the family. Harvester Wheatsheaf, Brighton

Health Development Agency (HDA) 2001 Summary of activities 2001/2. HDA, London

Health Promotion Wales (HPW) 1990 A health promotion strategy for Wales. HPW, Cardiff

HMSO 1998 Smoking kills, a white paper on tobacco. HMSO, London

Illich I 1977 Medical nemesis: the expropriation of health. Penguin, Harmondsworth

Katz J, Peberdy A, Douglas J 2000 Promoting health, knowledge and practice, 2nd edn. Open University Press, Buckingham

Kelly M, Charlton B 1995 The modern and the postmodern in health promotion. In: Bunton R, Nettleton S, Burrows R (eds) The sociology of health promotion. Routledge, London

Lalonde M 1974 A new perspective on the health of Canadians. Minister of Supply and Services. Ottawa, Canada

MacIntyre S et al 2001 Using evidence to inform health policy: case study. British Medical Journal 322:222–225

McKeown T 1979 The role of medicine – dream, mirage of nemesis. Basil Blackwell, Oxford

McKee M et al 1996 Preventing sudden deaths – the slow diffusion of an idea. Health Policy 37:117–135

McQueen D 2000 Perspectives on health promotion: theory, evidence, practice and the emergence of complexity. Health Promotion International 15(2):95–97

Rose R 1992 The strategy of preventive medicine. Oxford University Press, Oxford

Rosenstock IM, Strecher VJ, Becker MH 1988 Social learning theory and the health belief model. Health Education Quarterly 15:175–183

Scambler G, Scambler A 1995 Social change and health promotion among sex workers in London. Health Promotion International 10:17–24

Smith GD, Ebrahim S, Frankel S 2001 How policy informs the evidence. British Medical Journal 322:184–185

Tones BK 1996 The anatomy and ideology of health promotion: empowerment in context. In: Scriven A, Orme J (eds) Health promotion: professional perspectives. Macmillan, London

Tones BK, Tilford S 1994 Health education: effectiveness, efficiency and equity. Chapman Hall, London

WHO 1948 Constitution of the World Health Organization. WHO Regional Office for Europe, Copenhagen

WHO 1978 Alma Ata Declaration. WHO Regional Office for Europe, Copenhagen

WHO 1984 Report of the working group on concepts and principles of health promotion. WHO Regional Office for Europe, Copenhagen

WHO 1986 Ottawa charter for health promotion. WHO, Geneva

WHO 1997 Jakarta declaration on leading health promotion into the 21st century. Health Promotion International 12:261–264

WHO-EC-CE 1997 WHO European Commission Council for Europe. The European Network of Health Promoting Schools. WHO Regional Office for Europe, Copenhagen

Ziglo E, Hagard S, Griffiths J 2000 Health promotion development in Europe: achievements and challenges. Health Promotion International 15(2):143–154

Measuring Health Outcomes

Ray Fitzpatrick

During the twentieth century, health problems in the industrialized societies shifted steadily from the infectious diseases to chronic and degenerative diseases. Health services are now expected to have an impact on a diverse range of health problems that variously involve what can be called the 'five Ds': death, disease, disability, discomfort and dissatisfaction. The health services that have emerged to respond to such demands are of unprecedented size, diversity and complexity. Perhaps the greatest challenge now facing health services is to assess their impact on health problems. Now that public funds are an essential component of financial support for health care, governments of all political persuasions have begun to require evidence of the effectiveness of health services. At the same time, the health professions are also beginning to look more closely at the impact that their treatments and interventions might have. The common focus of such concerns is on assessing the outcomes of health care, that is, the impact on patients and populations of health services.

This chapter examines some of the different ways of conceptualizing and measuring health outcomes and some of the lessons to be gained from such evidence. In a discussion of the evaluation of health services, it is customary to distinguish between three different components of healthcare evaluation.

1. The structure of health care, which involves focusing on such matters as the numbers, distribution and qualifications of doctors, nurses and other health professionals.

2. The processes of health care, which are concerned with the therapeutic, diagnostic and other activities performed by health professionals for patients.

3. The outcomes of health care – these are the most important focus in evaluation and consider the ultimate results achieved for patients by health services.

MORTALITY

The first measure of outcome is important for a number of reasons. Most obviously, it is a central concern of clinicians and society to prevent deaths. From the perspective of measurement it is relatively simple to define compared with most other dimensions of health status. Moreover, particularly in industrialized societies, national recording systems have virtually complete information about deaths, something that cannot be said for most other measures of outcome.

Mortality rates can be used for a number of purposes. Thus, they indicate inequalities in health status between different parts of England and Wales. The highest standardized mortality ratios (SMRs) consistently occur in the northern Regional Health Authorities and the lowest in the south and west. The use of SMRs to examine inequalities between social and ethnic groups has been discussed in Chapter 8. Mortality rates can also be used to examine improvements over time. In England and Wales, life expectancy – a summary measure of the mortality rates prevailing at any time – increased for females from 42 years in 1841 to 80 years in 1997. Most of this improvement has occurred because of reductions in infant mortality; life expectancy at later ages has not improved so markedly: a woman aged 65 in 1841 could expect to live another 12 years; this figure had increased to 18 years by 1997. Nevertheless, mortality rates can be used to show significant progress in some areas in the recent past. Thus, among young men, there was a dramatic 44% reduction in lung cancer in the period 1975–87, a change almost entirely due to reductions in smoking and the tar content of cigarettes. Over the same period, mortality rates due to some other cancers, such as Hodgkin's disease, leukaemia and cancer of the testis, declined markedly as a result of medical interventions such as radiotherapy and chemotherapy. This is persuasive evidence that counterbalances the more pessimistic analyses of progress against cancer.

Infant mortality tends to be used as a particularly sensitive measure of the overall health of a country. Variations between countries in infant mortality are considered to be a reflection of social and economic conditions generally, as well as the quality of maternity and neonatal care.

Avoidable mortality

One important approach to mortality statistics is to focus on deaths from certain conditions considered amenable to health-service intervention. Maternal and infant mortality can be used as indicators of the quality of obstetric and infant care. This approach has been extended to other causes of death where variations in death rates might indicate limitations of healthcare provision, particularly if deaths below particular ages are the focus of attention. For example, cervical cancer is regarded as, in principle, avoidable by a combination of screening and early treatment by surgery or radiotherapy. Similarly, preventive immunization or drug therapy for established cases is highly effective against tuberculosis, so that most mortality is in principle avoidable. Hypertensive disease can be detected by screening and ought to be amenable to dietary and smoking advice together with drug management (Box 18.1). A study in Finland showed that over the period 1969–81, death rates for causes amenable to medical intervention declined by two-thirds for individuals aged 64 years or less (Poikolainen & Eskola 1986).

Hospital deaths

Deaths can nevertheless be an important alarm signal in health care and, as information systems become more effective and public concern over issues of quality increases, it can be expected that increasing attention will be given to hospital mortality data. A great deal of controversy followed the publication in the USA of the death rates for different hospitals of public sector (Medicare) patients. For example, mortality in a 30-day period following admission for pneumonia varied from 0 to 60% between different hospitals. It was argued that such evidence pointed to serious potential deficiencies in the quality of care of certain hospitals about which the public had a right to know. Similarly, death rates across all causes for admission in the NHS were found to vary across hospitals from 3.4% to 13.6% (Jarman et al 1999). However, technical objections can be raised regarding the quality of mortality data and incautious interpretations regarding their significance. In particular, account needs to be taken of the variation in the severity and complexity of illness of patients admitted to different hospitals. A study of patients admitted to NHS intensive care units found substantial and significant differences in death rates between units, with the worst mortality rate more than two-and-a-half times higher than the most favourable (Rowan et al 1993). However, when the study took account of severity of illness in the patients, variations in mortality were explained away for the majority of units, although 15% of units still had significantly higher death rates.

Of course, for many other kinds of hospital admissions, such as end-stage cancer, death will be the inevitable and accepted outcome and other criteria, such as the dignity of care, would be the most appropriate measure of quality. Again, as with avoidable mortality, there is a practical problem that death for particular hospital units are mercifully too infrequent an event to rely on for purposes of assessing outcomes and quality of care.

It is important to find explanations for why hospitals might have significantly different mortality rates after the severity of presenting illness has been taken into account. Studies of relatively simple-to-measure organizational factors such as whether a hospital has teaching or non-teaching status, is located in a rural or urban area and the number of hospital beds have not proved consistently important. For certain surgical procedures the greater the volume of the procedure performed, the lower the mortality rate, suggesting

BOX 18.1	Avoidable Deaths and the NHS

1. Avoidable death rates vary in different areas of Britain
   - Rates are influenced by social and environmental factors, e.g. deaths due to hypertensive/cardiovascular disease
   - Figures for health authorities, when controlled for social and environmental factors, show variation (Charlton et al 1983)
   - This variation is greater than could have occurred by chance
2. Are they due to the quality of health services?
   - The positions of health authorities on 'league tables' of avoidable deaths has remained stable (Charlton et al 1986)
   - Information on mortality is used as an indicator of quality of medical care, but have the social factors been properly allowed for in the analysis?

that experience and expertise acquired through practice improves the quality of outcomes. Other evidence shows that hospitals with more favourable mortality outcomes are more likely to use procedures (for example, thrombolytic agents, beta-blockers and aspirin for heart attacks) proven to be effective (Halm & Chassin 2001).

HEALTH STATUS AND QUALITY OF LIFE

For many health problems treated by health services, not only is death an uncommon and inappropriate measure of outcome but also, more importantly, the primary purpose of treatment is to improve patient's functioning and well-being. Consider, for example, drug treatment for rheumatoid arthritis, epilepsy or migraine, hospice care of the terminally ill, or surgery for ulcerative colitis. In all such instances the focus is on the broad, pervasive effects that health problems have on the patient in terms of pain, disability, anxiety, depression, social isolation, embarrassment or difficulties in carrying on daily life. From the patient's perspective, health care is judged largely in terms of impact on these broader aspects of personal well-being. Patients themselves advocate that more research be conducted into the impact of treatments on these aspects of their lives. In recent years, outcome measures have emerged in an attempt to capture such aspects of patients' experiences. Frequently termed quality-of-life measures, they can often also be referred to as health-status instruments.

An early attempt to assess quality of life in patients in a systematic way was the Karnofsky Performance Index (Karnofsky & Burchenal 1949) (Table 18.1). The scale was designed particularly for use in the field of cancer and involves the clinician making a simple rating of the patient. It is still one of the more frequently used 'quality-of-life' scales and is very useful in drawing attention to those factors that matter to patients. It also helps health professionals predict which patients on a ward will require more attention and need more time and resources. Some of its disadvantages are considered here:

1. Is quality of life unidimensional? There is a fallacy behind the use of a unidimensional scale. Such a scale requires the assumption that a bed-bound person must have a quite

TABLE 18.1	The Karnofsky Performance Index	
Description		**Score (%)**
Normal, no complaints		100
Able to carry on normal activities; minor signs or symptoms of disease		90
Normal activity with effort		80
Cares for self. Unable to carry on normal activity or to do active work		70
Requires occasional assistance but able to care for most of own needs		60
Requires considerable assistance and frequent medical care		50
Disabled; requires special care and assistance		40
Severely disabled; hospitalization indicated although death not imminent		30
Very sick; hospitalization necessary. Active supportive treatment necessary		20
Moribund		10
Dead		0

Reproduced with permission of Souvenir Press from Fallowfield (1990)

poor score even if, for example, he or she is well adjusted to illness, receives full social support and sees life as fulfilling. Conversely, someone ambulant but otherwise depressed, isolated, with low self-esteem and anxious about health status would, nevertheless, receive a favourable score. In other words, instruments such as the Karnofsky Performance Index do not allow for the multidimensional nature of quality of life.

2. Is the scale reliable? It is not surprising, in view of the complex nature of quality of life, that the index is deficient in a basic requirement for such instruments in that it is not reliable; different raters disagree in applying the scale to patients.

3. Is the scale valid? A serious deficiency is that clinicians sometimes disagree with patients' self-ratings on the scale. Indeed, it has more generally been found to be the case, across a wide range of healthcare settings, that health professionals make significantly different judgements of their patients' quality of life than patients themselves (Sprangers & Aaronson 1992). Such problems have underlined the need for instruments that patients can, whenever possible, complete themselves.

281

Health-status instruments

A large proportion of published clinical trials purporting to assess the impact of therapies on patients' quality of life rely on inaccurate evidence, such as the doctor's opinion or inappropriate laboratory measures. Where patients' perceptions of their health or quality of life are obtained in clinical trials, the questionnaires are often unvalidated or simplistic, and leave patients little scope for expressing their feelings. A review of quality of life measures in randomized controlled trials found a steady increase in the assessment of quality of life measures but, by 1997, still only 4.7% of trials overall included this dimension of outcome (Sanders et al 1998).

A number of instruments (variously termed 'health-status', or 'quality-of-life', instruments) have therefore emerged, designed to be used as questionnaires for self completion. One of the most widely used of such instruments is the Short-Form 36-Item (SF-36) Health Survey Questionnaire (McHorney et al 1994). The SF-36 contains 36 simple questions about the respondent's health. The items fall into one of eight scales addressing different aspects of subjective health: physical functioning, role limitations due to physical problems, role limitations due to emotional problems, social functioning, mental health, energy/vitality, pain and general health perception. The designers of the instrument have made considerable efforts to establish that the instrument is reliable (i.e. produces consistent responses if completed on different occasions not too far apart), and valid (for example, is able to distinguish individuals with different types and severity of health problem). The SF-36 has now been used to examine the impact on individuals' subjective health of a number of different healthcare interventions.

A large number of health-status or quality-of-life measures are now available. Although different in style, content and general approach to measuring patients' problems, they generally tend to focus on those aspects of patients' daily lives that are most affected by ill-health (Fitzpatrick et al 1992) (Box 18.2).

Instruments such as the SF-36 are ambitious in that they are intended to assess the impact on the patient's well-being and quality of life of a wide range of different health problems. It is often necessary to assess the patient's perspective with an instrument more specifically designed to be sensitive to one particular disease. One very typical and quite successful instrument of this kind is the Arthritis Impact Measurement Scale (AIMS), which, by means of simple questions, assesses the impact of rheumatic disease on patient well-being in areas such as mobility, dexterity, household activities, pain and depression.

| BOX 18.2 | Dimensions of Quality of Life Usually Assessed in Health Status Instruments |

- Physical function, for example, mobility, ability to look after self
- Emotional well-being, for example, depression, anxiety, self-esteem
- Social function, for example, close attachments, social support, social integration
- Roles, for example, paid work, housework, child care
- Pain, for example, severity, frequency
- Other symptoms, for example, nausea, stiffness, fatigue

Reproduced with permission from Fitzpatrick et al (1992).

The instrument has been shown to be sensitive to improvements in patients within just 4 weeks of treatment with non-steroidal anti-inflammatory drugs (Anderson et al 1989). In a chronic disease such as rheumatoid arthritis, where improvements to the patient's condition can be quite subtle and undramatic, such instruments have a vital role to play in improving our understanding of outcomes, especially in view of evidence in rheumatology that they might be no less reliable and accurate than conventional laboratory and radiological measures and often provide the clinician with more meaningful information on the impact of treatment. Box 18.3 gives an example of how a questionnaire to assess patients' quality of life has been constructed in one particular field of medicine. The instrument described in the box now provides a validated assessment of quality of life in Parkinson's disease. Such measures provide essential information on outcomes not attainable from conventional clinical assessments for use in trials of the increasing number of medical and surgical treatments emerging for Parkinson's disease (Koller et al 2000).

| BOX 18.3 | Constructing a Quality of Life Instrument |

- **Objective**: Parkinson's disease (PD) is a chronic degenerative disease mainly affecting individuals at older ages. There is no cure and treatment is designed to arrest the progression of symptoms and improve the quality of life. However, there is no specific measure of quality of life in PD.
- **Step one. Identify the problems**: interview individuals with the problem. Allow them to say in their own words how PD affects them. Content analysis of interviews (tape-recorded) draws out a rich variety of themes
- **Step two. Draw up questions**: put together a long list (65+) of questions based on the results of Step one. Ask individuals with PD in the community to complete the questionnaire. Ask for their comments on items. Analyse results to find redundant or difficult items. Statistical analysis found that 39 questionnaire items could be used to assess eight important areas of life: mobility, activities of daily living, emotional well-being, stigma, social support, cognitions, communication, bodily discomfort
- **Step three. Test the questionnaire**: Again ask individuals with PD in the community to complete the (39-item) questionnaire. Ask some to repeat the task. Examine the results for internal consistency and test–retest reliability. Also ask patients in neurological clinics to complete the questionnaire to check that patterns of answers agree with other evidence of neurological problems for purposes of validity
- **Result**. A questionnaire that patients find easy to complete, that emphasizes issues that matter to them and that can be used to assess the course of illness and impact of interventions.

Reproduced with permission by Oxford University Press from Peto et al (1995) and Jenkinson et al (1995).

Some observers argue that questionnaires such as those just described are still limited because they ask a standard set of fixed questions of everyone and do not leave much room for individuals' personal concerns or problems to be expressed if they happen not to be included as a questionnaire item (O'Boyle et al 1992). For this reason, several instruments have recently been developed in which respondents identify their own most important areas of life (family, religion, leisure activities or whatever) rather than respond to questionnaire items determined by the investigator. They can then rate how well they are doing in these personally nominated areas of life and also on subsequent occasions judge any changes for better or worse in these domains. Such approaches attempt to address the concern that quality of life is an essentially individualized and personal judgement.

Adverse consequences of health care

Many medical treatments have harmful side-effects. This is the case in, for example, cancer therapies, which are designed to prolong life but which can have a variety of adverse effects at the same time. Cytotoxic chemotherapies can produce nausea, vomiting, hair loss and tiredness, as well as mood effects such as depression. In some cases, the costs to the patient from treatments outweigh benefits gained in terms of longevity. Quality-of-life measures allow us to give some quantitative expression to such adverse effects. Thus, Croog et al (1986) used a battery of quality-of-life measures to assess the impact of three alternative drugs for controlling hypertension. They measured general well-being, physical symptoms, sexual function, work performance, emotional state, cognitive function (e.g. memory), social participation and life satisfaction. Although achieving similar levels of blood pressure control, one drug stood out from the other two as having less harmful effects on quality of life. They found that some of the harmful side-effects of drugs produced broadly equivalent effects on quality of life to those found by individuals who have just lost their jobs. Broadly based measures of quality of life make it possible to detect and assess harmful effects that might occur in any of a wide range of aspects of patients' lives.

Attaching values to health

All healthcare systems have to make choices between different healthcare interventions; resources are not available to fund and provide all of the treatments that, in principle, are available. This requires extremely difficult choices to be made between interventions for very different health problems, e.g. between coronary bypass surgery, renal transplant, lipid screening and day hospitals for psychiatric patients. One of the many problems complicating such choices is that there is no single numerical scale in terms of which to measure the diverse states of health and illness treated by different healthcare programmes. Utility measurement is an approach that can be used to produce numerical values on a scale between 0 and 1 for all possible health states by assessing their relative value to individuals. In principle, it then becomes possible to assess in a standard way the improvements to health that can result from otherwise widely differing medical interventions.

A number of techniques have been developed to elicit how desirable individuals regard one health state compared with another. One such technique is the so-called standard gamble technique in which a subject is asked to choose between a particular state of ill health on the one hand and a gamble on the other hand. The gamble involves a hypothetical treatment that can cure the individual of the state of ill health, but with a particular probability of death from the treatment. For states of ill health perceived by the subject to be very undesirable, one would expect the individual to prefer the gamble even with quite high probabilities of death. This probability is varied experimentally to reveal how ready the individual is to take the gamble rather than choose (hypothetically) to carry on living in the particular state of ill health being investigated. Data can be gathered from a sample of experimental subjects in such a way as to produce numerical values for a range of health states.

An alternative method (magnitude estimation) is to ask subjects to state how much worse they regard each of a number of ill-health states relative to one standard health state. One research group (Rosser & Kind 1978) asked subjects to rate the relative undesirability of 29 different states of illness produced by a matrix formed from combinations of two dimensions, varying degrees of distress and disability. The resulting relative values or 'utilities' of different health states are shown in Table 18.2. It is worth noting that some health states were rated as worse than 'dead' by judges. The research group found that values attached to different health states were reliable in the sense that individuals' responses were consistent over time.

QUALITY-ADJUSTED LIFE-YEARS

Some health economists have argued that the values attached to different states of health and illness by methods such as those outlined above can be combined with survival data on years lived as a result of medical treatments to produce a generic output measure, the 'quality-adjusted life-year' (QALY) (Williams 1985). This standard, unitary means of expressing the benefits of medical treatments permits comparisons across treatments. Typically, information on QALYs has been combined with information about the costs of different treatment programmes (cost–utility analysis) and comparisons between programmes expressed in terms of costs per QALY gained, as in Table 18.3. It is argued that health authorities, faced with a scarcity of resources to meet all health problems, need to maximize their use of resources. The methodology of QALYs identifies treatments that maximize the use of resources by obtaining the greatest gain in terms of health for a unit of resource. Table 18.3 indicates that general practitioners giving advice to stop smoking is a dramatically more effective use of resources than, say, hospital haemodialysis. Such

TABLE 18.2	Valuation matrix of different health states[a]			
	Distress rating			
Disability rating	**No distress**	**Mild**	**Moderate**	**Severe**
No disability	1.000	0.995	0.990	0.967
Slight social disability	0.990	0.986	0.973	0.932
Severe social disability and/or slight physical impairment	0.980	0.972	0.956	0.912
Physical ability severely limited (e.g. light housework only)	0.964	0.956	0.942	0.870
Unable to take paid employment or education, largely housebound	0.946	0.935	0.900	0.700
Confined to chair or wheelchair	0.875	0.845	0.680	0.000
Confined to bed	0.677	0.564	0.000	−1.486
Unconscious	−1.078	NA	NA	NA

Reproduced with permission by Oxford University Press from Drummond (1989).
[a] Healthy = 1.0, dead = 0.0. NA, not applicable.

TABLE 18.3	'League table' of costs and QALYs for selected healthcare interventions (1983–4 prices)

Intervention	Present value of extra cost per QALY gained (£)
GP advice to stop smoking	170
Pacemaker implantation for heart block	700
Hip replacement	750
CABG for severe angina LMD	1040
GP control of total serum cholesterol	1700
CABG for severe angina with 2VD	2280
Kidney transplantation (cadaver)	3000
Breast cancer screening	3500
Heart transplantation	5000
CABG for mild angina 2VD	12600
Hospital haemodialysis	14000

Reproduced with permission by Oxford University Press from Drummond (1989).
CABG, coronary artery bypass graft; GP, general practitioner; LMD, left main disease; 2VD, two vessel disease.

information appears to provide a more explicit and more rational basis for making decisions about the allocation of resources. However, the approach outlined above has generated intense debate (Box 18.4).

PATIENT SATISFACTION

The patient's perspective

One source of evidence about the outcomes of health care that has, until recently, been all too frequently neglected is the patient's view. This neglect was partly due to the widespread assumption that the patient is insufficiently well informed to comment on his or her health

BOX 18.4	Debate About QALYs

Arguments against
- There are no agreed methods – at least six methods have been developed (Froberg & Kane 1989)
- People's values differ and health means different things to different people
- Doctors' rate states of ill health as less desirable than do patients (Rosser & Kind 1978)
- Even if the principle of 'league tables' is accepted, the methods of assessing costs and outcomes varies, therefore the results are problematic
- Can moral judgements be made scientific?
- QALYs condone cutting healthcare resources
- QALYs have unfair consequences, systematically disadvantaging some social groups, e.g. the elderly and terminally ill

Arguments in favour
- The current system of resource allocation is worse
- QALYs make decisions more open and accountable

care. Undoubtedly, there is also a tendency in many large bureaucratic organizations such as the National Health Service (NHS) to pursue internally generated routines and objectives without seeking external evidence of their reception by users. It should be clear that a primary objective of any healthcare system is to provide services in a manner that is acceptable to the patient. The Griffiths NHS Management Inquiry was highly critical of the failure of the NHS to act on this principle by systematically obtaining consumer feedback about the quality of services (DHSS 1983). Since that report, most health authorities have made much more effort to conduct such surveys.

There is also ample evidence from social scientific research to indicate how important the issue of patient satisfaction is. Patients who are dissatisfied with their health care are more likely not to follow the medical advice or regimen that they receive. In a sample of patients attending a neurological clinic for chronic headache, those who were more dissatisfied with the consultation (when interviewed afterwards) were significantly less likely to take the medication that had been prescribed for them (Fitzpatrick & Hopkins 1981). Similar results have been obtained between satisfaction and compliance in hypertension and paediatric clinics, and in general practice; dissatisfied patients are less likely to reattend for further care (Orton et al 1991) or might change their doctor (Rubin et al 1993). Satisfaction might also be an indication of how successful a treatment has been (Fitzpatrick et al 1987).

A common distinction made in relation to health care is that between the technical and interpersonal aspects of care. Technical aspects of care refer to the technical competence with which treatment is provided. Interpersonal aspects focus on how doctors, nurses and other health professionals treat the patient – in other words, the degree of personal care and concern shown. Patient satisfaction is a particularly important indicator of interpersonal aspects of care. Thus, in a study of mothers attending a paediatric clinic with their children, the medical consultations were tape-recorded and analysed and mothers interviewed independently by researchers after the consultation to assess satisfaction (Korsch et al 1968). Satisfaction was higher when the doctor displayed a friendly manner to the mother. Satisfaction was also positively related to directly questioning mothers early in the consultation as to the main worries and concerns that had prompted the consultation. In a similarly designed study of general medical clinics in which analyses of tape-recorded consultations could be related to subsequent patient satisfaction, those patients who were given encouragement by the doctor to explain their medical problem in their own terms were significantly more satisfied than patients who reported their symptoms in response to more structured doctor-focused questioning (Stiles et al 1979). A study of patients attending primary care in England found that patients were significantly more satisfied after their consultations with the doctor if they felt that the doctor had showed sympathy, was interested in the patient's worries and discussed and agreed with the patient in partnership treatments for problems presented, behaviours all considered by the investigators to be examples of good 'patient-centred care' (Little et al 2001).

One of the more important of interpersonal skills in health care is giving information. Failures in this area are one of the most important sources of patient dissatisfaction. It can also be shown experimentally that efforts to improve the communication of information are appreciated by patients. Ley (1982) reported a study in which medical inpatients were allocated to one of three different patterns of communication. A 'placebo' group experienced the normal and routine pattern of communication from doctors. A 'control' group received in addition one visit from a junior doctor who discussed general matters not specifically related to the patient's admission. In the 'experimental' group the junior doctor, in the one visit to the patient, made a point of giving an explanation to the patient of the treatments and procedures he or she was receiving. All three groups subsequently completed questionnaires and the 'experimental' group produced significantly higher satisfaction scores.

Patient satisfaction studies also underline the importance of continuity and accessibility to patients. Women with breast cancer in remission were randomized between two alternative follow-up regimes, standard care requiring hospital-based check-ups at fixed intervals or primary-care-based follow-up by their own general practitioner. Although there were no differences in the detection of recurrences between the two groups, levels of satisfaction were significantly higher in the primary-care-managed group, women especially valuing speed and accessibility of primary care but also the advantages of seeing a doctor who knew them well and of consultations in which it was easier to discuss problems (Grunfeld et al 1999).

There are two distinct ways in which we can go about obtaining individuals' views in a survey on a subject like health care (Box 18.5). The choice will depend on circumstances. A general problem with all methods is that patients of different backgrounds tend to differ in readiness to express critical comments about health services. Younger patients, those with poorer health status and individuals with higher levels of education are more likely to express dissatisfaction.

Surveys of hospital care

To aid its deliberations, the Royal Commission on the NHS commissioned a survey of a sample of patients who had recently experienced either inpatient or outpatient treatment. The results of the national survey carried out by the Office of Population Censuses and Surveys are likely to be very similar to those that are obtained in local surveys of a particular hospital or district (OPCS 1978).

Table 18.4 shows that much of the dissatisfaction could be traced to problems of having to wait for outpatient appointments or hospital admission, and to the length of time waiting to see a doctor. Other complaints focused on amenities such as food and washing facilities in wards and the waiting room in outpatient clinics. A particularly large number in both patient groups were dissatisfied with information. A more recent survey of over 5000 patients attending 36 NHS hospitals found problems of communication still the main source of dissatisfaction, with 16% of patients receiving no explanation about their condition from the doctor and 60% receiving no advice about activities to do or not do after discharge (Bruster et al 1994).

BOX 18.5   Obtaining Views in a Survey

There are two basic strategies to finding the views of patients. Either respondents are given a questionnaire to complete themselves or personal interviews are conducted to ask the questions.

Advantages of the two approaches:

Self-completed questionnaire	Interview
Questions easy to standardize and process	More appropriate for sensitive or complex material
No interviewer bias	Easier to clarify ambiguous items
Low cost of data gathering	Rapport results in completion of questionnaire
Less need for trained staff	Scope to follow-up non-respondents

Reproduced with permission from Fitzpatrick (1991).

TABLE 18.4	Dissatisfaction with regard to aspects of the NHS			
Outpatients	**%**	**Inpatients**	**%**	
Information about progress	37	Woken too early	43	
Time waiting for hospital transport	28	Information about progress	31	
Waiting for first appointment	21	Food	21	
Length of time at hospital	19	Waiting for admission	20	
Adequacy of waiting room	18	Washing and bathing facilities	19	
Length of wait to see doctor	16	Toilet facilities	15	

Reproduced with permission of the Controller of HMSO and the Office for National Statistics from OPCS (1978).

It might be noted that absent from either study are any views from patients about the value in terms of outcomes of medical care. Indeed, a systematic review of a wide range of studies of patient satisfaction found that only 8% of studies included outcomes as a subject on which to elicit patients' views (Wensing et al 1994). Investigators appear to avoid this subject, either because of limited faith in patients' competence to judge the benefits of treatment or because this subject is perceived as a purely clinical matter to be assessed solely by professional criteria. As a result, we know far less than we should about patients' perceptions of the value of medical care.

It is surprising how similar are the results of surveys of patients' views of their hospital care across developed countries. Coulter & Cleary (2001) report the results of surveys using a standardized questionnaire with patients completed within a month of discharge from hospitals in UK, USA, Germany, Sweden and Switzerland. The problems that were most commonly reported by patients in all five countries were in the area of transition from hospital to community, such as advice about resumption of normal activities, about medication and danger signals to watch for at home. The area causing least problems as viewed by patients was physical comfort of the hospital. Importantly, when asked more general, global views of their hospital care, patients gave more positive ratings than might be predicted from their reports of specific problems, with the lowest level of dissatisfaction observed in Switzerland (3.7%) and the highest level of dissatisfaction (8.5%) in the UK.

OUTCOMES AND THE EVALUATION OF SERVICES

Evaluation and the medical profession

One of the features that can distinguish a profession from other kinds of occupation is that it retains a very high level of control in assessing the value and quality of the product it provides to the public (see Chapter 15). Historically, the medical profession has exercised this control by means of a number of methods, such as monitoring the content and standards of the training provided for new or established members of the profession or by penalizing individual doctors who fail to uphold required professional standards. In Britain, the General Medical Council (GMC) was established – after lengthy negotiations between the State and the newly emerging medical profession in the middle of the nineteenth century – as one of the main institutions to ensure satisfactory performance by doctors. However, health care has now become so complex and costly that traditional methods of upholding professional standards are no longer sufficient. Moreover, society has changed profoundly since the nineteenth century. The State is now intimately involved in health care through funding medical services with public money. It seeks evidence that such funds are well spent. In the USA, in addition to the federal government's concern about public healthcare spending, industry has become concerned about the value of medical services because so much is paid for from employers' insurance contributions. In other words, powerful forces such as government and business are seeking clearer evidence of the value of health care. In addition, consumers have also become more knowledgeable, more demanding and more sceptical in their dealings with health professionals.

The medical profession has not only faced external pressures to evaluate its activities. From within, epidemiologists such as Cochrane (1972) have argued that insufficient attention has been given to the scientific appraisal of the impact on health of medical interventions. The response of the medical profession to such pressures has been to take more seriously its responsibility to examine and monitor the quality and value of its services, in particular by practising medical audit. Medical audit has been defined as 'looking at what we are doing with the aim of making improvements in patient care and use of resources' (Difford 1990). It is conventional to distinguish between audit of process, in which the focus is the evaluation of medical activities (normally against agreed standards), and audit of outcome in which the question concerns the impact of activities upon illness. The latter is, as this chapter establishes, more difficult, so that most audit has been concerned with examining process, by methods such as reviewing samples of case notes, analysing hospital statistical data or comparing local use of procedures such as X-rays against published expert advice.

289

Evaluation and the future of health care

At least three different views can be taken of the impact that measurement of outcomes can have on health care. For many observers, the evaluation of outcomes will be a fundamental turning point in the history of medicine, allowing for explicit, rational, scientific answers to all the problems arising from current uncertainties as to the value of medical treatments. As is examined in Chapter 19, outcomes research must address the enormous variations in the rates at which many medical and surgical treatments are performed, even among populations with similar levels of medical need. The hope is that all parties – the doctor, the patient and the purchaser – will have access to clearer information as to the likely results of investigations and treatments, and will, therefore, be able to make more informed decisions about health care.

A second position about future developments in this area is to adopt a more cautious stance and to argue that, at present, the advocates of outcomes measurement are expressing something of an article of faith. Despite enormous advances in computers and information systems, we are a very long way from the kinds of integrated systems that can monitor the longer-term impact of medical interventions in populations, and the kinds of practical and valid measures of outcome that can be used on a large scale are only just now beginning to be developed and examined. To understand the outcomes of most procedures, long-term studies integrating hospital and community data, to an extent that is not yet feasible outside of very special research contexts, will be required.

There is also a third, longer-term view of these developments. Analysts of both British and American health care (Ham 1981) have suggested that two distinct interest groups have tried to shape the future of health care. One group – the 'professional monopolizers' – have sought to defend the traditional privileges and practices of the medical profession, particularly the clinical autonomy of the doctor. A second group – 'the corporate rationalizers'– emphasize the many irrationalities and inefficiencies that bedevil healthcare systems when traditional professional autonomy is left unchecked by planning and evaluation. According to such analyses there has for a very long time been a stalemate in health policy between these two conflicting philosophies, and the present debate over outcomes is unlikely to result in decisive shifts. According to this view, for the foreseeable future health services will defy precise measurement of their value because of the inherent uncertainties and complexities of medical practice. Whatever the future direction of medical care, the assessment of outcomes will remain a central concern of health services.

References

Anderson J, Firschein H, Meenan R 1989 Sensitivity of a health status measure to short term clinical changes in arthritis. Arthritis and Rheumatism 32:844–850

Bruster S et al 1994 National survey of hospital patients. British Medical Journal 309:1542–1546

Charlton J et al 1983 Geographical variation in mortality from conditions amenable to medical interventions in England and Wales. Lancet i:691–696

Charlton J, Lakhani A, Aristidou M 1986 How have 'avoidable death' indices for England and Wales changed? 1974–78 compared with 1979–83. Community Medicine 8:304–314

Cochrane A 1972 Effectiveness and efficiency. Nuffield Provincial Hospitals Trust, London

Coulter A, Cleary P 2001 Patients' experiences with hospital care in five countries. Health Affairs 20:244–252

Croog S et al 1986 The effects of antihypertensive therapy on the quality of life. New England Journal of Medicine 314:1657–1664

Department of Health and Social Security (DHSS) 1983 NHS management inquiry. HMSO, London

Difford F 1990 Defining essential data for audit in general practice. British Medical Journal 300:92–94

Drummond M 1989 Output measurement for resource allocation decisions in health care. Oxford Review of Economics and Politics 5:59–74

Fallowfield L 1990 The quality of life: the missing measurement in health care. Souvenir Press, London

Fitzpatrick R 1991 Surveys of patient satisfaction: I – Important general considerations. British Medical Journal 302:887–889

Fitzpatrick R, Hopkins A 1981 Patients' satisfaction with communication in neurological outpatient clinics. Journal of Psychosomatic Research 25:329–334

Fitzpatrick R et al 1987 Problems in the assessment of outcome in a back pain clinic. International Disability Studies 9:161–165

Fitzpatrick R et al 1992 Quality of life measures in health care. I: Applications and issues in assessment British Medical Journal 305:1074–1077

Froberg D, Kane R 1989 Methodology for measuring health-state preferences – III: Population and context effects. Journal of Clinical Epidemiology 42:585–592

Grunfeld E et al 1999 Comparison of breast cancer patient satisfaction with follow-up in primary care versus specialist care: results from a randomised controlled trial. British Journal of General Practice 49:705–710

Halm E, Chassin M 2001 Why do hospital death rates vary? New England Journal of Medicine 345:692–694

Ham C 1981 Policy making in the National Health Service. Macmillan, London

Jarman B et al 1999 Explaining differences in English hospital death rates using routinely collected data. British Medical Journal 318:1515–1520

Jenkinson C et al 1995 Self reported functioning and well-being in patients with Parkinson's disease. Age and Ageing 24:505–509

Karnofsky D, Burchenal J 1949 The clinical evaluation of chemotherapeutic agents in cancer In: MacLeod C (ed) Evaluation of chemotherapeutic agents. Symposium at New York Academy of Medicine. Columbia University Press, New York, p 191–205

Koller W et al 2000 Randomised trial of tolcapone versus pergolide as add-on to levodopa therapy in Parkinson's disease patients with motor fluctuations. Movement Disorders 16:858–866

Korsch B, Goszzi E, Francis V 1968 Gaps in doctor patient communications: 1. Doctor patient interaction and patient satisfaction. Paediatrics 32:855–871

Ley P 1982 Satisfaction, compliance and communication. British Journal of Clinical Psychology 21:241–254

Little P et al 2001 Observational study of effect of patient centredness and positive approach on outcomes of general practice consultations. British Medical Journal 323:908–911

McHorney C, Ware J, Lu J 1994 The MOS 36-Item Short Form Health Survey (SF-36): III Tests of data quality, scaling assumptions and reliability across diverse patient groups. Medical Care 32:40–66

O'Boyle C et al 1992 Individual quality of life in patients undergoing hip replacement. Lancet 339:1088–1081

Office of Population Censuses and Surveys (OPCS) 1978 Royal commission on the National Health Service: patients' attitudes to the hospital service. HMSO, London

Orton M et al 1991 Factors affecting women's response to an invitation to attend for a second breast cancer screening examination. British Journal of General Practice 41:320–323

Peto V et al 1995 The development and validation of a short measure of functioning and well-being for individuals with Parkinson's disease. Quality of Life Research 4:241–248

Poikolainen K, Eskola J 1986 The effect of health services on mortality: decline in death rates from amenable and non-amenable causes in Finland 1969–81. Lancet i:199–202

Rosser R, Kind P 1978 A scale of valuations of states of illness: is there a social consensus? International Journal of Epidemiology 7:347–358

Rowan K et al 1993 Intensive care society's APACHE II study in Britain and Ireland – II: outcome comparisons of intensive care units after adjustment for case mix by the American APACHE II method. British Medical Journal 307:977–981

Rubin H et al 1993 Patients' ratings of outpatient visits in different practice settings. Journal of the American Medical Association 270:835–840

Sanders C et al 1998 Reporting on quality of life in randomised controlled trials. British Medical Journal 317:1191–1194

Sprangers M, Aaronson N 1992 The role of health care providers and significant others in evaluating the quality of life of patients with chronic disease: a review. Journal of Clinical Epidemiology 45:743–760

Stiles W et al 1979 Interaction exchange structure and patient satisfaction with medical interviews. Medical Care 17:667–679

Wensing M, Grol R, Smits A 1994 Quality judgements by patients on general practice care: a literature analysis. Social Science and Medicine 38:45–53

Williams A 1985 Economics of coronary bypass grafting. British Medical Journal 291:326–329

Organizing and Funding Health Care

Ray Fitzpatrick

Over the course of the twentieth century, health care developed from a collection of small-scale and low-cost services to a complex, labour-intensive and diverse industry. In modern industrialized societies a large and generally growing proportion of resources is now devoted to health care. As the size and scope of this industry have expanded, so too have individuals' rights and expectations with regard to health. Governments have thus become increasingly committed to making health services available to their citizens. The very scale of modern health care has prompted governments of all political persuasions to raise fundamental questions. How effective are health services? How efficient are they in delivering health care? Ultimately, the common theme of such questions concerns the value of modern health care. The answers are often sought by looking for lessons from alternative systems of health care. The most striking feature of modern health care is the diversity of funding and organization in different countries. This chapter describes the different types of healthcare system that have emerged in industrialized societies and the ways they shape the practice of medicine, and then examines the strengths and weaknesses of different systems.

TYPES OF HEALTHCARE SYSTEM

A basic requirement for any product or service such as health care is that some method is needed to permit consumers to obtain the product from the producer. The simplest method to understand is the market, wherein the consumer purchases the product directly from the producer at a price agreed between the two parties at the time of the transaction. This is the basic principle behind many transactions in modern industrial societies, and indeed, until quite recently, was the dominant means of providing and obtaining health services. However, health services have tended to evolve away from basic market transactions in two respects. First, potential consumers of health services have increasingly preferred to take out insurance to cover possible costs of health care, rather than face unpredictable and often expensive costs incurred at the time of illness. Second, an additional party has mediated between the producer and consumer of health care to provide resources necessary for the provision of health care. This 'third party', very often the government, but also employers, trade unions, sickness funds, insurance societies and charities, has tended to become increasingly influential in the way services are provided. The more that third parties provide funds directly to the producers (hospitals, doctors and the pharmaceutical industry) to allow them to provide care to those entitled to services, either because of citizenship or an adequate record of insurance contributions, the further the system has evolved away from market mechanisms.

All healthcare systems can be understood in terms of the different ways in which transactions occur between these three key parties. In particular, systems differ in the extent to which market versus third-party mechanisms, particularly public provision, dominate transactions and, more specifically, in the ways that individuals obtain insurance against healthcare costs. A simple typology distinguishes four major alternative systems of health care that can be found in western industrialized societies (Field 1973) (Box 19.1).

The socialized systems of health care have probably experienced the most dramatic changes in recent years. In theory, these systems provided comprehensive care to all citizens without user charges. Services were planned centrally to maximize efficient and fair use of resources. It became increasingly clear, however, that behind this ideal model of health care there were major deficiencies, as the healthcare system of countries such as Russia received only 2% of gross national product, resulting in major shortages of basic drugs and other facilities (Field 1995). Moreover, unofficial bribing was often necessary for patients to obtain adequate care, and major inequalities existed in access to health care between political elites and other groups. As the former socialist societies have moved toward

---

BOX 19.1 Alternative Systems of Health Care

1. The pluralistic health system
   - A wide variety of coexisting schemes (insurance, fee-for-service) provide funds
   - Healthcare facilities owned by wide variety of institutions (private, State, federal)
2. The health insurance system
   - Resources gathered by third party as compulsory insurance from individuals and employers
3. The health service system
   - Most facilities owned by the State
   - Doctors independent but receive most of their income from the State
4. The socialized health system
   - All facilities owned by the State
   - Most healthcare personnel are salaried State employees

markets and privatization, their healthcare services have also changed, the preferred model now being based on health insurance contributions from employees and their employers, which insurance agencies pay as fees to clinics and hospitals (Curtis et al 1995).

An even greater diversity of forms of health care may be found in non-western societies. A full classification would need to include the traditional systems of healing that have developed in India and China over many hundreds of years. In both these countries traditional medicine has provided sophisticated diagnostic and therapeutic methods that have developed completely independently of western biomedical science. However, the rapid social and economic changes that these countries are currently experiencing are having dramatic impacts on their health care systems. For example, during its Socialist period, China evolved a comprehensive system of primary care to cover its largely rural population. 'Bare-foot doctors' with minimal medical training and facilities provided a simple but comprehensive primary care service, referring to secondary medical centres the problems that they could not address. The system was funded collectively by the rural commune. However, in the 1980s agriculture was privatized and this collective form of rural medical care virtually disappeared to be replaced by fee-for-service, with the result that illness creates major financial suffering to poorer families (Liu et al 1995). Meanwhile, the growing urban populations of China increasingly receive health care through insurance plans provided by the employer, with marked differences in coverage between plans. Social and economic growth has thus been accompanied by growing inequalities between regions and social groups in China (Hsiao 1995).

Payment mechanisms

In addition to the wide variety of organizational arrangements that have emerged in different western countries, there are also major differences in the methods of paying doctors and these can also exert considerable influence on the nature of medical care. We can distinguish three major types of method, although in most healthcare systems a mixture of the methods can coexist and, often, individual doctors are paid by more than one method.

Fee-for-service involves the patient paying the doctor a fee for each separate item or element of care for which the doctor wishes to charge. In its simplest and historically earliest form, this involves direct patient payments at the time of use. This is still one of the most important methods of paying for health bills in the USA, involving 28% of all personal health expenditure. Insurance systems have emerged in most western countries that reduce or eliminate the need for direct patient payments. However, very often the medical profession has insisted on retaining fee-for-service as their method of payment, with the fees being reclaimed from federal and provincial government (Canada), from the patient's private insurer (USA), or from sickness funds (Germany).

Capitation reimburses the doctor by paying a fixed, usually annual, sum for each patient under his or her care. It is most naturally a method employed in primary care where the doctor has a continuous list or 'panel' of patients for whom he or she is responsible. Britain and Holland are two of the main examples.

Salary is the last method and involves an employer paying the doctor an annual income in return for his or her services. It is the method for paying hospital doctors in Britain, Sweden and Germany.

Unfortunately, there is no perfect method of paying doctors. Each method is known to have certain potentially harmful effects on the provision of health care. The most serious and most clearly documented problems are those associated with fee-for-service. This system encourages doctors to perform those procedures specifically rewarded by fees, which in most systems tend to be technical investigations and more interventionist treatments. To put it bluntly, many fee-for-service systems do not recognize talking to the patient as a distinct item of service! Fee-for-service requires more mechanisms than other methods of payment to control potentially wasteful treatments or investigations. Another problem that tends to occur in countries where doctors are paid by fee-for-service is that doctors tend to be poorly distributed geographically, as economic incentives encourage concentrations in more affluent areas.

Capitation provides more financial incentives that encourage doctors into 'under-doctored' areas. Among its main limitations are that it does not provide financial rewards for good quality care (as income is unrelated to quality or amount of activity) and might encourage doctors to refer-on difficult medical problems.

Salaried payment is also not without problems. In principle, it requires the doctor to be more concerned about pleasing his or her superiors or employers, who determine rewards and promotions, and less concerned with pleasing the patient. Generally, the medical profession has been quite conservative, preferring to keep to the particular system of payment historically established in each country. However, an overall trend can be detected for more doctors to be paid on a salaried basis, typically as employees of an organization.

Health expenditure in different countries

Western countries vary not only in how they organize and fund health services, but also – most dramatically – in the amount of funds devoted to health care. Comparisons of levels of expenditure are not easy because of problems of what is included and excluded in the category of health care in different countries, and also because of unstable exchange rates for countries' currencies. Nevertheless, the most recent figures produced on a systematic standardized basis show differences in levels of expenditure between countries that have remained fairly stable over time (Table 19.1). It is clear that there are considerable differences between countries that might all be regarded as similarly advanced industrial societies, whether expressed as absolute amounts of expenditure or as proportions of the gross domestic product (GDP), used as the most reliable measure of countries' overall wealth. Table 19.1 shows that, for example, the USA spent more than 2.5 times as much per capita as the UK. It is also clear that some countries at very similar levels of wealth in terms of GDP (for example Denmark and Canada) spend quite different amounts of their wealth on health care.

A number of different explanations have been offered to account for the differences between countries in their levels of expenditure. One factor that can play a role is the level of health professionals' earnings, especially those of doctors, which are undoubtedly high in countries such as the USA. A very different explanation would point to the important role of the general practitioner in systems like the NHS in acting as a filter or gatekeeper and limiting access to more expensive hospital facilities. Another factor that clearly distinguishes systems like the USA and the UK is that the former is an open system in which no actor – the doctor, the patient, the hospital, the insurance company or the government – has the full capacity and incentives to control the volume of medical activities and the costs that ensue. Typically in the USA, doctors or hospitals bill patients' insurance companies, who ultimately recover their costs from patients' employers, who hope in turn to pass on these costs to the general public in prices to the consumer. The healthcare system in the USA has historically been a highly inflationary one because of this capacity of actors to pass on their costs, and this process stands in direct contrast to the UK, where a closed financial system operates in that the total amount of finance available to the NHS is set and controlled centrally by the Treasury and, to a large extent, cannot be expanded further.

However, the most general explanation offered to explain differences in countries' levels of healthcare expenditure is that the greater a country's wealth, the greater will be not only

TABLE 19.1	The per capita expenditure on health, the percentage of wealth (GNP) spent on health and the various mortality rates for selected countries for 1998					
Country	Per capita expenditure on health (US $)	Health expenditure as proportion of GNP (%)	GNP[a] per capita (US $)	Life expectancy (years), male	Life expectancy (years), female	Infant mortality (per 1000 live births)
USA	4080	13.9	29240	73.9	79.5	7
Germany	2727	10.7	26570	74.3	80.6	5
Denmark	2576	8.0	33040	74.2	78.5	5
France	2287	9.6	24210	75.2	83.1	5
Sweden	2220	8.6	25580	77.3	82.0	4
Holland	1988	8.5	24780	75.4	81.0	5
Canada	1855	9.2	19170	76.0	81.5	5
UK	1480	6.8	21410	74.8	79.9	6

Adapted from The World Bank (2000).
[a] GNP estimates differ slightly from those used to calculate proportions in column two.

the amount but also the proportion of the wealth devoted to health care. Support for this view comes from analyses of data (such as in Table 19.1) for a number of different countries that produce highly significant correlations between countries' GDP and the proportion of GDP allocated to health care (Maxwell 1981). Such analyses can also be used to predict the level of health care that might be expected for a particular country, given its GDP. It has been suggested that, for example, the USA consistently spends more than expected and the UK less than might be expected from its GDP. However, others have argued that such analyses are inappropriate and use misleading exchange rates to calculate standardized expenditures (Parkin et al 1989).

VARIATIONS IN MEDICAL CARE

It is not surprising, in view of these differences in funding, to discover that the extent of medical intervention also varies between countries. Thus the rate of surgery in the USA and Canada is at least twice that in the UK, once differences in population size and structure have been taken into consideration. A recent study of hysterectomy (McPherson 1990) showed the age-standardized rate per 100 000 women as 700 in the USA, 600 in Canada, 450 in Australia, 250 in the UK and 110 in Norway. Similar international variations could be shown for tonsillectomy, cholecystectomy and prostatectomy. These international differences are not confined to surgery. Aaron & Schwartz (1984) showed a wide range of differences between the USA and the UK. In the USA, twice as many X-ray examinations were carried out per person; there was six times greater computer tomographic scanning capacity; three times more kidney dialysis treatment was provided; and between five and ten times more hospital intensive-care beds were available.

Variations within countries

Much of the international variation in rates of medical treatments can be accounted for in terms of general differences in economic prosperity of different countries. There is also a tendency for fee-for-service systems of paying the doctor to be associated with higher use of technical procedures such as investigations, and greater resort to active treatments, such as surgery, because such forms of care tend to be more financially rewarding (Abel-Smith 1976). However, it has become increasingly apparent that there are variations in surgical and medical procedures within countries that are as great as those between countries. It is less easy to explain such variation in terms of gross economic incentives. Thus a six-fold variation in tonsillectomy rates and a four-fold variation in hysterectomy rates have been found for different areas within New England (Wennberg & Gittelsohn 1982). Two New England cities, which were socially and demographically similar – Boston and New Haven – were examined in more detail. Although Boston had 2.3 times higher rates for carotid endarterectomy, the rates for cholecystectomy and hysterectomy were two-thirds, and for coronary bypass surgery only half, of those in New Haven (Wennberg et al 1987). Similar variations have been found in different regions of the NHS. For example, rates for hysterectomy per 100 000 women have been found to vary between 181 in Mersey and 287 in North-East Thames, whereas rates for tonsillectomy varied from 144 in Trent to 251 in North-East Thames (McPherson et al 1981).

Explanations for medical variations

Studies showing variation in the performance of treatments between areas within a country raise fundamental issues. It is extremely unlikely that variation in morbidity in the populations served could explain very much, if any, of the wide variations found in such studies. Moreover, it is unlikely that differences in consumer demand could explain large amounts of the differences in treatment rates prevailing in populations of similar social composition. One factor that is clearly implicated is supply. It can be no coincidence that the two-fold differences in surgical rates in the USA compared with the UK is mirrored by there being twice the number of surgeons per capita in the USA. However, where studies have attempted systematically to examine the effects of supply (McPherson et al 1981) it has been found possible to explain only a small amount of the variation in rates of treatment this way. It is clear that, for many procedures, the main problem is inherent uncertainty about the appropriate indications for treatment and the precise value of treatment in terms of outcomes.

It is known that clinicians can vary enormously in the diagnostic and history-taking procedures used in making decisions about elective surgery (Bloor 1976). However, to produce large and consistent differences in rates between areas, such individual differences in clinical opinion and approach must also be influenced by local or regional preferences or customs, otherwise the effects on variations in treatment rates produced by individual differences in clinical style would be cancelled out. Therefore, at the heart of any explanation of variations in treatment rates are professional uncertainty, lack of agreement about the indications for intervention and the value of intervention. Local and international variation is known to be greater for procedures such as tonsillectomy, prostatectomy and hysterectomy, over which professional uncertainty is greater than for procedures such as cholecystectomy, where some degree of consensus has emerged (Wennberg et al 1982).

CRITERIA FOR EVALUATING HEALTH SYSTEMS

Healthcare expenditure and health status

The main reason why so much uncertainty surrounds many medical and surgical procedures is that they have not been evaluated properly. It is very difficult to distinguish specific effects of a medical therapy from other possible causes of change in the course of illness, such as placebo effects and spontaneous changes in the underlying disorder. For this reason it is often argued that only a randomized controlled trial (RCT), where patients are randomly allocated between the treatment group and a control group and differences in subsequent health status compared between the two groups, is adequate to distinguish real treatment effects. Very few medical interventions have been evaluated by means of such demanding methods (Cochrane 1971). Some would argue that, especially when RCTs might pose ethical problems because of the need to withhold treatment, medical treatments can still be reasonably evaluated by less exact methods such as, for example, longitudinal observational studies in which the impact of therapies on groups of patients are recorded and compared with untreated comparison groups. However, such studies are still all too rare (McPherson 1990).

Greater uncertainty surrounds the relationship between overall levels of healthcare expenditure and benefits in terms of health status. Table 19.1 compares the expenditure figures for health care in a range of western countries with a number of the most recently available health-status measures. Life expectancy is a global measure that summarizes the mortality rates prevailing at all ages. It is apparent from Table 19.1 that the USA, despite spending much more on health care than other countries, does not enjoy more favourable life expectancy than countries such as Denmark and the UK, with quite low per capita healthcare expenditure. The infant mortality rate is a quite widely used indicator not only of infant health status but also of whole populations. Again, it is clear that the USA does not enjoy infant mortality rates commensurate with its high healthcare expenditure.

Other analyses of the relationship between countries' levels of healthcare expenditure and mortality rates have similarly failed to find evidence of the negative correlation that might reasonably be expected (Cochrane et al 1978, Maxwell 1981). Indeed, the one variable that tends to predict mortality rates from such comparisons of national data is the gross national product (GNP) – the overall level of wealth of the country (Cochrane et al 1978). This would, of course, be consistent with the arguments of McKeown that, historically, social and economic factors have exerted far greater influence upon health than have medical measures (see Chapter 1). In view of the evidence that mortality rates are largely influenced by social, economic and environmental factors rather than medical care, it might well be argued that mortality rates are not appropriate measures of health status with which to compare countries' healthcare systems. Rather, it might be argued, the main impact of health services is intended to be upon morbidity. In particular, the objectives of health services are to reduce the impact of illness in terms of pain, discomfort, disability and other aspects of health status. However, as indicated in Chapter 18, instruments for measuring these outcomes of health services have only recently been developed and there are numerous logistic and methodological problems that would make the comparative assessment of different healthcare systems extremely difficult. At present, therefore, the only available data with which to evaluate the effectiveness, in terms of impact upon health, of different healthcare systems is mortality.

Efficiency

There are a number of different ways in which one might evaluate the quality of different health services. Box 19.2 lists the widely cited criteria of Maxwell (1984). From the above discussion it is clear that there are basic difficulties in examining the effectiveness of healthcare systems, particularly problems of measuring outcomes. The scope for using the other five criteria are examined briefly below.

BOX 19.2	Criteria to Assess the Quality of Health Services

- Effectiveness
- Efficiency
- Accessibility
- Equity
- Social acceptability
- Relevance to needs

Reproduced with permission from Maxwell (1984).

Efficiency is a term that is frequently applied to health care but seldom used with much clarity. The efficiency of an engine is the relationship between the actual and the theoretically possible amount of energy used to achieve a desired output. The closer the machine gets to the lowest level of energy use considered possible, the greater its efficiency. In human systems one normally compares the costs of two or more alternative ways of achieving the same output or result, with the less costly alternative being regarded as more efficient. The scope for increasing efficiency in health services is potentially enormous. For example, in a wide range of problems, outpatient or day-case care can be substituted for longer inpatient management; or the nurse or general practitioner can replace more costly hospital care. Efficiency is examined by health economists using techniques such as cost–benefit analysis, in which all the costs of two or more alternative therapies or ways of organizing care are compared. This requires taking into account the costs of alternative treatments, such as any additional burden imposed on the family or other carers, as well as formal healthcare costs.

The British government sought to achieve numerous 'efficiency savings' from the NHS during the 1980s. However, in practice, this often meant reducing levels of spending available, which should not be confused with real improvements in efficiency because saving money can often be associated with deteriorating efficiency.

Efforts have been made to measure efficiency more directly, but the exercise has proved particularly difficult. One solution has been the development of 'performance indicators' (such as average length of hospital stay, throughput of patients per annum and turnover interval between cases occupying a bed), which can be measured for different units, hospitals and districts. However, such measures can be quite misleading. A unit might appear to be performing more efficiently if patients' mean length of hospital stay is lower than other units. However, a full cost–benefit analysis might show that this short length of hospital stay involved transferring higher costs to the community by premature discharge, together with unresolved complications of treatment that actually led to many patients being readmitted. It is also possible that varying lengths of stay in different units are due to different levels of severity of disease in the patients admitted.

It is even more difficult to compare healthcare systems in terms of efficiency. In general, the length of stay in hospitals in the USA is considerably shorter than in Britain. Economic pressures have been the main factor driving down lengths of stay in the USA. Unfortunately, lengths of stay tend to be a matter of local practice and tradition, and optimum length of stay has rarely been subjected to the kind of scientific examination adopted by Deyo et al (1986), who were able to show from a randomized controlled trial that shorter lengths of bed rest were as effective in the management of back pain as longer stays.

Another aspect of efficiency would include consideration of 'bureaucracy' or adminis-tration costs of health care because such costs do not apparently make a direct contribution to patient care. The NHS fares particularly well compared with most other systems. For example, it has been estimated that the USA spends as much as 22% of its health expenditure on administration costs, compared with about 6% required by the NHS (Himmelstein & Woolhandler 1986). High administration costs arise from a combination of fee-for-service and the need to itemize and bill every procedure. It is of note that, as the NHS began to experiment with 'internal markets', both health authorities and hospitals required a great deal more information of this kind and administration costs rose sharply.

Accessibility

This criterion is concerned with how readily available health services are. The healthcare system with the most visible problem is the more market oriented one of the USA, in which some 15–20% of the population have inadequate healthcare insurance. No other western healthcare system permits this degree of financial inaccessibility. Given that, for those who are insured in the USA, out-of-pocket expenses at the time of seeking care are higher than in European systems, it is remarkable that consultation rates are no different between systems. A different kind of problem of access is the need to wait for admission for treatment. This would appear to be very much more of a problem for the publicly funded and provided services of Britain and Sweden and is one major reason why in both these countries proposals have been implemented to increase the incentives for hospitals to reduce waiting times by a more competitive structure of revenue.

Equity

Equity with regard to health involves addressing some very complex issues, especially when trying to compare the performance of different healthcare systems. Thus a distinction can be made between equality of access (the extent to which different social groups have access to health services) and equality of health status (the extent to which different social groups enjoy similar levels of health). As other chapters in this book have shown, social differences in health status can be caused by a wide range of social, economic and environmental factors and the scope for intervention by health services, no matter how broadly defined, can be modest. Some would therefore argue that it is more reasonable to confine attention to comparing the efforts of different healthcare systems to achieve equality of access, although even with this more modest criterion there could be substantial social and cultural factors influencing use of health services. Other problems complicating quantitative comparisons of inequalities are that the social groupings (such as classes) are not consistent between countries and that social and cultural factors can influence individuals' perceptions of their health status (see Chapter 3).

With regard to social differences in health status, it is clear that all European and North American societies continue to experience differences in mortality between social groups, and the view that social democratic welfare states or Socialist societies have eradicated such differences is misguided (Illsley 1990). Thus a comparative study of Denmark, Finland, Norway, Sweden, Hungary and England and Wales showed that in all countries mortality among men with the highest level of education was 40–60% lower than men of the lowest educational level (Lahelma & Valkonen 1990). In general, some of the lowest inequalities in health status appear to be found in Sweden, a country that has probably the strongest and most active commitment to welfare policies. Nevertheless, even in Sweden there are occupational and regional inequalities in mortality arising from work hazards, dietary- and alcohol-related diseases and other unexplained environmental factors (Diderichsen 1990).

All healthcare systems have taken some steps to reduce or eradicate differences of access by income. At one extreme, a substantial proportion of the population in the USA does not have full access to health care because of inadequate insurance. Such individuals have to resort to a 'second-class' system of publicly funded health care, which has experienced particularly tight financial restrictions in the last 10 years. At the other extreme, financial barriers to access are largely removed from most European systems, and further steps have tended to be taken centrally to reduce regional inequalities of access. Particularly successful was the impact on the NHS of the Resource Allocation Working Party (RAWP), which resulted in England and Wales having the least regional inequalities in the geographical distribution of doctors when compared to France, Germany and Holland (Townsend & Davidson 1982).

Social acceptability

In those healthcare systems where an attempt has been made to assess consumers' views about their health care, the majority of respondents have expressed positive satisfaction. Indeed, a standardized survey of consumers in a cross-national survey that included citizens of Canada, the USA, England, Finland and Yugoslavia found that only 5% of respondents expressed dissatisfaction with their doctor's care, and that rates of dissatisfaction did not appear to differ significantly from country to country (Kohn & White 1976). The most common complaint across systems focused on the length of time spent waiting to see the doctor. However, a more recent comparative study of patient satisfaction with primary care has found higher levels of satisfaction in cities in the UK and Greece than in Belgrade and Moscow (Calnan et al 1994). Generally, such studies suggest that dissatisfaction with information provided by health professionals is also a universal problem. Some healthcare systems generate unique complaints. It is unlikely that any other healthcare system than the NHS would continue to wake patients up so early that 43% of patients complain about this aspect of being in hospital. Conversely, American consumers focus more critically than the consumers of other healthcare systems on the high costs they face from medical care. Americans also differ fundamentally from citizens of other countries in that, although they are generally satisfied with their own care, they view the healthcare system as a whole as unsatisfactory and in need of fundamental change (Blendon & Donelan 1990).

Relevance to health needs

Relevance is the last important criterion emphasized in Maxwell's list for evaluating health services. At the extreme it is possible to conceive of a healthcare system that takes little or no account of the health needs of the population it served. Thus it has often been a key problem in third world countries that the healthcare system has developed largely to conform to the standards of western high-technology medicine and, although relevant to the needs of urban social and political elites, it has failed to address the often more basic health needs of the rural majority populations. Such stark failures of relevance are less easy to identify in western healthcare systems and involve major initial difficulties in defining the health needs of populations.

Nevertheless, one very promising line of research has begun to open up the more focused and manageable issue of appropriateness. To what extent are the treatments provided in a healthcare system appropriate to the patients who receive them? The methodology for addressing this question is complex and can take different forms, but one approach essentially involves asking representative samples of relevant clinicians to rate the appropriate indications for a particular medical or surgical intervention (for example, which test results, past medical history and other patient characteristics would be appropriate indications for someone to undergo coronary artery bypass graft (CABG)). These agreed indications are then used to analyse the characteristics of samples of patients who have actually undergone the particular procedure. This methodology has been largely used in the USA and has produced quite startling results. Retrospective analyses of case records showed that for patients who received carotid endarterectomy, about one-third were rated as appropriate, one-third equivocal and one-third inappropriate. Similarly, one-quarter of coronary angiographies and one-quarter of endoscopies were rated as equivocal or inappropriate (Brook 1990). These studies lend support to the view that a substantial proportion of the treatment provided in the USA might be of questionable value in terms of outcomes and could occur as much out of a more general optimistic bias and faith in technology in American culture or, more cynically, because of strong financial rewards built into fee-for-service medicine.

This methodology has now been applied cross-nationally. Two panels of physicians and surgeons, one from the USA and one from the UK, were asked to rate a large number of indications in the form of elements of case histories, in terms of appropriateness for coronary angiography and also for CABG (Brook et al 1988). The American panel rated a much larger number of case-history indications as being appropriate for either procedure. The sets of indications the two panels were then applied to real case histories. First, they were applied to two samples of American patients who had undergone coronary angiography. The American panel's ratings resulted in 17% and 27% being rated as inappropriate, whereas the British panel's ratings identified 42% and 60% as inappropriate. The ratings of indications were then applied to another sample – American patients who had undergone CABG. By the American criteria 11% of operations were inappropriate; by the British criteria this figure was 15%. There are, therefore, quite powerful differences of views about the scope for benefit from medical treatment in medicine, despite the fact that medical science and medical training are very similar in the two countries.

The World Health Organization reported a very ambitious programme to assess the performance of all healthcare systems comparatively and quantitatively (WHO 2000). The framework used to compare healthcare systems involved assessment against three criteria: (1) impact on health; (2) responsiveness; and (3) financial fairness. The first criterion is more self-evident and assesses impact of healthcare systems on health status. The other two criteria go beyond what has usually been assessed by bodies such as WHO. Responsiveness focuses upon how well healthcare systems have respect for users of the service and demonstrate a client orientation as reflected in measures such as patients' reports about being given appropriate information about their health problems (see Chapter 18). Financial fairness is considered to occur when all households contribute a similar proportion of income to health care regardless of health status or level of use of the health service (Murray & Frenk 2001).

The report that emerged from the WHO combined statistical evidence for all countries' healthcare systems in relation to the three criteria into a single rank-ordering of countries (WHO 2000). It caused considerable controversy, partly because the countries ranked as having the most successful healthcare systems (France, Italy and Spain; ranked 1st, 2nd and 3rd respectively) were unexpected. Just as controversial, the USA, which spends far the greatest proportion of its wealth on health, ranked only 37th. More importantly, the report received considerable methodological criticism. It was felt that insufficiently robust data existed to measure many of the properties of healthcare systems in a standardized way (Almeida et al 2001). Moreover, basic definitions were criticized. It was argued that the view of fairness that all households contribute the same proportion of spending on health failed to take account of countries' intentions to be fair by funding health care through some degree of progressive taxation (i.e. higher rates of taxes borne by those with higher incomes). The WHO definition of fairness did not acknowledge that different households had different levels of need. The approach was also criticized for exaggerating the role of health care in determining health (Navarro 2000). The response to such criticisms is to argue that governments and populations need comparative information on their healthcare systems to assess strengths and weaknesses and that only by the development of more valid methods can an evidence base for how to organise healthcare systems be developed (Murray & Frenk 2001).

MARKETS VERSUS REGULATION IN HEALTH CARE

In many respects the many complex difficulties faced by healthcare systems can be subsumed into two broad types of problem. First, healthcare systems need to obtain adequate funds to pay for the healthcare needs of the populations they serve and mechanisms are required to ensure that such funds do not outstrip the capacity of the funder to pay. Second, mechanisms are required to improve the effectiveness and efficiency of health services, particularly in the light of evidence of ineffectiveness and inefficiency of the kind briefly reviewed in this chapter. No healthcare system appears to have addressed either problem satisfactorily and there is a constant and increasingly international search for solutions to both problems. Again, to simplify the discussion, it is possible to detect two alternative strategies that have been pursued by governments, sickness funds, health providers and other agencies concerned with the provision of health care in attempts to address the twin problems just identified. One strategy has focused on competition. It has sought to intensify the scope of market forces in the field of health care. The hope has been that competition between providers of health care would force them to reduce their costs as well as maximize their efficiency and effectiveness in accordance with the logic of market competition in other spheres of commerce. The second and contrasting strategy has been to introduce regulation into the operations of the healthcare system. Faced with evidence or inefficiencies such as wide and unaccountable variations in clinical practice and use of resources, this solution has attempted to use methods of centralized planning and managerial control of health budgets. The competitive strategy is best characterized by the American system and the regulation/planning strategy is more typical of European systems.

The competitive strategy was pursued in the USA throughout the 1980s. Government finance for planning of health services was withdrawn and instead support was given to encourage competition, especially to promote the development of Health Maintenance Organizations (HMOs). HMOs were established in which a group of health providers offered a complete package of healthcare services to consumers at an annually agreed price. It was hoped that HMOs would compete with each other in terms of the attractiveness of the package of services offered and their price. Finally, competition was encouraged by increasing the proportion of health bills paid out-of-pocket by the patient in the hope that this would increase consumer sensitivity to costs. To date, there has been little evidence that procompetitive strategies have succeeded in the main objective of driving down the highly inflationary costs of American health care.

The planning and regulatory strategies of European health services are too diverse to encompass in a brief chapter. To varying degrees in each country, regulation has included efforts to set overall limits to expenditure on health care, particularly in the hospital sector, by setting doctors' fees, regulating the introduction of high-technology medicine. This strategy has been largely successful in containing costs, but analysts are less happy with the

303

evidence of continued inefficiencies and unexplained variations in most European systems, and countries such as Sweden and Britain continue to be concerned with the unresponsiveness of their healthcare systems to the consumer and the persistence of waiting lists as unresolved problems.

Partly because of their perceived lack of consumer responsiveness but more particularly to control costs, many European systems were, in the 1990s, subjected to major changes intended to induce greater market competitiveness. In the very different systems of the UK, Holland and Sweden, the distinction between purchasers and providers of care was sharpened and providers (particularly hospitals) were given greater incentives to compete for patients on whose behalf the health authorities in the UK and Sweden and the sickness funds in Holland purchased care (Ham & Brommels 1994). However, the benefits of competition predicted by neoclassical economic theory have not produced greater efficiency and effectiveness in the field of health care, whether in Europe or in the USA (Glaser 1993). Some of the problems exacerbated by greater competition, such as the perceived oversupply of hospitals in large cities, have needed traditional European mechanisms of planning and regulation to address them (Ham & Brommels 1994)

Convergence of healthcare systems?

Some observers (Enthoven 1990, Ham et al 1990) have argued that pure strategies of either market competition or central planning and regulation have failed to address the key problems of health services and have suggested that there is now evidence in many healthcare systems of a convergence towards a mixed approach combining elements of both strategies. Again, it is impossible to encompass all the varieties of strategy emerging in each country, but some commonly occurring themes can be detected. One theme is that of 'peer review', in which clinical decisions that could result in large use of resources, such as admission to hospital and decisions about surgery, are subject to external review by colleagues. This has gone much further in the USA, where peer review is current and intended to have a direct influence on the use of resources, than in Europe, where it has, to date, been largely retrospective and used more for educational purposes, as in medical audit.

The second theme is the development of information systems to monitor and measure the activities and outcomes of health care. The intention is to use increasingly sophisticated information technology to inform all the parties to health care – the doctor, the patient and the purchaser in particular – about the efficiency and effectiveness of healthcare activities (Ellwood 1988).

A third common theme emerging in healthcare systems to varying degrees is the desire to separate out the purchaser of health care (such as the health authority or sick fund) from the provider (such as hospitals) and to increase the degree of choice that the purchaser has between different providers. In systems such as those in the UK, Holland and Sweden, the intention is to induce competition within a publicly funded system. The hope is that a system that incorporates all three elements (peer review, increased attention to audit of outcomes and scope for funders to choose between providers who compete in terms of quality and price) will produce a solution to the many dilemmas of modern medical care.

The need to ration

One of the most controversial problems facing healthcare systems of all types is the need to decide mechanisms of allocating limited healthcare resources in relation to competing demands. 'Rationing' is an emotive short-hand term used in this context and suggests a process of explicit and deliberate decisions about resource allocation. In reality, many healthcare systems have implicitly rationed without formally deciding to do so, because, for example, low-income individuals are not able to purchase health care or because delays or queues discourage numbers of patients from obtaining care.

However, as medical technology continues to develop and new treatments and healthcare costs escalate, governments across Europe and North America have had to devise more morally explicit principles whereby healthcare resources are allocated. A number of alternative principles could be used (Box 19.3). Unfortunately, these principles can conflict with each other (Harrison & Hunter 1994). For example, patients for whom current treatments are ineffective would be denied health care if the criterion of effectiveness were applied strictly, whereas they would receive services under principles of need or equity. All of the principles are difficult to operationalize. There are, for example, no agreed ways of defining or determining need. Any healthcare system is therefore likely to have to make trade-offs or compromises between principles rather than rigorously adhere to one.

Health authorities are also increasingly consulting the public about how health services should be prioritized by means of postal surveys or public meetings. However, the results of such consultation exercises have served only to complicate decisions, partly because public responses are heavily influenced by the wording of the questions and partly because the principles on which the public makes its choices differ from those considered important by doctors or managers. The public appears more impressed by the acute and high technology services and to value less preventive interventions such as health education or services for mental illness (Brown 1995).

There are therefore no simple solutions to the problem of providing health services that meet every desirable objective for health. This chapter has illustrated the diversity of forms that advanced healthcare systems have adopted in the search for optimal solutions.

BOX 19.3 Alternative Principles for Allocating Healthcare Resources Between Conflicting Demands

1. Effectiveness
   - Resources are allocated to those treatments that have the greatest effect on outcomes in terms of health.
2. Cost-effectiveness
   - Resources are allocated according to the principle of effectiveness, but also take account of costs in relation to effectiveness (i.e. favouring treatment with the best cost–benefit ratio).
3. Need
   - Resources are allocated to those patients or patient groups with the greatest need.
4. Equity
   - Resources are allocated on a principle of a basis of fairness or equity between individuals and patient groups.
5. Chance or 'fair goes'
   - Resources are allocated by some form of random process so that everyone has a similar chance of care, or 'first come first served' principles.

Reproduced with permission by the Institute for Public Policy Research from Harrison & Hunter (1995).

References

Aaron H, Schwartz W 1984 The painful prescription. The Brookings Institution, Washington DC

Abel-Smith B 1976 Value for money in health services. Heinemann, London

Almeida C et al 2001 Methodological concerns and recommendations on policy consequences of the World Health Report 2000. Lancet 351:692–697

Blendon R, Donelan K 1990 The public and the emerging debate over national health insurance. New England Journal of Medicine 323:208–212

Bloor M 1976 Bishop Berkeley and the adenotonsillectomy enigma. Sociology 10:44–61

Brook R 1990 Relationship between appropriateness and outcome. In: Hopkins A, Costain D (eds) Measuring the outcomes of medical care. Royal College of Physicians, London

Brook R et al 1988 Diagnosis and treatment of coronary disease: comparison of doctors' attitudes in the USA and the UK. Lancet i:750–753

Brown S 1995 Assessing public opinion on investment in health services. International Journal of Health Services 6:15–24

Calnan M, Katsouyiannopoulos V, Ocharov V 1994 Major determinants of consumer satisfaction with primary care in different systems. Family Practitioner 11:468–478

Cochrane A 1971 Effectiveness and efficiency. Nuffield Provincial Hospitals Trust, London

Cochrane A, St Leger A, Moore F 1978 Health service input and mortality output in developed countries. Journal of Epidemiology and Community Health 32:200–205

Curtis S, Petukhova N, Taket A 1995 Health care reforms in Russia: the example of St Petersburg. Social Science and Medicine 40:755–766

Deyo R, Diehl A, Rosenthal M 1986 How many days of bed-rest for acute low back pain? A randomised clinical trial. New England Journal of Medicine 315:1064–1070

Diderichsen F 1990 Health and social inequalities in Sweden. Sociology, Science and Medicine 31:359–367

Ellwood P 1988 Outcomes management: a technology of patient experience. New England Journal of Medicine 318:1549–1556

Enthoven A 1990 What can Europeans learn from Americans? In: Health care systems in transition. Organization for Economic Cooperation and Development (OECD), Paris

Field M 1973 The concept of the 'health system' at the macrosociological level. Sociology, Science and Medicine 7:763–785

Field M 1995 The health crisis in the former Soviet Union: a report from the 'post-war zone'. Sociology, Science and Medicine 41:1469–1478

Glaser W 1993 The competition vogue and its outcomes. Lancet 341:805–812

Ham C, Brommels M 1994 Health care reforms in the Netherlands, Sweden, and the United Kingdom. Health Affairs 13:106–119

Ham C, Robinson R, Benzeval M 1990 Health check: health care reforms in an international context. Kings Fund Institute, London

Harrison S, Hunter D 1994 Rationing health care. Institute for Public Policy Research, London

Himmelstein D, Woolhandler S 1986 Cost without benefit: administrative waste in US health care. New England Journal of Medicine 314:441–445

Hsiao W 1995 The Chinese health care system: lessons for other nations. Sociology, Science and Medicine 41:1047–1056

Illsley R 1990 Comparative review of sources, methodology and knowledge. Sociology, Science and Medicine 31:229–236

Kohn P, White K 1976 An international study. Oxford University Press, Oxford

Lahelma E, Valkonen T 1990 Health and social inequalities in Finland and elsewhere. Sociology, Science and Medicine 31:257–266

Liu Y et al 1995 Transformation of China's rural health care system. Sociology, Science and Medicine 41:1085–1094

Maxwell R 1981 Health and wealth. Lexington Books, Lexington, MA

Maxwell R 1984 Quality assessment in health. British Medical Journal 288:1470–1472

McPherson K 1990 International differences in medical care practices. In: Health care systems in transition. Organization for Economic Cooperation and Development (OECD), Paris

McPherson K et al 1981 Regional variations in the use of common surgical procedures. Sociology, Science and Medicine 15A:273–288

Murray C, Frenk J 2001 World health report 2000: a step towards evidence-based health policy. Lancet 357:1698–1700

Navarro V 2000 Assessment of the world health report 2000. Lancet 356:1598–1601

Parkin D, McGuire A, Yule B 1989 What do international comparisons of health care expenditures really show? Community Medicine 11:116–123

Townsend P, Davidson N 1982 Inequalities in health: the Black report. Penguin, Harmondsworth

Wennberg J, Gittelsohn A 1982 Variations in medical care among small areas. Scientific American 246:120–134

Wennberg J, Barnes B, Zubkoff M 1982 Professional uncertainty and the problem of supplier-induced demand. Sociology, Science and Medicine 16:811–824

Wennberg J, Freeman J, Gulp W 1987 Are hospital services rationed in New Haven or overutilised in Boston? Lancet i:118

World Bank 2000 World development indicators 2000. The World Bank, Washington DC

World Health Organization (WHO) 2000 World health report 2000. WHO, Geneva

Index

311

328